Girt Reiman, M.D.
2514 Soma Ave.
Bellmore, N.Y. 11710
516-826-8469

Ultrasound in Urology

SECOND EDITION

Ultrasound in Urology

SECOND EDITION

Martin I. Resnick, M.D.

Professor and Chairman
Division of Urology
Case Western Reserve University
School of Medicine and
University Hospitals
Cleveland, Ohio

Roger C. Sanders, M.A., B.M., M.R.C.P., D.M.R.D., F.R.C.R.

Associate Professor of Radiology
and Radiologic Sciences
Associate Professor of Urology
Department of Radiology
Director of Abdominal Ultrasound
Johns Hopkins Medical Institutions
Baltimore, Maryland

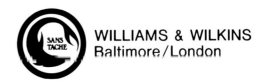

WILLIAMS & WILKINS
Baltimore / London

Editor: James L. Sangston
Associate Editor: Jonathan W. Pine, Jr.
Copy Editor: Deborah K. Tourtlotte
Design: Bert Smith
Illustration Planning: Reginald Stanley
Production: Carol L. Eckhart

Made in the United States of America

First Edition, 1979

Library of Congress Cataloging in Publication Data

Main entry under title:

Ultrasound in urology.

   Includes index.
   1. Genito-urinary organs—Diseases—Diagnosis. 2. Diagnosis, Ultrasonic. 3. Ultra-sonic waves—Therapeutic use. I. Resnick, Martin I. II. Sanders, Roger C. [DNLM:
1. Ultrasonics—Diagnostic use. 2. Urologic diseases—Diagnosis. WJ 141 U47]
RC874.U37   1984   616.6'07543   83-21633
ISBN 0-683-07219-6

Composed and printed at the
Waverly Press, Inc.
Mt. Royal and Guilford Aves.
Baltimore, MD 21202, U.S.A.

Vicki, Andy and Jeff
and
Angie and Nigel

Preface

With publication of the first edition of *Ultrasound in Urology*, the editors attempted to present an up-to-date, comprehensive text detailing the clinical application of ultrasound in urological practice. With the collaboration of a urologist and a radiologist, the book met the goals, emphasizing the proper utilization of this imaging technique to gain information related to specific clinical problems.

The editors realize that ultrasonography is a constantly changing discipline, and technological developments over the past 4 years have made portions of the first edition obsolete. The introduction and rapid acceptance and utilization of real-time imaging have greatly enhanced the diagnostic ability of this technique in the assessment of disorders of the genitourinary tract. In addition, there has been the continued development of biopsy techniques and percutaneous procedures that can be performed most successfully under ultrasonic guidance. New applications continue to arise, and it is expected that further improvements will continue in the future. The authors of the chapters have, therefore, attempted to present not only the most modern and up-to-date information but have also emphasized new developments and procedures that will be available in the future.

We wish to express our deep appreciation to the contributing authors who have greatly facilitated the development of this book. Most were cooperative in adhering to the guidelines and responding to our editorial comments and changes. We would also like to thank our secretaries, Barbara Roseman, Pamela Oliveri, and Joan Batt, who have assisted in correspondence and final manuscript preparation. Finally, we would like to thank Mr. James L. Sangston of Williams & Wilkins for his encouragement and cooperation.

Martin I. Resnick, M.D.
Roger C. Sanders, M.D.

Contributors

Peter H. Arger, M.D.
Radiology Department
Hospital of the University of Pennsylvania
Philadelphia, Pennsylvania

Diane S. Babcock, M.D.
Associate Professor of Radiology and Pediatrics
University of Cincinnati College of Medicine
Cincinnati, Ohio

John R. Babcock, M.D., F.A.C.S.
Assistant Clinical Professor of Surgery
Division of Urology
University of Cincinnati Medical Center
Cincinnati, Ohio

Damon D. Blake, M.D.
Professor of Radiology
Bowman Gray School of Medicine
Winston-Salem, North Carolina

Walter J. Bo, Ph.D.
Professor of Anatomy
Department of Anatomy
Bowman Gray School of Medicine
Winston-Salem, North Carolina

Donald Bodner, M.D.
Resident in Urology
Division of Urology
Case Western Reserve University
School of Medicine
Cleveland, Ohio

Patrick J. Bryan, M.D.
Associate Professor of Radiology
Department of Radiology
Case Western Reserve University
School of Medicine
Cleveland, Ohio

Daryl H. Chinn, M.D.
Department of Radiology
University of California
School of Medicine
San Francisco, California

Beverly G. Coleman, M.D.
Radiology Department
Hospital of the University of Pennsylvania
Philadelphia, Pennsylvania

Roy A. Filly, M.D.
Professor, Department of Radiology
University of California
School of Medicine
San Francisco, California

Floyd A. Fried, M.D.
Professor of Urology
University of North Carolina Medical Center
Chapel Hill, North Carolina

Barry H. Gross, M.D.
Assistant Professor
Department of Radiology
University of Michigan Medical Center
Ann Arbor, Michigan

Kazuya Harada, M.D.
Department of Urology
Tohoku University School of Medicine
Sendai, Japan

Hedvig Hricak, M.D.
Associate Professor
Department of Radiology
University of California
School of Medicine
San Francisco, California

Wayne A. Krueger, Ph.D.
Discipline of Anatomy
University of Osteopathic Medicine and Health
  Sciences
Des Moines, Iowa

Joseph P. LiPuma, M.D.
Associate Professor of Radiology
Department of Radiology
Case Western Reserve University
School of Medicine
Cleveland, Ohio

James F. Martin, M.D.
Director, Medical Sonics
Bowman Gray School of Medicine
Winston-Salem, North Carolina

Martin I. Resnick, M.D.
Professor and Chairman
Division of Urology
Case Western Reserve University

School of Medicine and University Hospitals
Cleveland, Ohio

Ward A. Riley, Ph.D.
Research Associate Professor of Neurology
  (Medical Ultrasound)
Department of Neurology
Bowman Gray School of Medicine
Winston-Salem, North Carolina

**Roger C. Sanders, M.A., B.M., M.R.C.P.,
  D.M.R.D., and F.R.C.R.**
Associate Professor of Radiology and Radiologic
  Sciences
Associate Professor of Urology
Department of Radiology
Director of Abdominal Ultrasound
Johns Hopkins Medical Institutions
Baltimore, Maryland

William Scheible, M.D.
Associate Professor of Radiology
University of California
San Diego, California

Thomas E. Sumner, M.D.
Associate Professor of Radiology
Associate Professor of Pediatrics
Department of Radiology
Bowman Gray School of Medicine
Winston-Salem, North Carolina

Rolfe D. White, M.D.
Assistant Professor
Department of Obstetrics and Gynecology
Eastern Virginia Medical School
Norfolk, Virginia

David L. Williams, M.D.
Assistant Professor
Department of Obstetrics and Gynecology
Eastern Virginia Medical School
Norfolk, Virginia

Hsu-Chong Yeh, M.D.
Associate Professor of Radiology
Department of Radiology
Mt. Sinai Hospital
New York, New York

Contents

CHAPTER 1

History of Ultrasound

JAMES F. MARTIN, M.D.

Ultrasound is a branch of acoustics which deals with the study and use of sound waves of frequencies above those within hearing range of the average person (frequencies above 20,000 cycles/second or 20 kHz). Many examples of the use of ultrasound are found in nature. Some animals—moths, porpoises, birds, dogs, and especially bats—use it for locating and identifying food, for navigational purposes, and for detecting danger. Lazzaro Spallanzini in 1794 demonstrated that insectivorous bats depend on hearing rather than vision to locate obstacles and prey. An excellent review of ultrasonics is presented by Ensminger and White (1) in which all of the various applications of ultrasound are described. Also included are the various contributions made by physicists and mathematicians beginning in the 17th and 18th centuries.

One of the most notable contributions made was by Jacques and Pierre Curie (2). Their studies of crystals, under the direction of and in cooperation with Charles Freidel, were primarily concerned with pyroelectricity, a phenomenon that had been known for some time and consisted of the appearance of electrical charges on certain crystals as they were heated. Research in symmetry of crystals led to the discovery of piezoelectricity, a property of nonconducting crystals that have no center of symmetry. Their first observations, published in 1880, discussed the physical characteristics of many different crystals, and in 1881, using quartz and tourmaline, they published information demonstrating that when an alternating electrical field was applied to their crystals, the piezoelectric plates of the two substances underwent either expansion or contraction and produced sound waves of very high frequency.

The first practical application of their phenomenon was the Galton dog whistle (1883) which was used to control a dog without producing audible sound. Little else was done until well after the turn of the century. The sinking of the Titanic in a collision with an iceberg in 1912 drew attention to the need for developing a technique to detect underwater obstructions, and this need became more evident in World War I when enemy submarines threatened the Allied Powers with defeat.

Paul Langevin, a former student of Pierre Curie, and Chilowsky (3) succeeded in producing the first piezoelectric ultrasound generator in 1917. They matched the frequency of the alternating field to the resonant frequency of the quartz crystal. The resonance thereby evoked in the latter produced powerful mechanical vibrations which were then transmitted through the surrounding medium as ultrasound waves. The crystal could serve as both generator and detector, since the latter causes mechanical vibrations in the crystal which, in turn, generates electrical charges on its surface.

Langevin lived to see the development of SONAR (Sound Navigation and Ranging) which played an important role in World War II. Although it is uncertain whether this technique contributed much toward submarine detection in the First World War, it certainly played a very important role in the Second World War. The initial generator used continuous ultrasound waves, but it was not until improvements in electronic technology permitted the generation of bursts of ultrasound waves that ranging and detection could be built. The technique is now widely used in determining the depth of waterway channels for navigation, in detecting underwater obstructions, and in locating schools of fish.

Other outstanding early work was done by Sergei Sokolov (4), a Russian scientist. His work at the Leningrad Electro-technical Institute emphasized the potential importance of ultrasound, and he envisioned the many different practical applications but was limited by the lack of technical advances. In 1929, he proposed the use of ultrasound to detect flaws in metals using the through transmission technique. He also proposed the use of ultrasound for use in microscopy, and he experimented with imaging systems using coherent light reflected from liquid surfaces which anticipated Gabon's later discovery of holography. He was awarded the Stalin prize for outstanding contributions to science and is regarded by many as the "Father of Ultrasonics."

The widespread application of ultrasound can be roughly divided into the use of sound waves of high or low intensity. High intensity application refers to those instances in which the purpose is to produce a change or an effect in the medium through which the wave passes. Such instances include: medical therapy, atomization of liquids, machining of brittle metals, welding, certain biological properties, and many others too numerous to list. The therapeutic applications have been described by Ensminger (1) but, unfortunately, have not been vigorously pursued in medicine to date. However, Fry et al. (5), using high intensity focused generators aimed by a stereotactic device, produced destructive lesions in the basal ganglia in cases of Parkinsonism.

The low intensity applications are those wherein the primary purpose is to learn something about the medium or to pass information through it without altering its state. Following the First World War the technology of electronics developed such that it became possible to amplify low amplitude electrical signals and to display these on the screen of a cathode ray oscilloscope. The practical applications include medical diagnosis, nondestructive testing, measurement of elastic properties of materials, livestock judging, underwater depth sounding, echo ranging, communication, and submarine detection, to mention only a few.

Technological advances by 1940 permitted Firestone (6) to develop the reflectoscope for the generation of brief pulses of energy for the detection of the reflections from flaws or fractures from within the castings. This secret device proved very important to the United States in the Second World War and became the basis of the Non-Destructive Flaw Detecting Technique which is used extensively throughout the world today. It is regarded by many as the one development which made medical ultrasound possible.

The first application of ultrasound in medical diagnosis was by a psychiatrist, Dr. Karl Dussik (7), and his brother at a hospital in Bad Ischl, Austria. He tried to locate brain tumors by using two opposing transducers and recording the through transmission of the sound beam. He also wanted to visualize the cerebral ventricles by measuring the attenuation of the ultrasound beam through the head and, in 1942, published the technique, "Hyperphonography of the Brain." Considerable controversy followed a study of his pictures because of the misinterpretation that the skull bone is thinner in the temporal area than elsewhere and thus could simulate the picture of the lateral ventricles (8). These objections led to the cessation of experiments with through transmission techniques. Similarly, a paper presented by Ballantine et al. (9) in 1954 indicated great difficulty in the interpretation of the returning echoes from the various organs and interfaces and claimed it had little value. The through transmission technique for echoencephalography appeared to be a failure following the early work of Dussik and Leksell. Leksell (10), in 1953, was faced with an emergency where there were reasons to suspect a subdural hematoma in a 16-month-old child. He borrowed a Siemens reflectoscope, and, due to the improvement in the performance of the instrument, he was able to detect a clear displacement of the midline echo. This was confirmed at surgery. He proved the usefulness of the shift in the midline echo for diagnosis of expanding processes in the brain which led to further publications with his collaborator, Stig Jeppson. His further work was published in *Acta Chirurgica* in 1956 following which midline echoencephalography was enthusiastically pursued in many centers.

Following Leksell's report in 1956, echoencephalography (M-mode) was investigated on both sides of the Atlantic with a reported high degree of accuracy. The largest series was reported by Schiefer et al. (11), who claimed an accuracy of 99.8% which was accomplished through the knowledge of the history and clinical findings. Kichuchi et al. (12) reviewed the use of the reflection technique to demonstrate reflected echoes from the excised brain and subsequently claimed it was possible to elicit echoes from tumors through the intact skull.

Ambrose (13), in 1964, was one of the first to measure the width of the lateral ventricles by the reflection technique. Ford and McRae (14) used the A-mode display to monitor and follow the width of the lateral ventricles following shunting. Further work in this period was challenged by the difficult technical problems inherent by the skull and the variable thicknesses encountered throughout. Considerable technical progress in overcoming these difficulties has been reported by Barnes et al. (15) from our institution with new instrumentation.

Since 1955, the clinical significance of estimation of the position of the midline echo has been confirmed and elaborated by many investigators, notably in England (Gordon, Jefferson, Ambrose, Taylor, Newell, Karvounis); in Sweden (Jeppson, Lithander); in Holland (de Vlieger, Ridder, Greebe); in Canada (White, Ford, Lee, Morley); in Japan (Juntendo University Research Group); in Switzerland (Müller); in France (Mikol, Fischer); in Germany (Schiefer, Kazner, Brückner, Kramer); and in the United States (Dreese, Grossman, McKinney, Barrows, Sugar).

The Doppler technique, "carotid echography," described by Buschmann in 1964 (16) had extensive application in neurology and has been a stimulus for current development.

It remained the method of study for several years following the introduction of a commercial unit by Spencer and Reid (Dopscan, Carolina Medical Electronics, Inc., King, NC). The interpretation of these studies was difficult, and new types of color-coded display have been developed by White and Curry (17).

The marked improvement in the resolution of real-time scanners and especially the small size of the sector scanner in the late 1970's led to the development of their use in the study of the neonatal brain (18–21). Because of the portability of instruments, its noninvasive nature, and the ease of examination, it has become an extremely useful clinical examination that has developed rapidly over the past few years.

The first published work on the pulse-echo technique was by Ludwig and Struthers (22) from the Naval Research Institute in 1949: "Considerations Underlying the Use of Ultrasound to Detect Gallstones and Foreign Bodies in Tissue." These early investigators were using available surplus war equipment and began to apply ultrasound to medicine and to develop equipment for medical diagnosis alone. By implanting gallstones in the gallbladder of a dog, they showed that this technique could successfully demonstrate the stones.

In the early 1950's there were three areas in the United States where development and research were being conducted. Studies were being conducted by Dr. Douglas Howry at the University of Colorado, Dr. John Wild at the University of Minnesota Medical School, and Dr. George

Ludwig at the University of Pennsylvania. All demonstrated that when ultrasound is sent into the body and reaches a tissue interface of different density, echoes will be reflected back to the transmitting transducer. The earliest work used the A-mode display on an oscilloscope.

Edler and Hertz had a very positive influence in Europe following their initial observations with the Siemens reflectoscope in 1953. Leksell, Donald, and Edler produced impressive results in their respective areas of interest. Similar work was done by many investigators in Japan, Austria, Sweden, France, and England, and all have made significant contributions too extensive to discuss here. There was extensive cross-communication between these groups of workers of varied backgrounds, such that each area of applications developed rapidly.

In 1947, Dr. Douglas Howry of Denver, Colorado, began developing forerunners of equipment in use today. He first started application of ultrasound in visualizing the soft tissue structures by displaying echoes from the various interfaces. Using discarded naval Sonar equipment, he developed his first piece of equipment in the basement of his home, which was later transferred to the University of Colorado School of Medicine. There, in 1949, in conjunction with an engineer, W. Roderic Bliss, he developed a successful pulse-echo system which could record echoes from tissue interfaces. In 1952, Howry and Bliss (23) published two-dimensional ultrasonic tomograms using a sector scan of various tissues in vitro and of the forearm in vivo. The principle of compound scanning was introduced in 1951 and consisted of two or more movements of the probe: the beam reached any point in the tissue from many positions of the probe, and the echoes were accurately recorded and integrated. Initial scans utilized the water immersion technique, and a variety of water containers were used, such as a laundry tub, a cattle-watering trough, and a gun turret of a B-29 airplane, which was purchased as scrap. The internal circular-toothed track rotated and carried the transducer smoothly around the subject. Howry tried to image the brain but was disappointed at the lack of echoes; however, he did produce a satisfactory scan of the neck, which is now quite well known. He called the device a "somoscope," because it appeared to be most effective in the study of soft tissues.

The marked disadvantages of the immersion technique soon became apparent and, in 1960,

Howry began experimenting with mechanical sector scanners applied to the body surface. This led to the development of a hand-held system with an articulated arm holding the transducer with freedom to scan in several planes. Howry left the University of Colorado in 1962 for reasons of health and worked as a radiologist at the Massachusetts General Hospital until his death in 1969. Much of the work in the development of the scanning arm and technique was carried out by Dr. Joseph H. Holmes. It became apparent that the reflection technique was a more practical method for medical diagnosis. Short bursts of sound were emitted from the transducer followed by a relatively long "listening time," where recordings were made of the amount of sound reflected by the tissue interfaces.

Wild and Reid, of St. Martin's Hospital in Minneapolis, Minnesota, began their work in 1949. In 1951, Wild and Neal (24) published their studies which were aimed primarily at determining the possibility of using ultrasound to detect the differences in normal and diseased tissue by an A-mode display. In 1952, Wild and Reid (25) published two-dimensional scans which included a breast carcinoma, normal kidney, and muscle tumor. Their findings indicated that, in general, cancerous tissue reflected more sound than normal tissue and that the tissue of nonmalignant tumors reflected less than normal tissue. Wild and Reid (26) were responsible for several other significant explorations in the clinical application of this technique. They demonstrated that there was a different echo pattern from the various layers of the intestine; they studied the walls of the sigmoid colon on withdrawal of a transducer placed via the sigmoidoscope and suggested the intragastric placement of a transducer to study the patterns of carcinoma of the stomach. Wild and Reid (27), in 1956, reported their results of examination of 77 palpable abnormalities of the breast. All but one of the 27 malignant tumors had typical echograms; of 50 benign lesions, 43 had an echogram of nonmalignant type and seven of malignant type. Most significantly, they reported a 90% accuracy in the diagnosis of cystic versus solid lesions of various organs using the B-scan technique.

The enthusiasm for the ultrasound technique received a temporary setback by a report published by the United States Atomic Energy Commission in 1955 (28). It concluded there was no possibility of adapting this method for study of intracranial lesions. This had a depressing effect upon workers in the United States, and progress in many areas was slowed considerably. This report was made with little consideration of the type of equipment and energy form used. However, workers in Europe, especially in Scotland and Sweden, were not adversely influenced, and in a brief period of time practically all advances and developments were reported by them. These early states of development in technique closely paralleled many other parameters of electronic technology. This continues even today with the development of digital display, computers, and new transducer materials.

In 1954, Ian Donald, upon accepting the appointment of Regius Professor of Midwifery of Glasgow, became interested in ultrasound and its application in obstetrics and gynecology. He, his engineer, and physician associates made great contributions using borrowed flaw detector instruments. His major interest initially was to compare A-scans to determine whether they could differentiate solid from cystic masses. He took two carloads of large abdominal tumors to the research laboratory of a large firm which built atomic boilers and used flaw detectors on them. He found that the patterns of the solid and cystic lesions were distinctly different, and on this basis the company loaned him a Mark 2 B flaw detector for further investigation. The problem with the unit was that it had an 8-cm "paralysis time" which blanked out the scan for the first 8 cm from the transducer.

Eventually, he contacted the firm making equipment for atomic boilers and convinced the directors to grant him money for his research. In 1955, Mr. Tom Brown, an engineer, began a long association with Dr. Donald. In 1957, they designed and constructed a prototype hand-operated two-dimensional contact scanner which is now used clinically for studies of the female pelvis and abdomen. The transducer probe was in direct contact with the skin and coupled with the use of olive oil. The main advantage of contact scanning was the elimination of the sound-transmitting water tank and its inconvenience. Photographs were made on Polaroid film, and the shutter of the camera remained open during the entire scanning period. The results were first reported in 1958 in the *Lancet* (29). This, he admits, was probably the most important paper that he had written.

Dr. Donald's primary interest was not in obstetrics, but in the differentiation of the truly massive abdomen due to either ovarian cysts or ascites. He had a very dramatic experience with a patient who was thought to have massive ascites due to obstruction from a radiologically demonstrated carcinoma of the stomach. He was called to see the patient and, after the clinical examination, suggested that she be examined by the A-scan ultrasound technnque. When he applied the probe to the most protuberant part of the patient's abdominal wall, there were no bowel echoes seen in the area, and only a large echo-free space with a well-defined posterior wall was evident. Following this, the patient was removed to his department for laparotomy, and a massive ovarian tumor was removed. She recovered nicely and remained a lifelong friend. This case marked the beginning of abdominal ultrasonography.

In 1957, pregnancy studies started when Dr. Donald became impressed by the very strong echoes coming from the fetal skull. His engineers provided electronic cursors which could be displayed on the cathode ray tube (CRT) and used to measure the fetal head size electronically. In 1960, he developed the first automatic scanner and demonstrated it, but it proved to be a very expensive instrument. It was developed because overscanning performed by the operator could occasionally produce artifacts. In 1961 (30), he published a paper on the hydatidiform mole and emphasized the extreme importance of the proper scanning technique and the avoidance of artifacts. About this time, Campbell (31) from his group began working on the growth patterns of the fetus as measured by serial biparietal diameters. In 1961 (30), the first diasonograph was demonstrated before the British Institute in Radiology. Donald was largely responsible for developing the contact scanning technique and for pioneering the extensive application of ultrasound in obstetrics and gynecology; to this day, despite extensive cardiac surgery, he remains quite active in this field.

It became important for Dr. Donald to develop his one-dimensional display into a two-dimensional sonogram, which was done with the help of Tom Brown and was first published in 1958 (29). Sunden, in 1958, visited Donald and the Smith Industrial Division in Glasgow where T. G. Brown had built Donald's first machine. His publication in 1964 (32) of a study of more than 400 patients demonstrated the clinical usefulness of the method in obstetrics and gynecology.

His report and that of Thompson et al. (33) were of great influence leading to the general acceptance for clinical use today.

Donald's experience emphasized that abdominal scanning can be very informative, and it was widely pursued by many workers. The presentation and recording from the CRT were referred to as "bi-stable," which meant that only strong reflections were recorded, and the picture was white on black with no graduations. This type of presentation, along with the fact that they represented only a thin slice or body section, was initially not attractive to physicians because it was a new presentation to which they were unaccustomed. Nevertheless, many workers made numerous contributions and developed great enthusiasm for the technique.

The introduction of the gray-scale presentation in 1971 (34, 35) proved to be a real stimulus for clinical development. The display was now a little more understandable to physicians for it was no longer white dots on a black background, but rather a pleasant picture with varying shades of gray. This was made possible by the use of the scan converter through which high and low level echoes were displayed as various levels of gray. The introduction of gray-scale echography marked the beginning of clinical acceptance for an ever-increasing variety of techniques. In 1973–1974, considerable attention was given to the visualization of the liver and kidneys. One of the major applications was the visualization of the vasculature of the upper abdomen, which, in 1976, led to a more positive identification of the pancreas.

Wild and Reid attempted transrectal studies of the prostate early in their work, but the scans were so poor they did not report on them. Japanese urologists in 1963 reported A-mode scans of the prostate gland which were somewhat difficult to interpret. Earlier reports by Takahashi and Ouchi (36) in 1963 and 1964 were far from being of practical use because of poor picture quality. Watanabe et al. (37), in 1971, reported ultrasonograms of the prostate using transrectal Plan-Position-Indication (PPI) scanning with a specially prepared concave transducer. Their paper illustrated a wide variety of prostatic disease with good picture quality. His transducer was covered with a water-filled balloon which assured good contact with the rectal wall. The patients were done in the sitting position. The bladder was filled with water and he demonstrated scans of the bladder, prostate, uterus, and seminal vesicles. Holm and Northeved (38) described a transurethral scanner in 1974 which was interchangeable with the optical system of a resectoscope.

King et al. (39) were the first to use the prostate scanner in the United States with good clinical results, and it was further reported by Resnick et al. (40). Initially, the scanning was done in the lithotomy position, but because of problems with air bubbles, most scanning is now done in the prone position. More recently, Hileman (personal communication) has developed transrectal scanning equipment which envelop two transducers in a single probe. He used 3.5 and 7.0 mHz transducers optomized for a range of 10 cm. His unit permits rapid recording on 35-mm film.

More recently, Henneberry et al. (41) and Abu-Yousef et al. (42) have demonstrated the value of B-scans of the prostate gland from the anterior abdominal wall through a full urinary bladder. Prostate size, contour, and margins are readily studied. Real-time scanning has proved to be a rapid and accurate method of prostate gland scanning.

THE DOPPLER EFFECT

A physicist, Christian Johann Doppler, in 1842, predicted that light emitted from a moving source would be changed in frequency and hence in color. Satomura (43) reported using the ultrasound Doppler technique in the study of flow patterns in peripheral arteries in 1959. Franklin et al. (44) in 1961, using two transducers to study arterial flow noninvasively, demonstrated the frequency spectrum of the returned beam to be broadened and used this method to measure the instantaneous flow of blood. These devices measured only amplitude of the returned signal. McLeod (45) (1967) and Pourcelot (46) (1971) designed directional systems which processed the backscattered ultrasonic signals in two separate channels, in which the respective Doppler shift signals are distinguished by a phase shift of 90°. These developments allowed the measurement of blood velocity in a localized area of the vessel lumen and made it possible to measure instantaneous profiles without interfering with flow.

The ultrasonic pulsed Doppler method has been the subject of various developments since 1968. It allows the measurement of blood velocity in a localized area of the lumen of the vessel, and it became possible to measure profiles of instantaneous blood velocity without interfering with flow (47).

Physicians throughout the world recognized and used this new technique to study the cardiovascular system and provided much new information in a noninvasive way. Much of the clinical experience has been related to peripheral vessels as described by Strandness et al. (48), Sigel et al. (49), and Lavenson et al. (50). Their studies on the peripheral arteries and veins have been found to be very useful in many clinical problems.

Continuous wave Doppler has been used by Tajik et al. (51) and Yoshida et al. (52) to examine the heart. The early work was used to obtain signals from the heart wall and valves by Kostis et al. (53) Huntsman et al. (54) have found this technique to be useful in studying the velocity of blood flow in the aorta and relating it to cardiac output.

Obstetrical Doppler applications were reported by Callagan et al. (55) in 1964, when they detected the movement of the fetal heart. Others found it possible to hear the fetal heart at about 12 weeks, and it was also found to be helpful in the localization of the placenta. It is used to detect fetal death as well as in the new area of continuous fetal monitoring.

Buschmann (16) (1964) decribed "carotid echography" for the diagnosis of carotid thromboses. The two walls of the carotid artery could be demonstrated and registered continuously; however, development of such ultrasonic Doppler has been slow since it proved difficult to separate and identify signals originating from the carotid and its branches. In 1971, Hokanson (56) first made spatial displays of the carotid bifurcation by means of a pulsed Doppler system. Reid and Spencer (Dopscan, Carolina Medical Electronics, Inc., King, NC) developed the first commercially available instrument with which it was possible to find occluded segments of the carotid bifurcation which do not appear on the image.

White and Curry (57) have reported a system which directly displays those regions from which higher frequency Doppler shifted signals are recorded with an appropriately coded color display. Additional techniques have used the real-time scanners and superficial scanners recently developed by several companies.

One of the most interesting developments was by Baker and Johnson (58) with the introduction of the pulsed Doppler cardiac technique.

This permitted the recording of valve movements as usually seen in routine echocardiography with the addition of a superimposed display and location of the Doppler signal. This technique, with simultaneous display of the two signals, provides for echo ranging and the location of various cardiac structures as well as sampling specific areas within the heart.

Considerable attention has been given the combination of a real-time cross-sectional system coupled with pulsed Doppler (59). Although this system was designed with cardiac studies in mind, it has found many other areas of application, especially in the abdomen where positive identification of arteries and veins can be made. Although this combination has only recently been developed and become available commercially, it is highly probable that this type of instrument will become the instrument of the future in certain areas.

The most recent development using the Doppler principle is the development of an instrument (MAVIS) (60) using 30 channels of pulsed Doppler simultaneously in order to differentiate arteries and veins by a simultaneous color-coded readout. It uses microcomputers to calculate mean blood flow in milliliters per minute and velocity profiles in selected portions of the artery during the cardiac cycle.

REAL-TIME

Real-time imaging probably originated with the advent of "compounding" which was really intended to add new information to the scan. Such a unit was built by Homes and his group at the University of Colorado to produce compound scanning in 1962. They used a small motor to rock the transducer five times per second back and forth on the patient's skin. The long phosphordecay left enough image on the screen to see the entire field as the brain swept back and forth. This represented a primitive real-time scanner and led to the development of several different instruments.

Kretztechnik of Austria in 1965 was commissioned by Dr. Werner Buschmann (16), an ophthalmologist, to build a 10-element phased array transducer. It was used to scan the eye, arteries, and other structures, but like all systems of that period it suffered from lack of sensitivity and poor video processing. This probably represents the first effort to build a dedicated real-time scanner. The resolution, however, was poor.

Kichuchi et al. (61), in 1966, introduced "synchronized ultrasonocardiotomography" which was used to obtain studies in nine different phases of the cardiac cycle. This system used a mechanically rotating transducer and a water path to obtain sector scans of the heart.

Somer (62), in 1968, reported the development of an electronic scanner for ultrasonic diagnosis. He used a 21-element array, of 1.2 MHz capacity, made of lead zirconate titanate. The array could be excited as a single unit, or each transducer could be excited in a sequential manner or in many combinations. The frame rate was 30 per second, and it produced a "real-time" image. The pulsations and the vessels of the brain could be demonstrated, but, because this was only a minor part in the diagnosis of intracerebral disease, it was not exploited. His system did, however, present a real-time image which was the first with a reasonable display.

Patzold et al. (63), in 1970, employed a rotating two-transducer sound source and a cylindrical parabolic mirror to produce images at about 15 frames per second. The unit was used extensively in Europe despite the flicker in the display.

Hertz and Lundstrom (64) also described a fast ultrasonic scanning system for heart investigations using a mirror system.

Bom et al. (65), in 1971, introduced a fast scanning system for the heart having good resolution and producing images in real-time which could be directly observed on the screen of a CRT. His transducer contained 20 small ultrasonic elements approximately 3 mm in diameter which were fired in rapid sequence.

Griffith and Henry (66), in 1974, developed a mechanical scanner which oscillated a standard transducer through either a 30° or 45° sector with a display frame rate of 30 per second. The quality of the scans obtained was considerably better than the multielement systems.

Other units have been developed, but probably the most sophisticated is the phased array principle developed by Thurstone and von Ramm (67). This technique employs multiple elements in the transducer, fired in a rather complicated sequence by a computer, to sweep electronically through a sector. New aditions are being made continually to improve range, focus, resolution, etc.

Real-time scanners are classified either as (a) mechanized or (b) electrical. The mechanical scanners have transducers which are either fixed and reflected from a rotating mirror or moved in some fashion. The electronic scanners use multiple transducers which are fired in a linear or phased array fashion. These more sophisticated systems provide better resolution but also are more expensive.

The many different techniques developed in the clinical use of ultrasound appear complimentary to one another and are often used together to provide better information. The early static B-scanner provided a great deal of useful clinical information but required considerable time to complete the examination. More recently, it has been used to produce static images which are stored in memory and then subjected to various processing techniques. In general, the B-scan is being mostly replaced by the real-time scanners, but some physicians feel both types of scans are necessary for a complete examination. However, because the real-time examination requires much less time to perform than does the B-scan and with the improved resolution in the systems, it seems logical that it will greatly reduce the use of the B-scanner.

Clinically, real-time scanners have had a rapid expansion in clinical applications in many areas of medicine because of accuracy and ease of application; in some areas, i.e., the gall bladder, this has become the examination of choice and, with more experience, may replace other routine examinations. Certain combinations of the ultrasound presentation have become extremely useful. For example, in the eye it has become important to combine the real-time with simultaneous A-mode and possibly Doppler techniques in the study of tumors; in obstetrics it has become important to combine the real-time with the M-mode to study the fetal heart; and in cardiology the combination of real-time and the M-mode provides a more complete study. Furthermore, the carotid artery study requires a real-time study as well as pulsed and continuous wave Doppler study. Many physicians studying the abdomen prefer a real-time survey scan followed by B-scans focused on the areas of abnormality.

Further development of real-time instruments has been made possible by the development of the digital technique of display and the extensive use of microcomputers to process the signal. The larger drug companies which recently acquired some smaller ultrasound companies have envisioned the many different significant clinical applications and have added present-day innovations in their instruments. This represents a marked change in the industry and provides greater support for further research and development. Their efforts have provided the clinician with a wide variety of high quality real-time instruments, each with variable processing capabilities.

The recent progress in the development and application of ultrasound has been possible by the combined efforts of a diversified and enthusiastic group of workers. Further progress can be expected from those involved in (a) transducer development and technology, (b) video signal processing, (c) the development of a solid state scan converter, (d) computer control of circuitry and techniques, and (e) recording and laser beam display techniques, just to mention a few.

Certain other areas of clinical use of the ultrasound technique have been omitted, i.e., use in radiation therapy, orthopaedics (congenital hip disorders, tendons, and muscles), the testicle, dentistry, the penis and urethra, neck masses, certain intrathoracic masses, the paranasal sinuses, etc. The widespread clinical application is only limited to one's interest and dedication.

The clinical application in medicine is being pursued vigorously with the rapid appearance of many new textbooks and training programs, as well as the increasing general recognition of the present capabilities and future applications of this technique. This brief history serves only as a small tribute to those dedicated workers in medicine and industry who have given their energy and effort to the field to this time. It should not be regarded as an all-inclusive review, because new applications are being developed and revised constantly.

References

1. Ensminger D: *Ultrasonics: The Low- and High-Intensity Applications.* New York, Marcel Dekker, 1973.
2. Curie J, Curie P: Sur l'electricite polaire dans cristaux hemiedres a face inclinees. *C R Seances Acad Sci* 91:383, 1880.
3. Chilowsky C, Langevin MP: Procedes et appareils pour la production de signaux sous-marins diriges et pour la localisation a distance d'obstacles sous-marins. French Patent No. 502913, 1916.
4. Sokolov SY: The ultra-acoustic microscope. *Zh Tekh Fiz* 19:271, 1949.
5. Fry WJ, Meyers R, Fry FJ, Schultz DF, Dreyer LL, Noyes RF: Topical differentia of pathogenetic mechanisms underlying Parkinsonian tremor and rigidity as indicated by ultrasonic irradiation of

the human brain. *Trans Am Neurol Assoc* 83:16, 1958.

6. Firestone FA: Flaw detecting device and measuring instrument. United States Patent No. 2,280,226, 1940.
7. Dussik KT: Uber die Moglichkeit hochfrequente mechanische Schwingungen als diagnostisches Hilfsmittel zu verwenden. *Z Ges Neurol Psych* 174:153, 1942.
8. Guttner W, Fielder G, Patzold J: Uber ultraschallabbildungen am menslichen Schadel. *Acustica* 2:148, 1952.
9. Ballantine HT Jr, Hueter TF, Holt RH: On the use of ultrasound in tumour detection. *J Acoust Soc Am* 26:581, 1954.
10. Leksell L: Echo-encephalography: detection of intracranial complications following head injury. *Acta Chir Scand* 110:301, 1956.
11. Schiefer W, Kazner E, Kunze ST: *Clinical Echo-Encephalography*. New York, Springer-Verlag, 1968, p 85.
12. Kichuchi Y, Uchida R, Tanaka K, Wagai T: Early cancer diagnosis through ultrasonics. *J Acoust Soc Am* 29:824, 1957.
13. Ambrose J: Pulsed ultrasound. Illustrations of clinical applications. *Br J Radiol* 37:165, 1964.
14. Ford R, McRae: Echoencephalography—a standardized technique for measurement of the width of the third and lateral ventricles. In *Diagnostic Ultrasound*. New York, Plenum Press, 1966, pp 117–129.
15. Barnes RW, Brinkley RP, McGraw CP: R-wave to intracranial artery echo activity time interval measurements using moving target indicator techniques. *Ultrasound Med Biol* 4:283–285, 1977.
16. Buschmann W: Zur diagnostic der carotisthrombose. *Albrecht Von Graefes Arch Ophthalmol* 166:519–529, 1964.
17. White DV, Curry GR: A comparison of 424 carotid bifurcations examined by angiography and the Doppler echoflow. *Ultrasound Med Biol* 4:363–375, 1977.
18. Pape KE, Cusick G, Houang MTW, et al: Ultrasound detection of brain damage in preterm infant. *Lancet* 1:1261–1264, 1979.
19. Grant EG, Schellinger D, Borts FT, McCullough DC, Friedman GR, Sivasubramanian KN, Smith Y: Real-time sonography of the neonatal and infant head. *AJNR* 1:487–492, 1980.
20. Ben-Ora A, Eddy L, Hatch G, Solida B: The anterior fontanelle as an acoustic window in the neonatal ventricular system. *J Clin Ultrasound* 8:65–67, 1980.
21. Deleted in proof.
22. Ludwig GD, Struthers FW: Considerations underlying the use of ultrasound to detect gallstones and foreign bodies in tissue. Project MN004-001. *Naval Med Res Inst* 4:1, 1949.
23. Howry DH, Bliss WR: Ultrasonic visualization on soft tissue structures of the body. *J Lab Clin Med* 40:579, 1952.
24. Wild JJ, Neal D: Use of high frequency ultrasonic waves for detecting changes of texture in living tissues. *Lancet* 260:655, 1951.
25. Wild JJ, Reid JM: Application of echo-ranging techniques to the determination of structure of

biological tissues. *Science* 115:226, 1952.
26. Wild JJ, Reid JM: Further pilot echographic studies on the histological structure of tumors of the living intact human breast. *Am J Pathol* 28:839, 1952.
27. Wild JJ, Reid JM: Diagnostic use of ultrasound. *Br J Phys Med* 19:248, 1956.
28. United States Atomic Energy Commission: *Studies in Methods and Instruments to Improve the Localization of Radioactive Materials in the Body with Special Reference to the Diagnosis of Brain Tumours and the Use of Ultrasonic Techniques.* AECU-3012. Minneapolis, University of Minnesota Press, 1955.
29. Donald I, Brown TG: Investigation of abdominal masses by pulsed ultrasound. *Lancet* 1:1188, 1958.
30. Donald I, Brown TG: Demonstration of tissue interfaces within the body by ultrasonic echo sounding. *Br J Radiol* 34:539, 1961.
31. Campbell S: An improved method of fetal cephalometry by ultrasound. *J Obstet Gynecol Br Commow* 75:568, 1968.
32. Sunden B: On the diagnostic value of ultrasound in obstetrics and gynecology. *Acta Obstet Gynecol Scand* 43 (suppl 6), 1964.
33. Thompson HE, Taylor ES, Holmes JH, et al: Ultrasound diagnostic techniques in obstetrics and gynecology. *Am J Obstet Gynecol* 472, 1964.
34. Kossoff G: Improved technques in ultrasonic cross sectional echography. *Ultrasonics* 10:221, 1972.
35. Kossoff G, Garrett WJ, Carpenter DA, Jellins J, Dadd MJ: Principles and classification of soft tissues by grey scale echography. *Ultrasound Med Biol* 2:89, 1976.
36. Takahashi H, Ouchi T: The ultrasonic diagnosis in the field of biology. In *Japanese Medicine and Ultrasonics*. The First Report, 7, 1968. The Second Report, 35, 1964.
37. Watanabe H, Igari D, Tanahasi Y, Harada K, Saitoh M: Development and application of new equipment for transrectal ultrasonography. *J Clin Ultrasound* 2:91, 1974.
38. Holm HH, Northeved A: A transurethral ultrasonic scanner. *J Urol* 111:238, 1974.
39. King WW, Wilkiemeyer RM, Boyce WH, McKinney WM: Current status of prostatic echography. *JAMA* 266:444, 1973.
40. Resnick MI, Willard JW, Boyce WH: Recent progress in ultrasonography of the bladder and prostate. *J Urol* 117:444, 1977.
41. Henneberry M, Carter MF, Neiman HL: Estimation of prostate size by suprapubic ultrasonography. *J Urol* 121:615, 1979.
42. Abu-Yousef, Monzer M, Narayana AL, Ambati S: Transabdominal ultrasound in the evaluation of prostate size. *J Clin Ultrasound* 10:275–278, 1982.
43. Satomura S: Study of the flow patterns in peripheral arteries by ultrasonics. *J Acoust Soc Am Jpn* 15:151, 1959.
44. Franklin DL, Schlegal WA, Rushmer RF: Blood flow measured by Doppler frequency shift of back scattered ultrasound. *Science* 134:564, 1961.
45. McLeod FD Jr: A directional Doppler flowmeter. In Jacobson B: *Digest 7th International Conference on Medical and Biologic Engineering.* Stockholm, The Royal Academy of Engineering Sci-

ences, 1967.

46. Pourcelot L: Nouveau debitmetre sanguin a effet Doppler. In Bock J, Ossoinig K: *Ultrasonographia Medica.* Vienna, Verlag der Wiener Medizinischen Akademie, 1971, p 125.

47. Peronneau O, Deloche A, Bui-Mong-Hung, Hinglais J: Debitmetrie sanguine par ultasons. Deveolppements et application experimentales. In *Third Congress of the European Society for Experimental Surgery,* Munich, 1968.

48. Strandness DE, McCutheon EP, Rushmore RF: Application of a transcutaneous Doppler flowmeter in evaluation of occlusive arterial disease. *Surg Gynecol Obstet* 122:1039, 1966.

49. Sigel B, Popley GL, Boland JP, Wagner DK, Mopp EMcD: Augmentation flow sounds in the ultrasonic detection of venous abnormalities. *Invest Radiol* 2:256, 1967.

50. Lavenson GS, Rich NM, Baugh JH: Value of ultrasonic flow detection in the management of peripheral vascular disease. *Am J Surg* 120:522, 1970.

51. Tajik AJ, Gau GT, Shattenberg TT: Echocardiographic pseudo IHSS pattern in atrial septal defect. *Chest* 62:324, 1972.

52. Yoshida, et al: Analysis of heart motion with ultrasonic Doppler and its clinical application. *Am Heart J* 61:61, 1961.

53. Kostis JB, Fleishmann D, Bellet S: Use of ultrasonic Doppler method for the timing of valvular movement. *Circulation* 40:197, 1969.

54. Huntsman LL, Gams E, Johnson CC, Fairbanks E: Transcutaneous determination of aortic bloodflow velocities in man. *Am Heart J* 89:605, 1975.

55. Callagan DA, Rowland TC, Goldman DE: Ultrasonic Doppler observation of the fetal heart. *Obstet Gynecol* 23:637, 1964.

56. Hokanson DE: Ultrasonic arteriography: a new approach to arterial visualization. *Biomed Eng* 6:420, 1971.

57. White DN, Curry GR: A comparison of 424 carotid bifurcations examined by angiography and the Doppler echoflow. *Ultrasound Med Biol* 4:363, 1977.

58. Baker DW, Johnson SL: Doppler echocardiography. In Gramiak R, Waag RC: *Cardiac Ultrasound.* St Louis, CV Mosby, 1974, p 24.

59. Griffith IM, Henry WI: An ultrasound system for combined cardiac imaging and Doppler blood flow measurement in man. *Circulation* 57:925, 1978.

60. Fish PJ: Pulse Doppler Angiography. In *Proceedings of the 2nd European Congress on Ultrasonics in Medicine,* Munich, 1975.

61. Kichuchi Y, Uchida R, Tanaka K, Wagai T: Early cancer diagnosis through ultrasonics. *J Acoust Soc Am* 29:824, 1957.

62. Somer JC: Principles and technical development of utlrasonics in medicine. *Electronic Sector Scanning in Cerebral Diagnosis.* The Second World Congress, Rotterdam, June 1973. New York, American Elsevier, 1974, pp 304–308.

63. Patzold J, Krause W, Kresse H, Soldner R: *IEEE Trans Biomed Eng* 17:263, 1970.

64. Hertz CH, Lundstrom K: A fast ultrasonic scanning system for heart investigators. In *3rd International Conference on Medical Physics.* Gotenburg, Sweden, August, 1972.

65. Bon N, Lancee CT, Honkoop J, Hugenholtz PG: Ultrasonic viewer for cross-sectional analyses of moving cardiac structures. *Biomed Eng* 6:500, 1971.

66. Griffith JM, Henry WL: A sector scanner for real-time two-dimensional echocardiography. *Circulation* 51:283, 1975.

67. Thurstone FL, von Ramm OT: A new ultrasound technique employing two-dimensional electronic beam steering. In Green PS: *Acoustical Holography.* New York, Plenum, 1974, vol 5.

Suggested Readings

Babcock DS, Bokyung KH, LeQuesne GW: B-mode gray scale ultrasound of the head in the newborn and young infant. *AJR* 134:457–468, 1980.

Baum G: A reappraisal of orbital ultrasonography, series II. *Trans Am Acad Ophthalmol Otolaryngol* 943–958, 1965.

Baum G: *Fundamentals of Medical Ultrasonography.* New York, GP Putnam and Sons, 1975.

Baum G: In White D, Lyons EA: *Ultrasound in Medicine.* New York, Plenum Press, 1978, vol 4, pp 299–318.

Baum G, Greenwood I: The application of ultrasonic locating techniques to ophthalmology. II. Ultrasonic slit lamp in the ultrasonic visualization of soft tissues. *Arch Ophthalmol* 60:263–279, 1958.

Blau JS, Mandell J: Real-time ultrasound evaluation of the breast. *Conn Med* 43:625, 1979.

Blum M, Goldman AB, Herskovic A, et al: Clinical applications of thyroid echography. *N Engl J Med* 287:1164–1169, 1972.

Bronson NR: Technqiues of ultrasonic localization and extraction of intraocular and extraocular foreign bodies. *Am J Ophthalmol* 60:596–603, 1965.

Carson PL, Dick DE, Thieme GA, Dick ML, Bayly EJ, Oughton TV, Dubuque GL, Bay HP: In White D, Lyons EA: *Ultrasound in Medicine.* New York, Plenum Press, 1978, vol 4, pp 319–322.

Ching J, Martin JF: Real time breast ultrasound. Presented at AIUM Meeting, New Orleans, September 1980.

Coleman DJ: Reliability of ocular and orbital diagnosis with B scan ultrasound. Part I. Ocular diagnosis. *Am J Ophthalmol* 73:501–516, 1972.

Coleman DJ: Reliability of ocular and orbital diagnosis with B scan ultrasound. Part II. Orbital diagnosis. *Am J Ophthalmol* 74:704–718, 1972.

Coleman DJ, Konig WW, Katz L: A hand-operated ultrasound scan system for ophthalmic evaluation. *Am J Ophthalmol* 68:256–263, 1969.

Coleman DJ, Weininger R: Ultrasonic M-mode technique in ophthalmology. *Arch Ophthalmol* 82:475–479, 1969.

Damascelli B, Cascinelli N, Livraghi T, Veronesi U: Pre-operative approach to thyroid tumors by a two-dimensional pulsed echo technique. *Ultrasonics* 6:242–243, 1968.

Ebina T, Oka S, Tanaka M, Kosaka S, Terasawa Y, Unno K, Kikuchi D, Uchida R: The ultrasonotomography of the heart and great vessels in living human subjects by means of the ultrasonic reflection technique. *Jpn Heart J* 8:331, 1967.

Edler I, Hertz CH: The use of ultrasonic reflectoscope for the continuous recording of movements of heart walls. *Kungl Frysiogr Sallsk Lund Forhandl* 24:5, 1954

Edler I, Hertz CH: The early work on ultrasound in medicine at the University of Lund. *J Clin Ultrasound* 5:352, 1977.

Effert S: Der derzeitige stand der ultraschallkardiographie. *Arch Kreislaufforsch* 30:213, 1959.

Eggleton RC, Townsend C, Herrick J, Templeton G, Mitchell JH: Ultrasonic visualization of left ventricular dynamics. *IEEE Trans Sonics Ultrasonics. SU* 17, 1970.

Feigenbaum H: *Echocardiography*, ed 3. Philadelphia, Lea and Febiger, 1976.

Feigenbaum H, Stone JM, Lee DA, Nasser WK, Chang S: Identification of ultrasound echoes from the left ventricle using intracardiac injections of Indocyanine green. *Circulation* 41:615, 1970.

Freund HJ: In *Electronic Sector Scanning in Cerebral Diagnosis*. The Second World Congress, Rotterdam, June 1973. New York, American Elsevier, 1974, pp 314–317.

Fry EK: *A Study of Ultrasonic Detection of Breast Disease*. 1st Quarterly Report. Bethesda, MD United States Public Health Service, 1968a.

Fry EK: *A Study of Ultrasonic Detection of Breast Disease*. 2nd Quarterly Report. Bethesda, MD, United States Public Health Service,

Fry EK: *A Study of Ultrasonic Detection of Breast Disease*. 3rd Quarterly Report. Bethesda, MD, United States Public Health Service, 1969.

Fry EK: *A Study of Ultrasonic Detection of Breast Disease*. Progress Report. Bethesda, MD, United States Public Health Service, Cancer Control Program, PH-86-68-193, 1970.

Fujimoto Y, Oka A, Omoto R, Hirose M: Ultrasound scanning of the thyroid gland as a new diagnostic approach. *Ultrasonics* 5:177–80, 1967.

Garrett WJ, Kossoff G, Jones RFC: Ultrasonic cross-sectional visualization of hydrocephalus in infants. *Neuroradiology* 8:279–288, 1975.

Gernet H, Franceschetti A: Ultrasound biometry of the eye. In Oksala A, Gernet H: *Ultrasonics in Ophthalmology*. Basel, S Karger, 1967, pp 175–206.

Gramiak R, Shah PM: Echocardiography of the aortic root. *Invest Radiol* 3:356, 1968.

Greenleaf JF, Johnson SA: Measurement of spatial distribution of refractive index in tissues by ultrasonic computer assisted tomography. *Ultrasound Med Biol* 3:327–339, 1978.

Greenleaf JF, Rajagopalan B, Kenue SK, Johnson SA, Bahn RC: *Third International Symposium on Ultrasonic Imaging and Tissue Characterization*. Gaithersburg, MD, National Bureau of Standards, 1978, pp 9–11.

Houry DH, Stott DA, Bliss WD: The ultrasonic visualization of carcinoma of the breast and other soft tissues. *Cancer* 73:354, 1954.

Jannson F: Measurements of intraocular distance by ultrasound. *Acta Ophthalmol* 74 (suppl):1–51, 1963.

Johnson ML, Mack LA, Rumack CM, Frost M, Rashbaum C: B-mode echoencephalography in the normal and high risk infant. *AJR* 133:375–381, 1979.

Joyner CR, Reid JM: Application of ultrasound in cardiology and cardiovascular physiology. *Prog Cardiovas Dis* 5:482, 1963.

Joyner CR, Reid JM, Bond JP: Reflected ultrasound in the assessment of mitral valve disease. *Circulation* 27:506, 1963.

Kamphuisen HAC: II. Space occupying processes and hydrocephalus. In *Electronic Sector Scanning in Cerebral Diagnosis*. The Second World Congress, Rotterdam, June 1973. New York, American Elsevier, 1974, pp 309–313.

Keidel WD: Uher eine Methode zur registrierung der Volumanderungen des Herzens am Mensche. *Z Kreislaufforsch* 39:257, 1950.

Kikuchi Y: Way to quantitative examination in ultrasonic diagnosis. *Med Ultrasonics* 5:1, 1968.

Kikuchi Y, Uchida R, Tanaka K, Wagai T: Early cancer diagnosis through ultrasonics. *J Acoust Soc Am* 29:824–833, 1957.

Kisslo J, Griedman G, Johnson M, von Ramm O: Two-dimensional echocardiographic assessment of normal mitral leaflet motion. *Circulation* 52 (suppl II):32, 1975.

Kobayashi T: Echographic diagnosis of breast tumor—current status of sensitivity graded method of ultrasonotomography and its clinical evaluation (in Japanese). *J Jpn Soc Cancer Ther* 9:310–323, 1974.

Kobayashi T, Hayashi M: Manual contact scanning in gray scale breast echography. *Univ Occup Environ Health (Jpn)* 2: 1980.

Kossoff G: Improved techniques in ultrasonic cross sectional echography. *Ultrasonics* 10:221–227, 1972.

Kossoff G, Garrett WJ, Radavanovich G: Ultrasonic atlas of normal brain of infant. *Ultrasound Med Biol* 1:259–266, 1974.

Laustela E, Kermine T, Lieto J, Tala P: Studies of the ultrasonic diagnosis of breast tumors. *Ann Chir Gynecol Fenn* 55:173–175, 1966.

Lees RF, Harrison RB, Sims TL: Gray scale ultrasonography in the evaluation of hydrocephalus and associated abnormalities in infants. *Am J Dis Child* 132:376–378, 1978.

Medical news. *JAMA* 248: 1982.

Morgan CL, Trought WS, Rothman SJ, Jimenez JP: Comparison of gray-scale ultasonography and computed tomography in the evaluation of macrocrania in infants. *Radiology* 132:119–123, 1979.

Mundt GH, Hughes WF: Ultrasonics in ocular diagnosis. *Am J Ophthalmol* 41:488–498, 1956.

Nassani SN, Bard R: In White D, Lyons EA: *Ultrasound in Medicine*. New York, Plenum Press, 1978, vol 4, pp 323–324.

Oksala A, Lehtinen A: Diagnostics of detachment of the retina by means of ultrasound. *Acta Ophthalmol* 35:461–467, 1957.

Ossoinig K: Ultrasonic diagnosis of the eye: an aid for the clinic. In Oksala A, Gernet H: *Ultrasonics in Ophthalmology*. Basel, S Karger, 1967, pp 116–133.

Ossoinig K: Clinical echo-ophthalmolography. In Blodi FC: *Current Concepts in Ophthalmology*. St Louis, CV Mosby, 1972, pp 110–130.

Purnell EW: Ultrasound in ophthalmological diagnosis. In Grossman CC, et al: *Diagnostic Ultrasound: Proceedings of the First International Conference, Pittsburgh, 1965*. New York, Plenum Press, 1966, pp 95–130.

Purnell EW: Ultrasonic interpretation of orbital disease. In Gitter KA, et al: *Ophthalmic Ultrasound.* St Louis, CV Mosby, 1969. pp 249–259.

Shkolnik A: B-mode scanning of the infant brain. A new approach case report. Craniopharyngioma. *J Clin Ultrasound* 3:229–231, 1975.

Skolnick ML, Rosenbaum AE, Matzuk T, Guthkelch AN, Heinz ER: Detection of dilated cerebral ventricles in infants. A correlative study between ultrasound and computed tomography. *Radiology* 131:447–451, 1979.

Somer JC: Electronic sector scanner for ultrasonic diagnosis. *Ultrasonics* 6:153–159, 1968.

Tajik AJ, Seward JB, Hagler DJ, Mar DD, Mair, DD Lie JT: Two-dimensional real-time ultrasonic imaging of the heart and great vesels. Technique, image orientation, structure. identification, and validation. *Mayo Clin Proc* 53:1978.

Taylor KJW, Carpenter DE, Barrett SS: Gray scale ultrasonography in the diagnosis of thyroid swellings. *J Clin Ultrasound* 2:327, 1974.

Tenner MS, Wodraska GM: *Diagnostic Ultrasound in Neurology: Methods and Techniques.* New York, John Wiley & Sons, 1975.

Vlieger M de, Sterke A, deMolin CE, Van der Ven C: Ultrasound for two dimensional echoencephalography. *Ultrasonics* 1:148–151, 1963.

von Ramm OT, Smith SW, Kisslo JA: Ultrasound tomography of the adult brain. *Ultrasound Med Biol* 4:261–268, 1977.

von Ramm OT, Thurstone FL: Cardiac imaging using a phased array ultrasound system. *Circulation* 53:258, 1976.

Waag RC, Gramiak R: Computer-controlled two-dimensional cardiac motion imaging. In *Proceedings of the 1974 Ultrasonics Symposium*, Milwaukee, 1974. IEEE Cat. No. 74CHO 896–ISU:12.

Wagai T, Takahashi S, Ohashi H, Ichikawa H: A trial for quantitative diagnosis of breast tumor by ultrasono-tomography. *Med Ultrasonics* 5: 39–40, 1967.

Wells PTN, Evans KT: An immersion scanner for two-dimensional ultrasonic examination of the human breast. *Ultrasonics* 6:220–223, 1968.

Wild JJ, Crawford HD, Reid JM: Visualization of the excised human heart by means of reflected ultrasound or echography. *Am Heart J* 54:903, 1957.

Yamakowa K, Naito S: Ultrasound diagnosis in Japan. IV. Application for the disease of the thyroid. In Grossman CC, Holmes JH, Joyner C, Purnell E: *Diagnostic Ultrasound: Proceedings of the First International Conference, Pittsburgh, 1965.* New York, Plenum Press, 1966.

CHAPTER 2

Basic Physics and Instrumentation

THOMAS E. SUMNER, M.D.
WARD A. RILEY, Ph.D.

A brief discussion of the basic physics and instrumentation of diagnostic ultrasound will be given in this chapter. A more detailed treatment of the topics discussed can be obtained from several widely used references (1–9). Our objective is to provide a concise summary of some of the important principles required for the clinician entering the field of diagnostic ultrasound. As experience is gained in the field, a considerably greater depth of understanding of these principles should be achieved in order to adequately perform and interpret studies covering a broad range of clinical applications.

ULTRASOUND AND X-RAYS

Prior to the development of diagnostic ultrasound over the last two decades, the primary form of radiation used in diagnostic imaging was x-radiation, a form of *electromagnetic* radiation. Ultrasound, by contrast, is a form of *mechanical* (or acoustical) radiation, which propagates through tissues at a much slower speed and interacts with these tissues in a fundamentally different way. Table 2.1 highlights several important differences between these two forms of radiation and gives several examples of both types. While a detailed discussion of these differences is beyond the scope of this text, an initial consideration of the possible biological effects of ultrasonic radiation must begin with an appreciation of these fundamental differences. In addition, one should approach ultrasonic imaging without too great a preconception as to how such images should be interpreted since they are directly related to the *mechanical* properties of tissues rather than the *charge density* properties associated with conventional x-rays.

ULTRASONIC WAVE TERMINOLOGY

Ultrasound is an acoustic wave that propagates through soft tissues, advancing about 1.5 mm in one millionth of a second (1 μs). The ultrasonic frequencies (number of vibrations per second) encountered in diagnostic imaging cover the range of 1 million cycles/second (1 MHz) to 10 million cycles/second (10 MHz). These mechanical waves propagate in two basic modes, longitudinal and transverse, and their characteristics are summarized in Table 2.2.

In imaging applications, short acoustic pulses approximately two to three cycles long are generated by highly damped piezoelectric crystals. Three common types of transducers are illus-

Table 2.1.
Mechanical and electromagnetic radiation

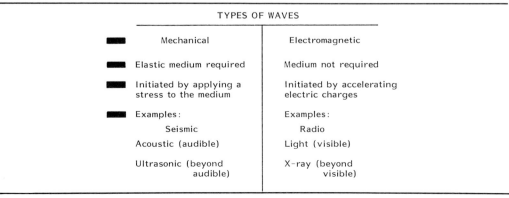

TYPES OF WAVES	
Mechanical	Electromagnetic
Elastic medium required	Medium not required
Initiated by applying a stress to the medium	Initiated by accelerating electric charges
Examples:	Examples:
Seismic	Radio
Acoustic (audible)	Light (visible)
Ultrasonic (beyond audible)	X-ray (beyond visible)

Table 2.2.
Mechanical wave propagation

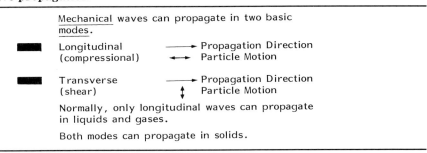

Mechanical waves can propagate in two basic modes.

Longitudinal (compressional) — Propagation Direction — Particle Motion

Transverse (shear) — Propagation Direction — Particle Motion

Normally, only longitudinal waves can propagate in liquids and gases.

Both modes can propagate in solids.

trated in Figures 2.1 to 2.3: the single element circular faced transducer, the multiple element linear array transducer, and the multiple element array used in sector scan images. The short pulses will extend through a distance of approximately 1 mm along the direction of travel (axis), and typically this is a good estimate for the ultimate axial resolution capability of the system. Since the length of the pulse gets shorter and the beam can be more highly focused as the frequency of the transducer is increased, the resolution capability increases, in general, with frequency. However, tissues extract more energy per unit distance from the ultrasonic pulse at higher frequencies, and to image deeper structures it may be necessary to compromise on resolution. The fundamental mechanisms by which energy is extracted from an ultrasonic beam are shown in Figure 2.4.

THE MOST COMMON ULTRASOUND IMAGE

The image obtained with a diagnostic ultrasound instrument is a map of the differences in mechanical properties of the adjacent tissues. Specifically, the acoustic impedance of a tissue is of primary importance. The acoustic impedance is the product of the mass density and speed of sound propagation in the tissue. The intensity of the reflection of an ultrasonic pulse at the interface of two tissues is proportional to the square of this difference in acoustic impedances of the tissues. The intensity of the reflection between soft tissue interfaces is relatively weak. The reflection between air-soft tissue or bone-soft tissue interfaces is very strong. Most two-dimensional images (called B-scans for brightness) are *acoustic impedance difference maps of internal body structures. The brightness* of the spot on the cathode ray tube (CRT)

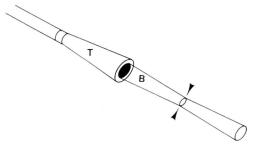

Figure 2.1. Circular face medical ultrasound transducer (*T*) commonly used in static B-scan systems. The transmitted beam (*B*) is shaped to its narrowest diameter (*arrows*) at the depth of major importance to a particular application.

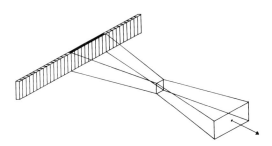

Figure 2.2. Linear array medical ultrasound transducer used to obtain reticilinear real-time B-scan images. The transmitted beam is formed by electronically exciting multiple elements as a group. The returning echoes can also be electronically processed to shape further the width of the ultrasonic beam.

corresponds to the intensity of the original echo reflection from the interface. Display of the echoes as dots on the CRT is called a B-mode display. The image can be displayed either as a gray-scale image, in which the dots are varied in

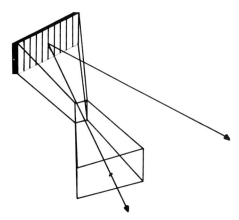

Figure 2.3. Linear array medical ultrasound transducer used to obtain sector format B-scan images. The transmitted beam is electronically scanned through an arc to interrogate a pie-shaped region. The returning echoes can also be electronically processed to shape further the width of the ultrasonic beam.

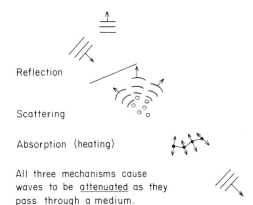

Waves lose energy as they travel through a medium due to

Reflection

Scattering

Absorption (heating)

All three mechanisms cause waves to be attenuated as they pass through a medium.

Figure 2.4. Principal methods by which ultrasonic beams lose energy as they travel through tissue. It is typical for ultrasonic beams to lose very significant fractions of their total energy after traveling only a few centimeters into soft tissue.

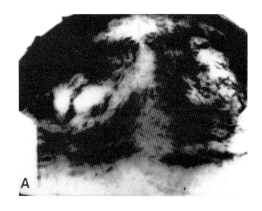

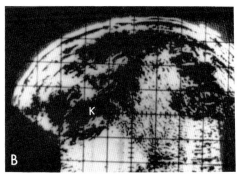

Figure 2.5. Comparison prone transverse scans of hydronephrotic left kidney (*K*). *A*, Gray-scale. *B*, Bi-stable. (Note: Scans are of historical interest and are not meant to represent current sonographic quality.)

intensity according to the signal level (Fig. 2.5*A*), or in a bi-stable image, in which the dots are all presented at the same intensity regardless of signal level (Fig. 2.5*B*). In general, gray-scale imaging affords display of soft tissue interfaces, whereas bi-stable processing is characterized by enhanced delineation of mass borders.

OTHER TYPES OF INFORMATION DISPLAYS

M-Mode

When the motion of rapidly moving structures is of interest, an M-mode (Motion-mode) may provide valuable information. This mode is also called TM-mode for time-motion display. In this display format, the B-mode trace moves as a function of time to show the dynamics of tissue interfaces. This method is currently used for echocardiography, since echoes emanating from ventricular, valvular, and pericardial interfaces can be displayed and their motion studied. An example of clinical importance is shown in Figure 2.6.

A-Mode

When a semiquantitative relative comparison of the amplitudes of the ultrasonic pulses arriving from a region as a function of distance is

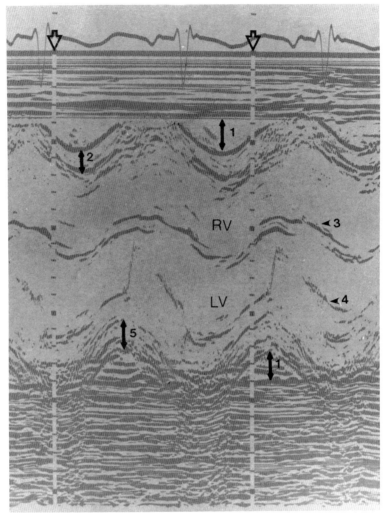

Figure 2.6. M-mode. TM- or M-mode stands for time-motion mode. Motion of the echo sources toward and away from the transducer with respect to time is depicted. Centimeter markers (*open arrows*) are displayed each second. This image reveals a periardial effusion (*1*); *2*, right ventricular wall; *3*, septum; *4*, mitral valve; *5*, left ventricular wall; *RV*, right ventricle; *LV*, left ventricle.

desired, an A-mode (Amplitude-mode) may provide useful information. The high amplitude distal echoes characteristic of cystic masses are easily shown on an A-mode tracing (Fig. 2.7). In addition, no echoes will be seen between the near and far walls of a cyst. A-mode displays are limited in their utility, because of their small sampling volume and lack of anatomical landmarks in establishing exactly where the ultrasound beam is directed. At present, clinical application is primarily in evaluating cystic lesions, such as renal cysts. The range of an area for aspiration or biopsy, as well as needle loca-

tion, can be assessed. These procedures will be described in more detail in Chapter 16.

Doppler

Another means of observing moving objects is by use of the well-known Doppler effect, which is an apparent change in frequency of a sound source with motion, such as a train whistle as it approaches and passes a stationary listener. Doppler instruments contain separate sending and receiving transducers that can detect a change in frequency of the reflected pulse resulting from motion of the reflecting target (Fig. 2.8). When, for example, ultrasound is scattered from moving red blood cells, the frequency of the wave is slightly changed (Fig. 2.9).

Real-Time

Another type of B-mode display is real-time or dynamic imaging. Real-time imaging employs a transducer array consisting of several small transducers or a single transducer that moves along a prescribed track and is able to perform a set of rapid B-scans so quickly that the echo

sources can be followed. Several examples of real-time scans obtained in urology applications are shown in Figures 2.10 to 2.12. Due to its widespread urological application and continually changing instrumentation, the instrumentation segment of this chapter will focus on real-time imaging.

REAL-TIME INSTRUMENTATION

The computer term "real-time" describes any computative process performed instantaneously

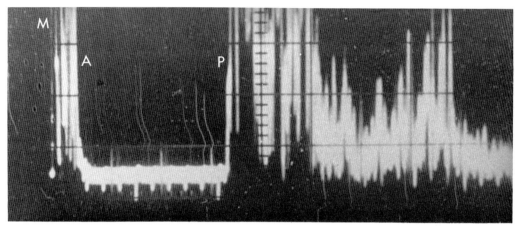

Figure 2.7. A-mode. A stands for amplitude. This tracing was obtained during scanning of a mesenteric cyst. The initial pulse or "main bang" (*M*) appears as a peak; the height of the peak corresponds to the amplitude of the echo. Echo peaks are recorded arising from the anterior (*A*) and posterior (*P*) walls of the cyst; no echoes are seen between the proximal and distal walls of the cyst.

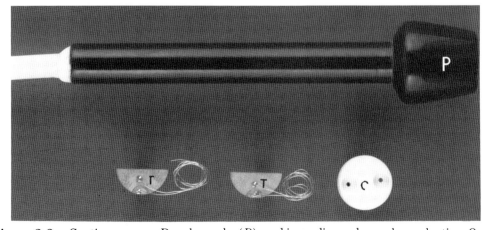

Figure 2.8. Continuous wave Doppler probe (*P*) used in cardiac and vascular evaluation. Quartz sending and receiving transducers (*T*) are positioned behind cover (*C*). (Courtesy of Steven Meads, Carolina Medical Electronics.)

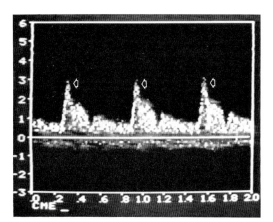

Figure 2.9. Common carotid Doppler spectral display depicting peak frequency (*open arrows*) of red blood cell flow velocity. (Courtesy of Carolina Medical Electronics.)

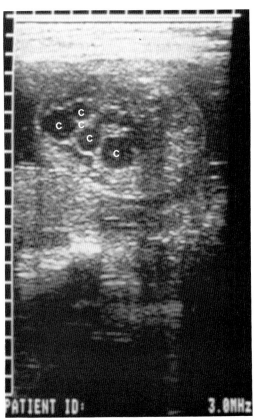

Figure 2.10. Multicystic kidney (in utero scan). Multiple cysts (*C*) are separated by linear septa. Linear array real-time scan with rectilinear format. (Courtesy of L. Nelson, M.D.)

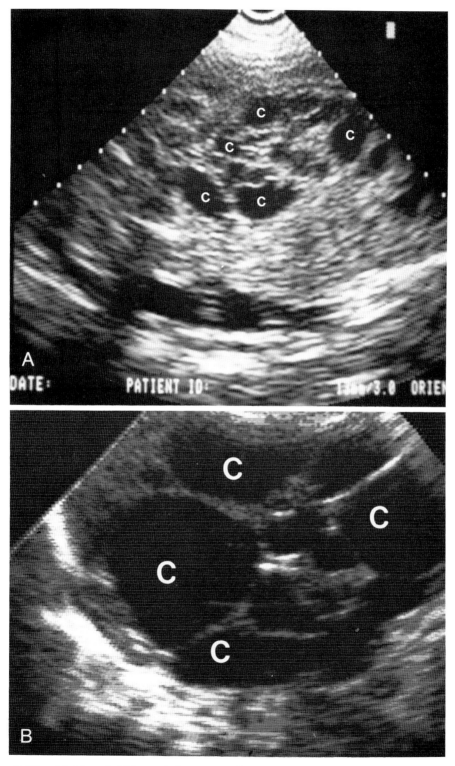

Figure 2.11. Multicystic kidney. *A,* In utero real-time scan with sector format. (Courtesy of L. Nelson, M.D.) *B,* Supine longitudinal scan of same kidney in vivo using a sector real-time scanner with sector format.

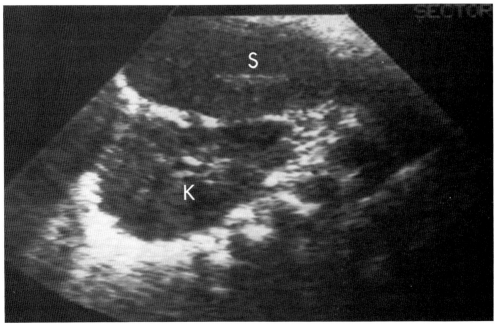

Figure 2.12.   Normal neonatal kidney (*K*) (supine longitudinal). *S*, spleen.

without storage and data manipulation. When applied to ultrasound instrumentation, "real-time" refers to scanners that instantaneously image and display internal body structures. As a result, the sonographer can both scan areas of interest and study moving structures. This feature of real-time sonography is analogous to fluoroscopy.

The two main categories of real-time scanners are *mechanically steered* and *electronically steered*. Mechanical beam steering can be accomplished by either moving the transducer itself or by reflecting the beam from a moving mirror. To ensure adequate acoustic coupling, most mechanically steered scanners have a fluid-filled compartment with an acoustically transparent window containing the moving parts. Variations of mechanically steered scanners include *oscillating transducer scanners* (Fig. 2.13), *stationary transducers with oscillating acoustic mirror* (Fig. 2.14), and *rotating wheel transducers* (Fig. 2.15). Oscillating transducer scanners include linear oscillating "small parts" scanners (Fig. 2.16) and "wobbling" single transducer scanners (Fig. 2.17). As an alternative to oscillating transducers, stationary transducers with oscillating mirrors are available (Fig. 2.18). Advantages of the oscillating mirror design include elimination of the need to move an oscillating transducer and the fact that the oscillat-

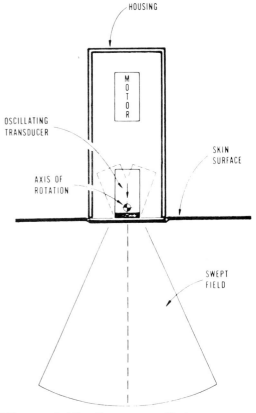

Figure 2.13.   Contact oscillating system. (Adapted with permission from Winsberg (9).)

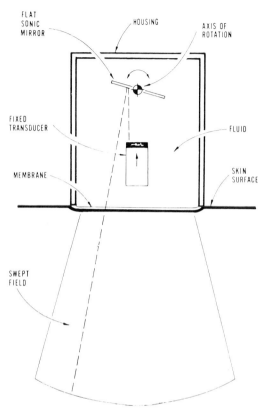

Figure 2.14. Stationary transducer with reflecting, moving-mirror system. (Adapted with permission from Winsberg (9).)

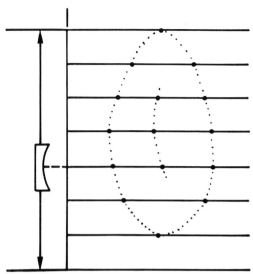

Figure 2.16. Linear oscillating "small parts" system. (Courtesy of A. Fleischer, M.D.) ·

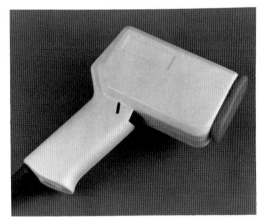

Figure 2.17. "Wobbling" single transducer system. (Courtesy of Diasonics.)

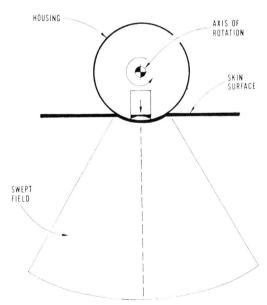

Figure 2.15. Rotating wheel transducer system. (Adapted with permission from Winsberg (9).)

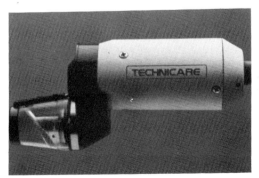

Figure 2.18. Stationary transducer with oscillating mirror system. (Courtesy of Technicare.)

ing mirror is usually lighter, thus it is more easily and rapidly moved than the transducer itself. *Rotating wheel transducers* are the most common types of mechanically steered transducers. In one popular model, three transducers are mounted 120° apart on a wheel; the wheel is rotated by an external motor (Fig. 2.19). Both the wheel and transducers are housed in a fluid-filled case with an acoustic window at the lower end to facilitate good transducer-patient acoustic coupling. Ultrasonic beam output is sequentially switched from one transducer to the next, depending upon which transducer rotates in front of the acoustic window. Rapid framing (30 frames/second) results from this design. With the exception of the linear oscillating "small parts" scanner with its rectilinear field of view, the mechanically steered scanners have a sector (pie-shaped) image format.

Electronically steered scanners include linear phased arrays (Fig. 2.20), multielement linear sequence arrays (Fig. 2.21), and multielement annular arrays (Fig. 2.22). These instruments create a composite ultrasonic beam by proper phasing of the transmit-receiving timing of their transducers. Electronic focusing is accomplished by precise superposition of ultrasonic waves individually generated by transducer arrays. *Linear phased arrays* are often called electronic sector scanners since their format is pie shaped. The transducer array is variably activated and delayed, resulting in specific wave depth and

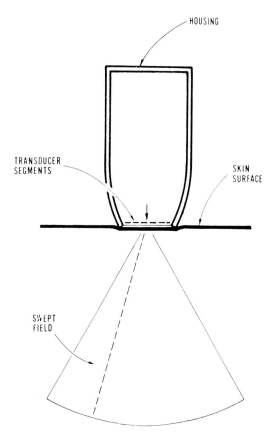

Figure 2.20. Linear phase steered array system. (Adapted with permission from Winsberg (9).)

focus (Fig. 2.23). Electronic switched linear arrays have proved useful for abdominal, obstetrical and gynecological, and pediatric cardiac applications. The linear format lends itself to fetal imaging, but transducer size and shape limit subcostal examinations of organs such as liver and kidney. *Multielement linear sequence arrays* are pulsed so as to produce a wave front that moves normal to the transducer face, thus yielding a rectangular field (Fig. 2.24). Transducer length is often approximately 20 cm. Clinical applications include abdominal, obstetrical, and gynecological.

Annular phased arrays combine features of both mechanical and electronic scanners. Beam formation and focusing are electronically accomplished, whereas beam steering is mechanical, using an oscillating mirror within a fluid-filled housing (Fig. 2.25). Transducer size, often 10 cm or larger, is a limitation, but excellent focusing and larger field of view result. Variable

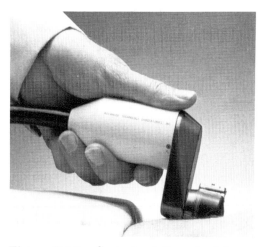

Figure 2.19. Contact rotating wheel transducer. (Courtesy of Advanced Technological Laboratories, © copyright 1981, ATL. Reproduced with permission.)

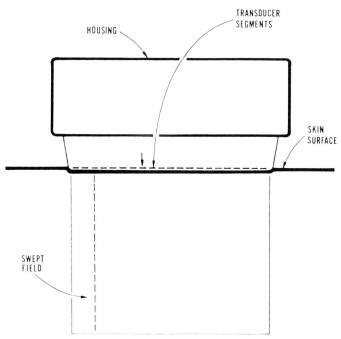

Figure 2.21. Multielement linear sequenced array system. (Adapted with permission from Winsberg (9).)

ANNULAR PHASED ARRAY

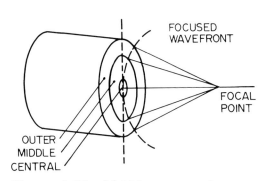

Figure 2.22. Multielement annular array system. (Courtesy of A. Fleischer, M.D.)

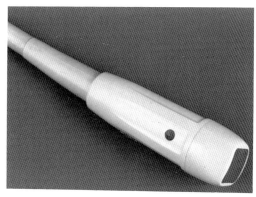

Figure 2.23. Linear phased array transducer. (Courtesy of Hewlett-Packard.)

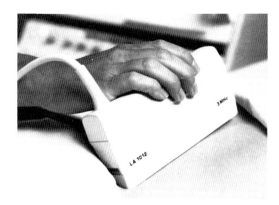

Figure 2.24. Multielement linear sequenced array transducer. (Courtesy of Philips.)

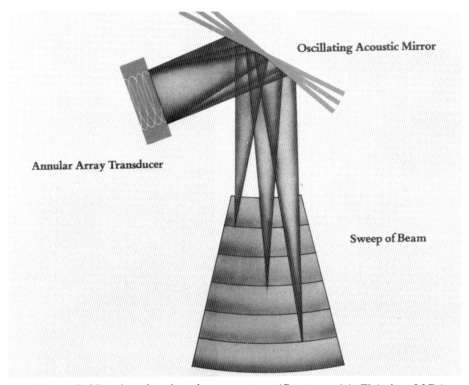

Figure 2.25. Annular phased array system. (Courtesy of A. Fleischer, M.D.)

focal zones are available, permitting operator selection of optimum depth after a survey scan. Breast scanning often utilizes annular phased arrays. Recently, smaller annular array probes have been manufactured with applications in obstetrics, abdominal, and carotid artery scanning (Fig. 2.26, *A* and *B*). Both types of phased arrays afford excellent lateral and axial resolution.

CHOOSING A REAL-TIME SCANNER

None of the described real-time scanners is ideal for all applications. Particular clinical sit-

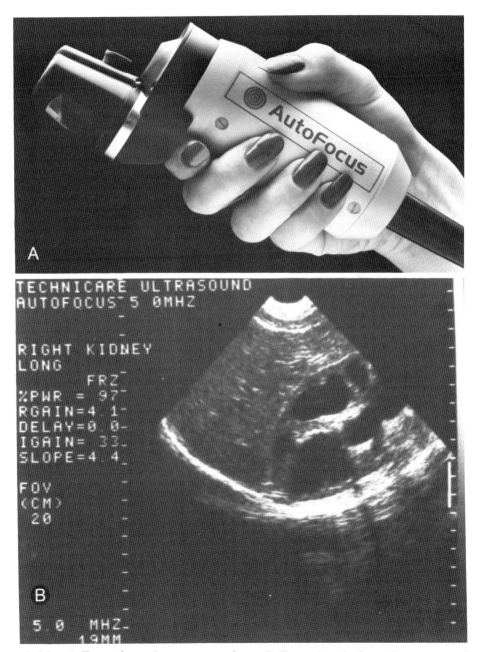

Figure 2.26. *A*, Focused annular array transducer. *B*, Example of hydronephrosis scanned with this transducer. (Courtesy of Technicare.)

uations may dictate a particular type, but many factors warrant consideration—scanner size and cost, resolution, field of view size.

In general, mechanical sector scanners have smaller transducer sizes, thereby requiring only small contact areas; also they may be angled to scan less accessible areas. In particular, these transducers allow scanning through the ribs (Fig. 2.27). This feature is important for renal evaluation. Linear array transducers, due to the relatively large size, are less easily maneuvered between ribs and in subcostal regions (Fig. 2.28). Their advantages, however, derive from the capability of depicting a large rectangular field of view as opposed to the smaller pie-shaped mechanical sector image. Recently, certain manufacturers have offered scanners with both sector and linear scanning in one system (Fig. 2.29).

Most annular array transducers are relatively large because they need a long fluid path within the transducer aperture to permit optimal focusing. Although its field of view is large, this type

of scanner is usually less maneuverable compared to mechanical sector scanners.

Phased arrays are the most expensive due to the computer control necessary for beam syn-

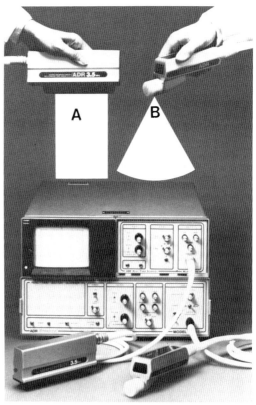

Figure 2.29. Separate linear array (*A*) and mechanical sector (*B*) transducers in a single system. (Courtesy of ADR, © copyright 1979. Reproduced with permission.)

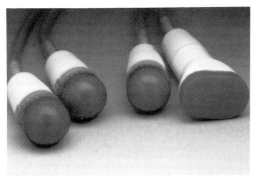

Figure 2.27. Varying frequency mechanical sector transducers. (Courtesy of Philips.)

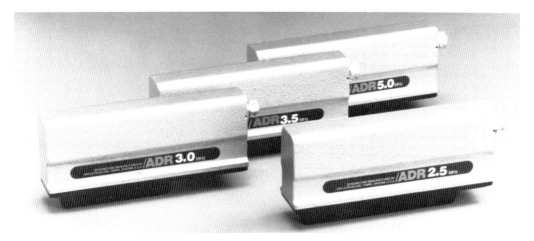

Figure 2.28. Varying frequency linear array transducers. (Courtesy of ADR, © copyright 1979, ADR. Reproduced with permission.)

thesis and steering. However, their lateral and axial resolution is superior due to computer-controlled focusing throughout the entire field of view. Cardiac evaluation often employs phased arrays since they require only a small contact area for imaging deep structures.

Specialized transducers have been developed. As discussed in later chapters, custom-designed transducers are available for prostate (Fig. 2.30) and scrotal scanning, intraoperative sonography, and renal puncture or biopsy (Fig. 2.31).

REAL-TIME VERSUS STATIC B-SCANNING

Real-time sonography has advantages of speed, portability, and dynamic evaluation of structures. In many instances, real-time scanning permits a rapid "survey scan" before concentrating upon a selected area.

The limited field of view may require further evaluation with static scanning to image a large area of interest fully. In this way, these two techniques are often complementary. In addition to global depiction, static scans best document abnormalities in relation to surrounding areas. The dynamic evaluation of physiological motion of structures afforded by real-time is a mixed blessing—it requires instantaneous recognition of normal and abnormal anatomy without the luxury of leisurely viewing static scans. Real-time portability is a major advantage, especially when scanning is required in the operating room or at the bedside. Table 2.3 summa-

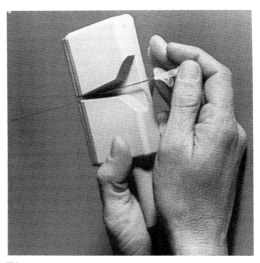

Figure 2.31. Biopsy transducer with needle guide attached to real-time transducer. (Courtesy of General Electric.)

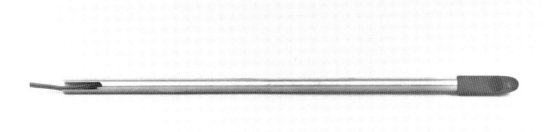

Figure 2.30. Transrectal prostate probe. (Courtesy of Caroline Medical Electronics.)

Table 2.3.
Comparison of real-time and "static" sonography[a]

Real-time	Static
1. Depicts limited field of view	1. Global depiction of an area of interest
2. Requires instantaneous recognition of normal and abnormal anatomy	2. Can be viewed after images are obtained
3. Motion of structures apparent	3. Motion not depicted
4. Portable	4. Not portable
5. Faster examination time	5. Slower examination time

[a] Modified and adapted with permission from Fleischer and James(2).

rizes the features of real-time scanning as compared to static scanning.

References

1. Fleischer AC, James AE: *Introduction to Diagnostic Sonography.* New York, John Wiley & Sons, 1980.
2. Fleischer AC, James AE: *Real-Time Sonography: Textbook and Teaching Tape.* New York, Appleton-Century-Crofts, 1983.
3. Keil O: Ultrasound and its various modes in use. Part I. *Med Instrument* 16:27–30, 1982a.
4. Keil O: Ultrasound and its various modes in use. Part II. Real-time scanners. *Med Instrument* 16:107–110, 1982b.
5. Kremkau FW: *Diagnostic Ultrasound: Physical Principles and Exercises.* New York, Grune and Stratton, 1980.
6. McDicken WN: *Diagnostic Ultrasonics: Principles and Use of Instruments,* ed 2. New York, John Wiley & Sons, 1981.
7. Rose JL, Goldberg BB: *Basic Physics in Diagnostic Ultrasound.* New York, John Wiley & Sons, 1979.
8. Wells PNT: *Biomedical Ultrasonics.* New York, Academic Press, 1977.
9. Winsberg F: Real-time scanners: a review. *Med Ultrasound* 3:99–106, 1979.

CHAPTER 3

Cross-sectional Anatomy of the Male Urogenital System*

WALTER J. BO, Ph.D.
WAYNE A. KRUEGER, Ph.D.

The purpose of this chapter is to present the gross morphology of the male urogenital system that is applicable to the ultrasonography which is presented in the following chapters. In addition to the descriptive anatomy, cross coronal and sagittal sections in the regions of the kidneys and prostate are included; the cross- and coronal sections were cut 1 cm apart. The cross-sections are viewed from below, similar to ultrasonographs, since this has been the conventional approach adopted, whereas the coronal sections are viewed from the anterior surface. The sagittal sections are viewed from the right.

KIDNEYS

The kidneys are paired structures which lie in the paravertebral gutters of the posterior abdominal wall opposite the bodies of the last thoracic and upper three lumbar vertebrae. Since the gutters pass inferiorly and laterally along the lateral margin of the psoas major muscles, the longitudinal axis of the kidneys is in the same direction. The transverse axis is directed laterally and slightly posteriorly. Each kidney is approximately 10 cm long, 5 cm wide, and 2.5 cm thick. The left kidney is at a slightly higher level than the right.

On examination, the kidneys present anterior and posterior surfaces, superior and inferior poles, and lateral and medial borders (Figs. 3.1 to 3.24). The relationships of the viscera to the kidneys can be seen in the cross-sections (Figs.

* This work was supported by a Venture Grant from Richard Janeway, M.D., Dean of the Bowman Gray School of Medicine. The authors are indebted to Mr. Robert Bowden, Anatomy Technologist, for helping in the preparation of the sections. The photographs of the cross-sections and sagittal sections in this chapter are reproduced with permission from Bo WJ, Meschan I, Krueger WA: *Basic Atlas of Cross-Sectional Anatomy*. Philadelphia, WB Saunders, 1980.

3.3 to 3.14), in the coronal sections (Figs. 3.15 to 3.21), and in the sagittal sections (Figs. 3.22 to 3.24).

The anterior surface of each kidney faces anterolaterally, and their relationships differ as indicated in Figure 3.1. The kidneys originally lie posterior to the peritoneum; however, due to development of the suprarenal gland and changes that occur during the development of the duodenum, pancreas, and colon, the peritoneal relations are altered. Although the kidneys are retroperitoneal, there are certain areas that are not covered with the peritoneum; on the left side, the areas related to the suprarenal gland, pancreas, and descending colon are devoid of peritoneum. For the right kidney, the areas related to the suprarenal gland, duodenum, and colon are devoid of peritoneum. Certain large vessels are related to the anterior surface of the left kidney: the splenic vein passes between the pancreas and kidney (Fig. 3.5), the splenic artery crosses the lower portion of the gastric area, and the superior colic vessels cross the jejunal area.

The posterior surface of each kidney is directed posteromedially, and they have similar relations, as indicated in Figure 3.2. Due to the lower level of the right kidney, the diaphragmatic area is larger on the left. The diaphragm separates the kidneys from the pleural sacs. Passing inferior and laterally between the quadratus lumborum and the kidney are the subcostal, iliohypogastric, and ilioinguinal nerves.

The superior pole of each kidney is approximately 2.5 cm from the midline, and the inferior poles are approximately 7.5 cm from the midline. The right kidney is usually at a lower level than the left kidney, and the inferior pole is approximately 2.5 cm from the iliac crest.

There are no specific viscera related only to the lateral border.

The medial border presents at its center a

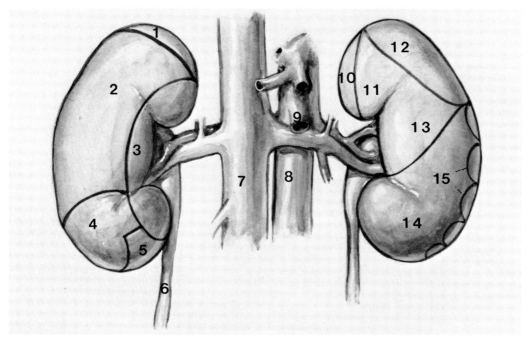

Figure 3.1. Structures related to the anterior surface of the kidneys. *1*, Right suprarenal gland; *2*, liver; *3*, duodenum; *4*, right colic flexure; *5*, small intestine; *6*, ureter; *7*, superior vena cava; *8*, aorta; *9*, superior mesenteric artery; *10*, left suprarenal gland; *11*, stomach; *12*, spleen; *13*, pancreas; *14*, jejunum; *15*, descending colon.

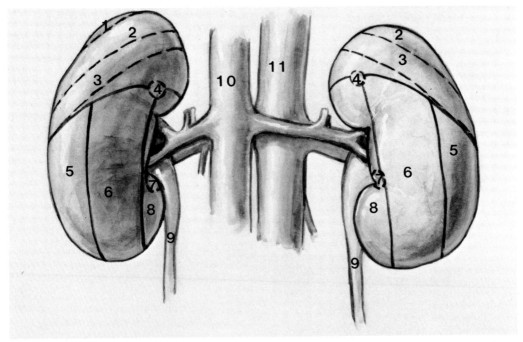

Figure 3.2. Structures related to the posterior surface of the kidneys. *1*, Eleventh rib; *2*, diaphragm; *3*, twelfth rib; *4*, transverse process of first lumbar vertebra; *5*, transversus abdominis muscle; *6*, quadratus lumborum muscle; *7*, transverse process of second lumbar vertebra; *8*, psoas major muscle; *9*, ureter; *10*, aorta; *11*, inferior vena cava.

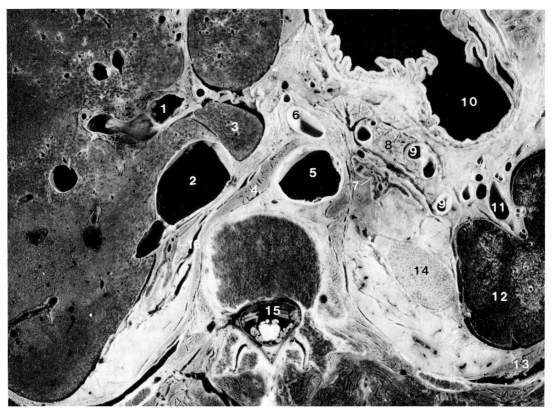

Figure 3.3. Cross-section through the body of the twelfth thoracic vertebra. *1*, Portal vein; *2*, inferior vena cava; *3*, caudate lobe of the liver; *4*, crus of the diaphragm; *5*, aorta; *6*, celiac artery; *7*, left suprarenal gland; *8*, pancreas; *9*, splenic artery; *10*, body of the stomach; *11*, splenic vein; *12*, spleen; *13*, diaphragm; *14*, superior pole of the left kidney; *15*, vertebral canal; *16*, right suprarenal gland.

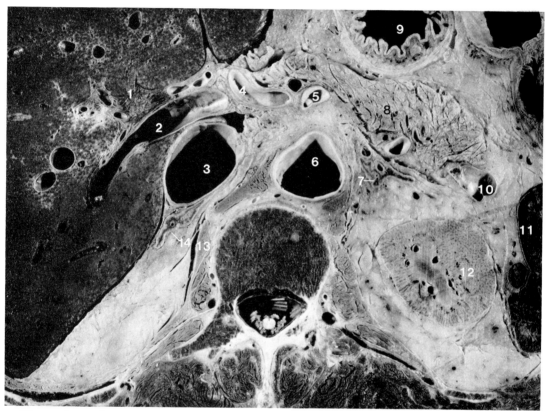

Figure 3.4. Cross-section through the lower portion of the body of the twelfth thoracic vertebra. *1,* Liver; *2,* portal vein; *3,* inferior vena cava; *4,* hepatic artery; *5,* splenic artery; *6,* aorta; *7,* left suprarenal gland; *8,* pancreas; *9,* body of the stomach; *10,* splenic vein; *11,* spleen; *12,* left kidney; *13,* diaphragm; *14,* right suprarenal gland.

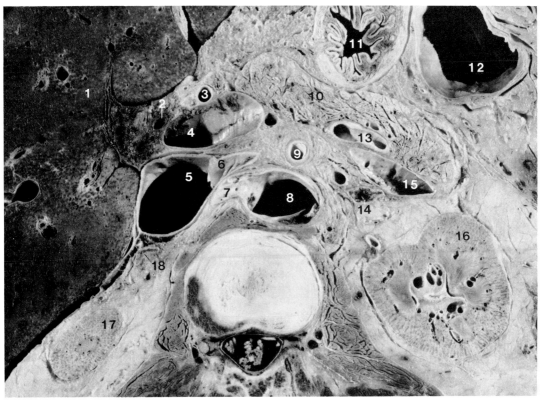

Figure 3.5.   Cross-section through the intervertebral disc between the twelfth thoracic and first lumbar vertebrae. *1*, Liver; *2*, common hepatic duct; *3*, hepatic artery; *4*, portal vein; *5*, inferior vena cava; *6*, left renal vein; *7*, right renal artery; *8*, aorta; *9*, superior mesenteric artery; *10*, pancreas; *11*, stomach; *12*, transverse colon; *13*, splenic artery; *14*, left suprarenal gland; *15*, splenic vein; *16*, left kidney; 17, superior pole of the right kidney; 18, right suprarenal gland.

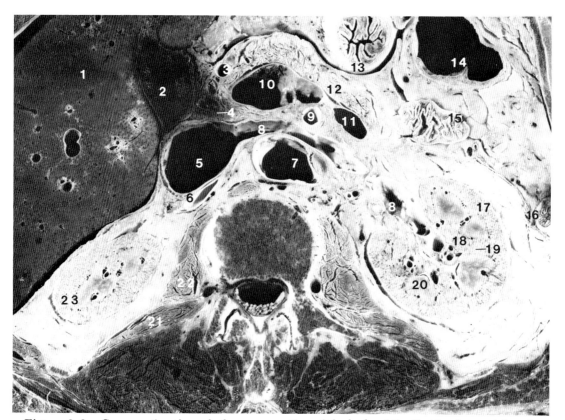

Figure 3.6. Cross-section through the upper portion of the body of the first lumbar vertebra. *1*, Liver; *2*, gallbladder; *3*, hepatic artery; *4*, hepatic duct; *5*, inferior vena cava; *6*, right renal artery; *7*, aorta; *8*, left renal vein; *9*, superior mesenteric artery; *10*, portal vein; *11*, splenic vein; *12*, pancreas; *13*, pylorus; *14*, transverse colon; *15*, jejunum; *16*, descending colon; *17*, renal cortex; *18*, renal medulla; *19*, renal column; *20*, renal papilla; *21*, quadratus lumborum muscle; *22*, psoas major muscle; *23*, right kidney.

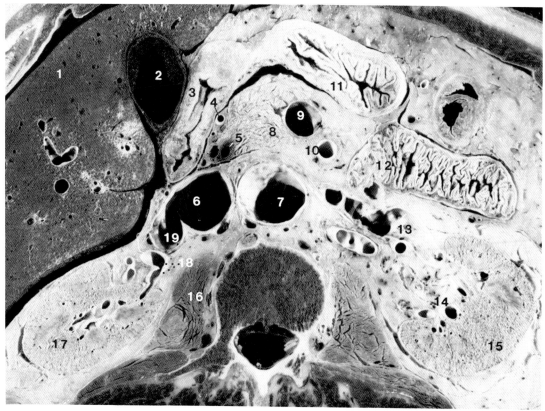

Figure 3.7. Cross-section through the body of the first lumbar vertebra. *1*, Liver; *2*, gallbladder; *3*, descending portion of the duodenum; *4*, superior pancreaticoduodenal artery; *5*, hepatic duct; *6*, inferior vena cava; *7*, aorta; *8*, pancreas; *9*, superior mesenteric vein; *10*, superior mesenteric artery; *11*, pylorus; *12*, jejunum; *13*, left renal vein; *14*, left renal artery; *15*, left kidney; *16*, psoas major muscle; *17*, right kidney; *18*, right renal artery; *19*, right renal vein.

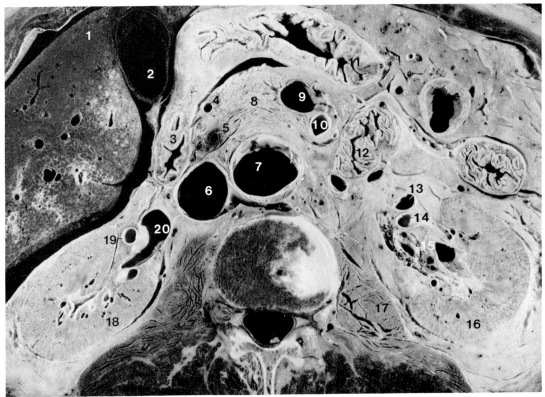

Figure 3.8. Cross-section through the lower portion of the body of the first lumbar vertebra. *1,* Liver; *2,* gallbladder; *3,* descending portion of the duodenum; *4,* superior pancreaticoduodenal artery; *5,* bile duct; *6,* inferior vena cava; *7,* aorta; *8,* pancreas; *9,* superior mesenteric vein; *10,* superior mesenteric artery; *11,* pylorus; *12,* jejunum; *13,* left renal vein; *14,* left renal artery; *15,* left renal pelvis; *16,* left kidney; *17,* psoas major muscle; *18,* right kidney; *19,* right renal artery; *20,* right renal vein.

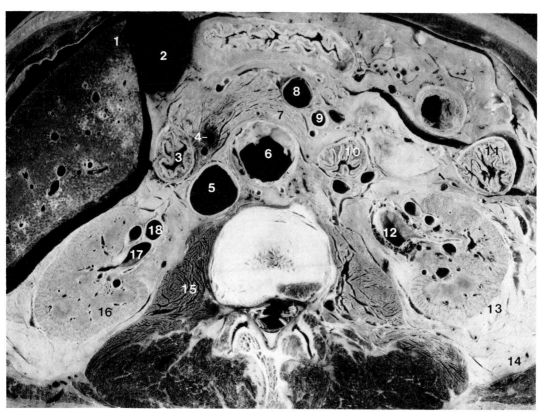

Figure 3.9. Cross-section through the intervertebral disc between the first and second lumbar vertebrae. *1*, Liver; *2*, gallbladder; *3*, descending portion of the duodenum; *4*, bile duct; *5*, inferior vena cava; *6*, aorta; *7*, pancreas; *8*, superior mesenteric vein; *9*, superior mesenteric artery; *10*, ascending portion of duodenum; *11*, jejunum; *12*, renal pelvis; *13*, perirenal fat; *14*, pararenal fat; *15*, psoas major muscle; *16*, right kidney; *17*, renal vein; *18*, renal artery.

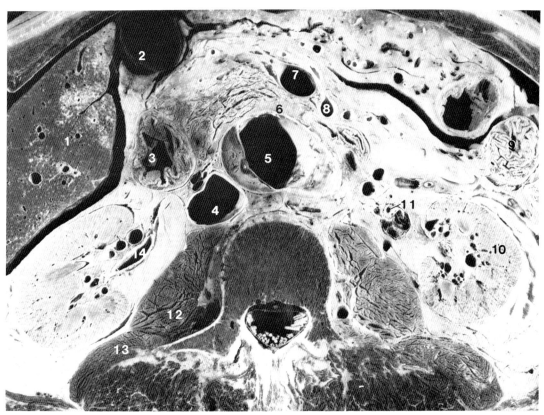

Figure 3.10.   Cross-section through the upper portion of the second lumbar vertebra. *1*, Liver; *2*, gallbladder; *3*, descending portion of the duodenum; *4*, inferior vena cava; *5*, aorta—greatly enlarged; *6*, pancreas; *7*, superior mesenteric vein; *8*, superior mesenteric artery; *9*, jejunum; *10*, left kidney; *11*, left ureter; *12*, psoas major muscle; *13*, quadratus lumborum muscle; *14*, right renal pelvis.

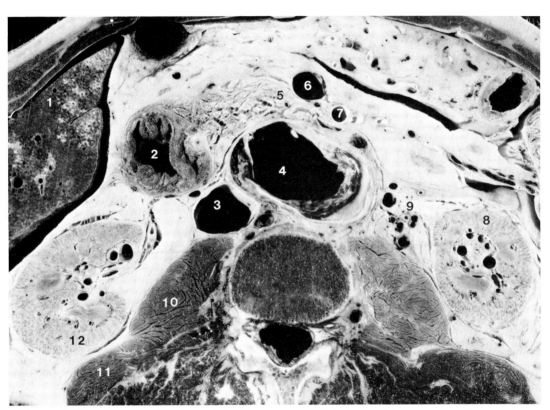

Figure 3.11. Cross-section through the lower portion of the body of the second lumbar vertebra. *1*, Liver; *2*, descending portion of the duodenum; *3*, inferior vena cava; *4*, aorta—greatly enlarged; *5*, pancreas; *6*, superior mesenteric vein; *7*, superior mesenteric artery; *8*, left kidney; *9*, left ureter; *10*, psoas major muscle; *11*, quadratus lumborum muscle; *12*, right kidney.

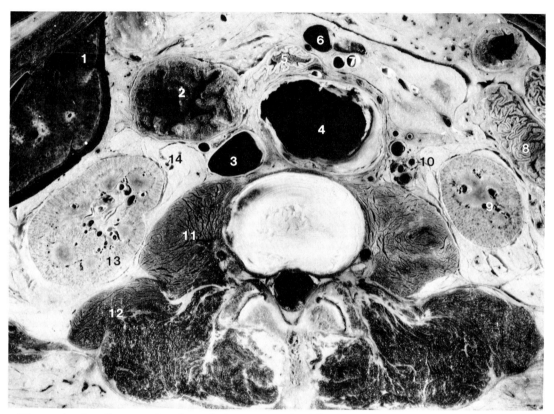

Figure 3.12.   Cross-section through the intervertebral disc between the second and third lumbar vertebrae. *1*, Liver; *2*, descending portion of the duodenum; *3*, inferior vena cava; *4*, aorta; *5*, transverse portion of the duodenum; *6*, superior mesenteric vein; *7*, superior mesenteric artery; *8*, jejunum; *9*, left kidney; *10*, left ureter; *11*, psoas major muscle; *12*, quadratus lumborum muscle; *13*, right kidney; *14*, right ureter.

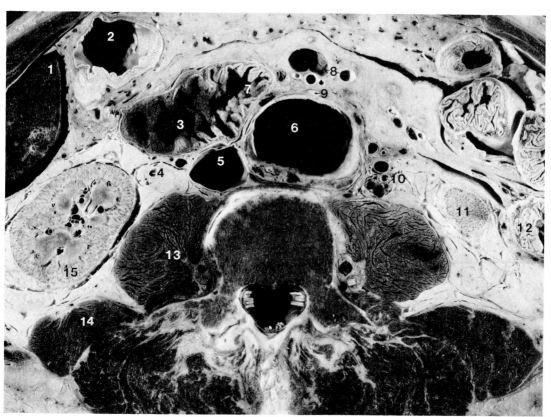

Figure 3.13. Cross-section through the upper portion of the body of the third lumbar vertebra. *1*, Liver; *2*, hepatic flexure; *3*, descending portion of the duodenum; *4*, right ureter; *5*, inferior vena cava; *6*, aorta; *7*, transverse portion of the duodenum; *8*, superior mesenteric vessels; *9*, inferior mesenteric artery; *10*, left ureter; *11*, inferior pole of left kidney; *12*, jejunum; *13*, psoas major muscle; *14*, quadratus lumborum muscle; *15*, right kidney.

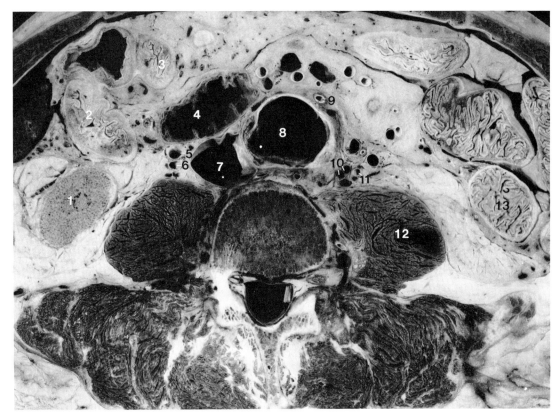

Figure 3.14. Cross-section through the body of the third lumbra vertebra. *1*, Inferior pole of right kidney; *2*, ascending colon; *3*, transverse colon; *4*, transverse portion of the duodenum; *5*, testicular vein; *6*, right ureter; *7*, inferior vena cava; *8*, aorta; *9*, inferior mesenteric artery; *10*, testicular vessels; *11*, left ureter; *12*, psoas major muscle; *13*, jejunum.

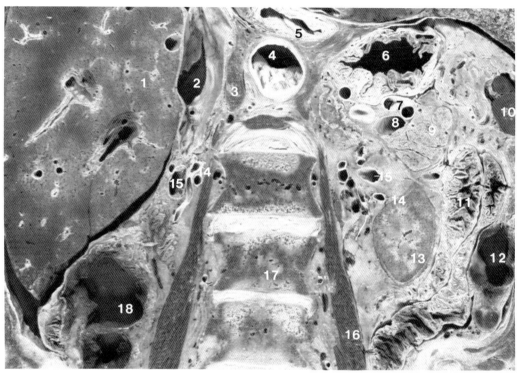

Figure 3.15. Coronal section through the anterior aspect of a portion of the left kidney. *1*, Liver; *2*, inferior vena cava; *3*, crus of the diaphragm; *4*, aorta; *5*, esophagus; *6*, stomach; *7*, splenic artery; *8*, splenic vein; *9*, pancreas; *10*, spleen; *11*, jejunum; *12*, descending colon; *13*, kidney; *14*, renal artery; *15*, renal vein; *16*, psoas major muscle; *17*, body of vertebra L3; *18*, ascending colon.

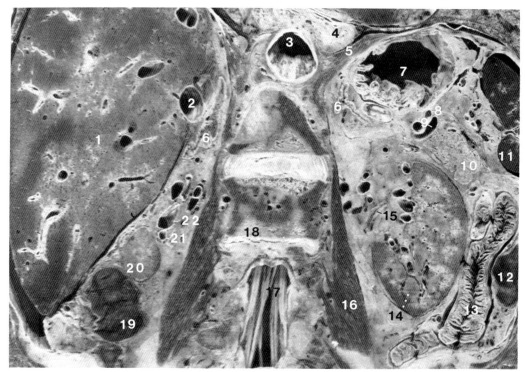

Figure 3.16. Coronal section through the anterior aspect of a portion of both kidneys. *1,* Liver; *2,* hepatic vein; *3,* aorta; *4,* esophagus; *5,* diaphragm; *6,* suprarenal gland; *7,* stomach; *8,* splenic artery; *9,* splenic vein; *10,* pancreas; *11,* spleen; *12,* descending colon; *13,* jejunum; *14,* renal pyramid; *15,* ureter; *16,* psoas major muscle; *17,* spinal nerve rootlets; *18,* body of vertebra L2; *19,* ascending colon; *20,* kidney; *21,* renal artery; *22,* renal vein.

vertical slit, the hilus, which leads into the renal sinus. Passing through the hilus (Figs. 3.17 and 3.22) are the renal vessels and the funnel-shaped continuation of the ureter, the renal pelvis (Fig. 3.9). The hilus of the right kidney is below the transpyloric plane, and in the left kidney the hilus is above it.The transpyloric plane is drawn around the body through the midpoint of a line joining the suprasternal notch to the upper border of the pubic symphysis. This plane passes through the vertebral column at the inferior border of the first lumbar vertebra. Although the relations of the structures that pass through the hilus may vary, the usual pattern is that the renal vein is anterior, the renal pelvis is posterior, and the renal artery is between the vein and the pelvis (Fig. 3.15).

The renal arteries arise from the lateral aspect of the aorta below the level of the superior mesenteric artery between the lower one-third and the middle one-third of the second lumbar vertebra. Due to the position of the aorta, the right renal artery is approximately 1 cm longer

than the left and passes posterior to the inferior vena cava. The renal arteries are large structures, and frequently there are accessory renal arteries because of the relative ascent of the kidney during development and because of the segmental supply to the developing kidney. In many instances the renal arteries separate into two divisions, a large anterior and a smaller posterior (Fig. 3.7). The anterior division supplies the entire ventral surface and a small portion of the dorsal surface along the convex margin of the kidney. The posterior division supplies the dorsal surface of the kidney. The line where the anterior and posterior divisions meet on the dorsal surface is Brodel's line. This line should not be confused with Brodel's white line which overlies the white longitudinal column of Bertin and may appear anteriorly or posteriorly, depending upon the degree of extension of the renal parenchyma. The renal veins are large structures; the left is longer than the right, and it passes ventral to the aorta just inferior to the origin of superior mesentric artery (Fig. 3.6).

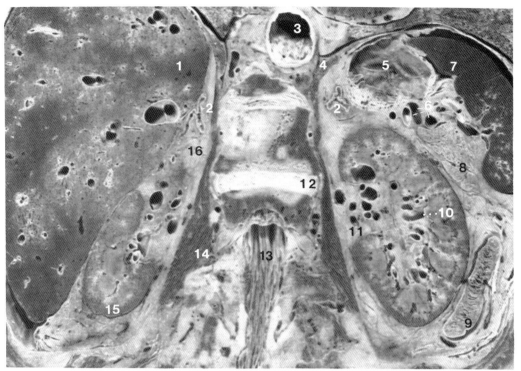

Figure 3.17. Coronal section through the hilus of the left kidney. *1*, Liver; *2*, suprarenal gland; *3*, aorta; *4*, diaphragm; *5*, wall of stomach; *6*, splenic vessels; *7*, spleen; *8*, pancreas, *9*, jejunum; *10*, minor calyx; *11*, renal hilus; *12*, intervertebral disc; *13*, spinal nerve rootlets; *14*, psoas major muscle; *15*, renal cortex; *16*, perirenal fat.

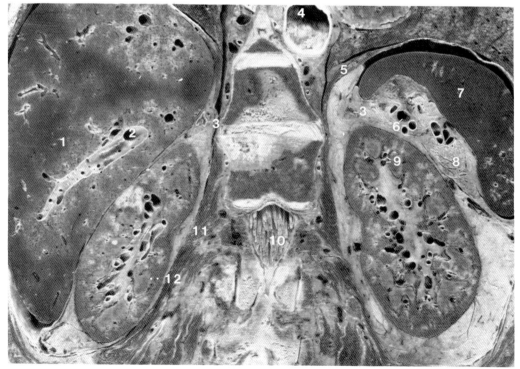

Figure 3.18. Coronal section through the kidneys 1 cm posterior to the preceding section. *1*, Liver; *2*, sublobular vein; *3*, suprarenal gland; *4*, aorta; *5*, diaphragm; *6*, splenic vessels; *7*, spleen; *8*, pancreas; *9*, interlobar vessels; *10*, spinal nerve rootlets; *11*, psoas major muscle; *12*, renal pyramid.

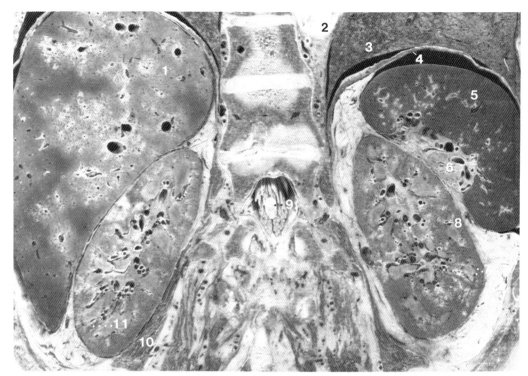

Figure 3.19. Coronal section through the kidneys 1 cm posterior to the preceding section. *1*, Liver; *2*, wall of aorta; *3*, lung; *4*, diaphragm; *5*, spleen; *6*, pancreas; *7*, arcuate vessels; *8*, interlobular vessels; *9*, spinal cord; *10*, psoas major muscle; *11*, renal column.

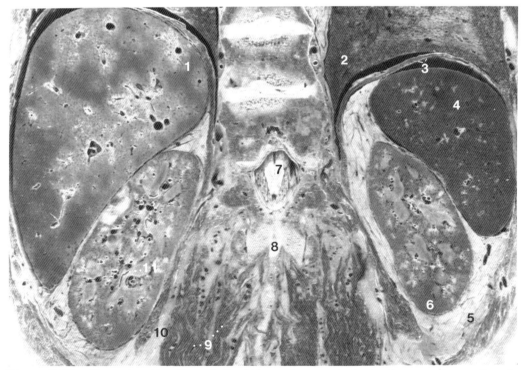

Figure 3.20. Coronal section through the kidneys 1 cm posterior to the preceding section. *1*, Liver; *2*, lung; *3*, diaphragm; *4*, spleen; *5*, pararenal fat; *6*, renal cortex; *7*, spinal cord; *8*, spinous process; *9*, transversospinal muscles; *10*, psoas major muscle; *11*, minor calyx.

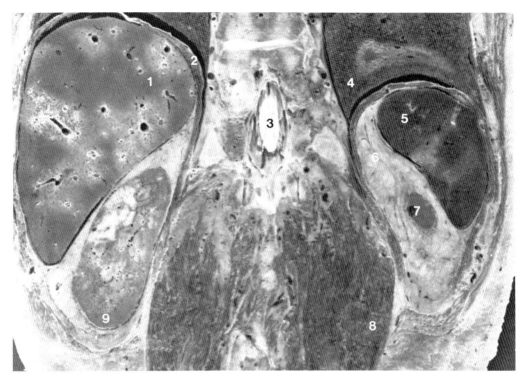

Figure 3.21. Coronal section through the kidneys 1 cm posterior to the preceding section. *1*, Liver; *2*, diaphragm; *3*, spinal cord; *4*, lung; *5*, spleen; *6*, pararenal fat; *7*, kidney; *8*, sacrospinalis muscle; *9*, renal cortex.

Because of the position of the two kidneys, the left renal vein opens into the inferior vena cava at a higher level than the right.

The capsule of the kidney is continuous with the renal sinus at the hilus. The sinus contains the renal pelvis and the vessels. The renal pelvis outside the sinus becomes continuous with the ureter (Fig. 3.16). Within the sinus the pelvis divides to form two or three major calices, and these in turn divide into minor calices. Each minor calyx (Figs. 3.17 and 3.20) is molded around one to three renal papillae (Fig. 3.6) which receive the openings of the collecting ducts of the kidney.

The renal fascia, which is distinct from the capsule, surrounds the entire organ and divides the retroperitoneal fat into two compartments. Between the renal fascia and the capsule is the perirenal fat (Fig. 3.17), and external to the fascia is the pararenal fat (Figs. 3.20 and 3.21). Superior to the suprarenal gland, the two layers of renal fascia fuse and become continuous with the diaphragmatic fascia. Inferiorly, the layers enclose the ureter; the anterior layer is lost in the retroperitoneal tissue of the pelvis, and the

posterior layer blends with the iliac fascia. The anterior layer of the renal fascia crosses the aorta to meet the same layer on the opposite side, and the posterior layer blends in with the fascia of the psoas major muscle. The origin of the renal fascia is not clear. Whether it is continuous with transversalis fascia or arises from the subserous fascia has not been completely established.

URETERS

The ureters are paired retroperitoneal structures which lead from the kidneys to the urinary bladder. Each begins as a continuation of the renal pelvis which is partly within the renal sinus (Figs. 3.16, 3.23, and 3.24). The ureter is approximately 25 to 30 cm long and is divided into two portions; the upper half is in the abdominal cavity, and the lower half is in the true or lesser pelvis.

In the abdomen the ureters pass inferiorly and medially on the anterior surface of the psoas major muscles (Figs. 3.10 to 3.14). The psoas fascia forms a paraurethral sheath around each ureter. On each side the ureters are crossed by

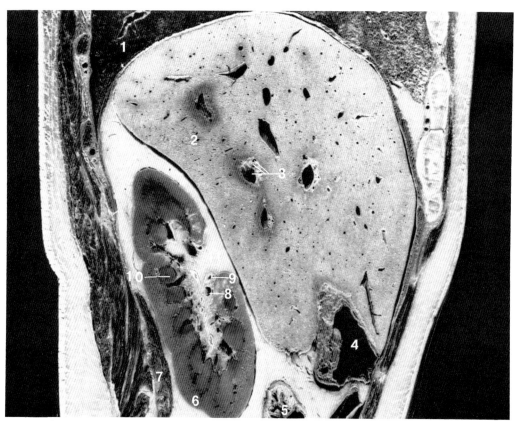

Figure 3.22. Sagittal section through the right kidney. *1*, Lower lobe of the lung; *2*, right lobe of the liver; *3*, hepatic triad; *4*, gallbladder; *5*, ascending colon; *6*, renal cortex; *7*, quadratus lumborum muscle; *8*, renal vein; *9*, renal artery; *10*, renal pyramid; *11*, renal hilum.

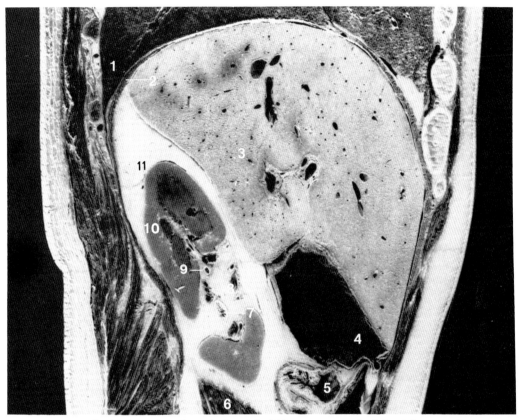

Figure 3.23. Sagittal section through the right kidney, 1 cm to the left of the preceding section. *1*, Lower lobe of the lung; *2*, diaphragm; *3*, right lobe of the liver; *4*, gallbadder; *5*, ascending colon; *6*, psoas major muscle; *7*, ureter; *8*, renal vein; *9*, renal artery; *10*, renal cortex; *11*, perirenal fat.

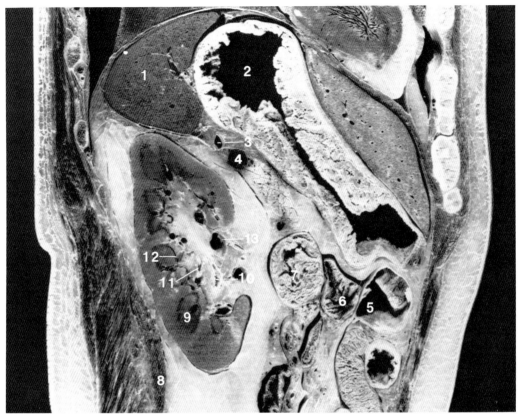

Figure 3.24. Sagittal section through the left kidney. *1,* Spleen; *2,* body of the stomach; *3,* splenic artery; *4,* splenic vein; *5,* transverse colon; *6,* jejunum; *7,* duodenojejunal flexure; *8,* quadratus lumborum muscle; *9,* renal pyramid; *10,* ureter; *11,* renal artery; *12,* renal papilla; *13,* renal vein.

the testicular arteries. From superior to inferior the right ureter is related anteriorly to the descending portion of the duodenum, right colic and ileocolic vessels, and the root of the mesentery. The left ureter is crossed anteriorly by the left colic vessels and the root of the sigmoid mesocolon.

The ureters cross the common iliac or the external iliac arteries to enter the lesser pelvis (Figs. 3.36 and 3.37). They pass along the lateral wall of the pelvis, ventral to the internal iliac vessels and medial to the levator ani muscles. At the level of the spine of the ischium, they pass medially to enter the bladder at the lateral margin of the junction between the superior surface and the posterior surface.

The ureters reach the urinary bladder approximately 5 cm apart and pierce the wall in an oblique fashion. They are embedded in the wall of the urinary bladder for approximately 2 cm prior to opening into the organ.

The ureters undergo constriction at the ureteropelvic junction, at the point where they cross the iliac vessels, and where they join the urinary bladder.

The blood supply to the ureters is derived from the renal, testicular, internal iliac, and inferior vesical arteries. In the abdomen the arteries approach the ureters from the medial side, whereas in the pelvis they approach the ureters from the lateral side.

In the pelvis each ureter is surrounded by a dense plexus of veins which communicates with the vesical plexus of veins and the internal iliac vein. In the upper portion of the ureter, the veins follow the arteries and join tributaries of the renal vein.

URINARY BLADDER

The size and relations of the urinary bladder (Figs. 3.25 to 3.29, 3.33 to 3.37, and 3.39) depend on the amount of distention. In the contracted

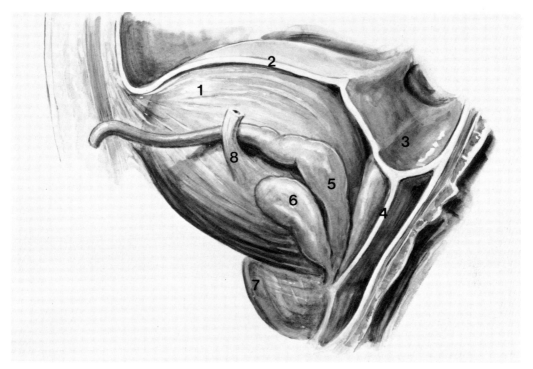

Figure 3.25. Posterolateral view of the urinary bladder. *1*, Urinary bladder; *2*, peritoneum; *3*, rectovesical pouch; *4*, Denonvillier's fascia; *5*, ampulla of the ductus deferens; *6*, seminal vesicle; *7*, prostate; *8*, ureter.

state it is located in the true or lesser pelvis. However, on distention it may expand superiorly and anteriorly into the abdominal cavity.

The empty bladder presents for examination a superior surface, two inferolateral surfaces, a base or fundus, and a neck. The distended bladder presents a posterosuperior surface, anteroinferior surface, two lateral surfaces, a fundus, and a summit. Only the relations of the empty bladder will be described.

The superior surface of the empty bladder is covered by peritoneum which is continuous with the parietal layer of the anterior abdominal wall (Figs. 3.25 and 3.33 to 3.37). Posteriorly, the peritoneum continues and covers the ureters, the ductus deferens, and the superior portion of the seminal vesicles. It then passes inferiorly to form the rectovesical pouch before the peritoneum continues on to the anterior surface of the rectum (Fig. 3.25). Anteriorly, the superior surface continues and forms the apex of the urinary bladder. The apex is continuous with the median umbilical ligament, which is a remnant of the urachus. Posteriorly, the superior surface is continuous with the fundus of the bladder. The

posterior border of the bladder is formed at the junction of the superior surface and the fundus. At the lateral ends of the border, the two ureters enter the bladder. The superior surface is related to the sigmoid colon and the termination of the ileum.

The inferolateral surfaces are related to the levator ani (Figs. 3.36 and 3.39) and the obturator internus muscles (Fig. 3.35). The surfaces form the boundaries of the retropubic space which is located between the bladder and pubis (Fig. 3.29). These two surfaces are directed posteriorly and inferiorly to form the neck of the bladder.

The fundus is triangular in shape and is directed posteriorly and inferiorly. It is separated from the rectum by the rectovesical pouch, seminal vesicles, and ductus deferens. The portion of the bladder between the two ductus deferens is separated from the rectum by Denonvillier's fascia (Fig. 3.25).

The neck is the lowest and the most fixed portion of the bladder. It is in continuity with the base of the prostate gland.

The pelvic fascia is divided into a parietal

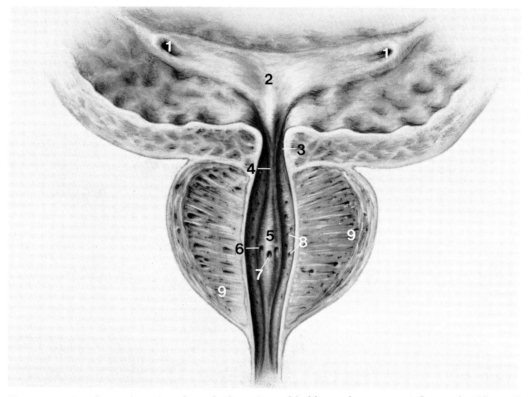

Figure 3.26. Coronal section through the urinary bladder and prostate. *1*, Internal orifices of the ureters; *2*, trigone of the urinary bladder; *3*, internal urethral opening; *4*, urethral crest; *5*, colliculus seminalis; *6*, opening of the ejaculatory duct; *7*, opening of the prostatic utricle; *8*, openings of the prostatic ducts; *9*, lateral lobes of the prostate gland.

layer which covers the pelvic muscles and a visceral layer which surrounds the organs. The visceral layer surrounds the bladder, and at the neck it is continuous with the parietal layer of the pelvic fascia. The condensation of the fascia in the area of the neck passes laterally to the arcus tendineus of the levator ani muscles to form the true ligaments of the bladder. Anteriorly, a thickening of the fascia of the pelvis forms the lateral and median puboprostatic ligaments. The lateral puboprostatic ligament passes from the anterior portion of the arcus tendinous to the sheath of the prostate gland. The median puboprostatic ligament extends from the pubic bone near the mid-portion of the pubic symphysis to the sheath of the prostate. This latter ligament forms the floor of the retropubic space. A condensation of the connective tissue surrounding the vesical veins as they pass to the internal iliac vein forms the posterior ligament of the bladder. The peritoneum on the

anterior surface of the bladder is thrown into folds as it passes laterally and forms the false ligaments of the bladder.

The mucous membrane of the bladder is thrown into folds except over a triangular area, the trigone of the bladder (Fig. 3.26), where the membrane is tightly bound to the underlying muscle layer. The trigone is bounded by the two orifices of the ureters and the internal urethral opening. Between the openings of the ureters is located the interureteric crest (Fig. 3.26). The orifices of the ureters are approximately 2 to 3 cm apart and are approximately the same distance from the internal urethral opening. The median lobe of the prostate gland may cause a slight elevation (uvula of the bladder) posterior to the urethral orifices.

The bladder is supplied primarily by the superior and inferior vesical arteries. The superior vesical artery arises from the umbilical artery which is a branch of the internal iliac, and the

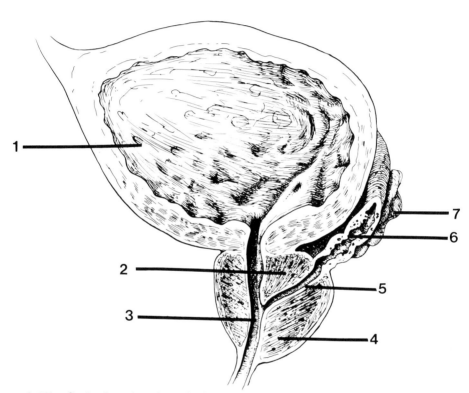

Figure 3.27. Sagittal section through the urinary bladder and prostate. *1,* Urinary bladder; *2,* median lobe of the prostate; *3,* prostatic urethra; *4,* lateral lobe of the prostate; *5,* ejaculatory duct; *6,* ampulla of the ductus deferens; *7,* seminal vesicle.

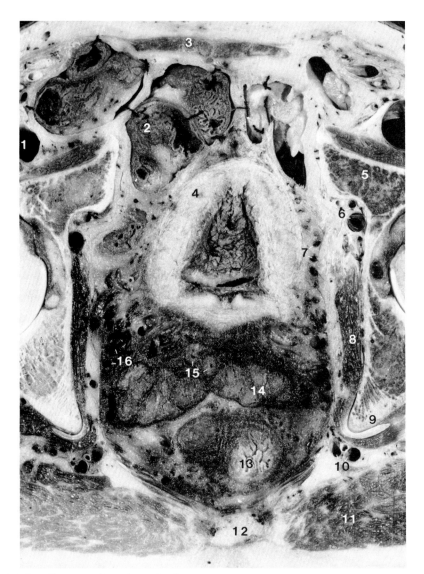

Figure 3.28. Cross-section through the coccyx. *1*, External iliac vein; *2*, ileum; *3*, rectus abdominis muscle; *4*, urinary bladder; *5*, pubis; *6*, obturator vessels; *7*, vesical veins; *8*, obturator internus muscle; *9*, spine of the ischium; *10*, internal pudendal vessels; *11*, gluteus maximus muscle; *12*, coccyx; *13*, rectum; *14*, seminal vesicles; *15*, ductus deferens; *16*, venous plexus.

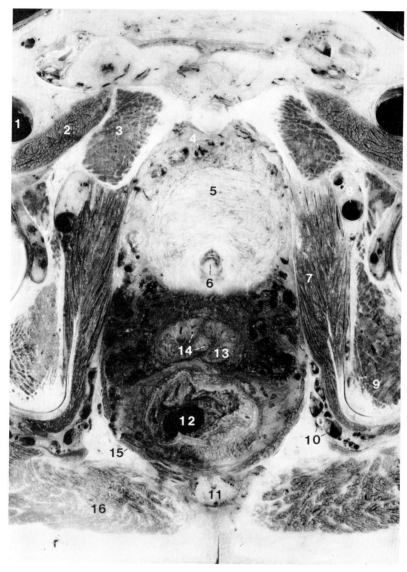

Figure 3.29. Cross-section through tip of coccyx. *1*, Femoral vein; *2*, pectineus muscle; *3*,pubis; *4*, prostatic venous plexus; *5*, apex of the urinary bladder; *6*, urethral crest; *7*, obturator internus muscle; *8*, obturator vessels; *9*, ischium; *10*, internal pudendal vessels; *11*, tip of the coccyx; *12*, rectum; *13*, seminal vesicles; *14*, ductus deferens; *15*, levator ani muscle; *16*, gluteus maximus muscle.

inferior vesical artery arises for the most part from the internal iliac artery. Other branches which occasionally supply the bladder arise from the obturator and the inferior gluteal arteries.

The veins of the bladder do not correspond to the arteries. They drain inferiorly toward the base and neck of the bladder to form a plexus of veins. This vesical plexus of veins (Fig. 3.28) is found within the fascial sheath and communicates with the prostatic plexus of veins. In ad-

dition to receiving the blood from the bladder, the vesical plexus also receives blood from the seminal vesicles and the ductus deferens. The vesical plexus drains primarily into the internal iliac veins.

PROSTATE

The prostate (Figs. 3.25 to 3.27, 3.30 to 3.32, and 3.34 to 3.39) is located in the pelvis between the urinary bladder and the urogenital dia-

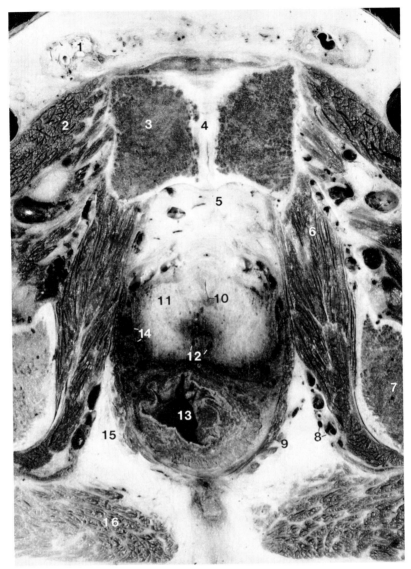

Figure 3.30.   Cross-section through the upper portion of the symphysis pubis. *1*, Spermatic cord; *2*, pectineus muscle; *3*, body of the pubis; *4*, interpubic disc; *5*, retropubic space (cave of Retzius); *6*, obturator internus muscle; *7*, ischium; *8*, internal pudendal vessels; *9*, levator ani muscle; *10*, prostatic urethra; *11*, lateral lobe of the prostate; *12*, ejaculatory ducts; *13*, rectum; *14*, prostatic venous plexus; *15*, ischiorectal fossa; *16*, gluteus maximus muscle.

phragm, posterior to the symphysis pubis and pubic arch and anterior to the ampulla of the rectum. The latter structure is separated from the prostate by Denonvillier's fascia or the rectovesicle fascia (Fig. 3.25).

The gland presents a base, apex, and three surfaces for examination.

The base of the prostate is united to the neck of the bladder by muscular tissue at the orifice of the urethra. A vesical groove separates the rounded border of the base from the bladder. The apex is in contact with the deep fascia of the urogenital diaphragm.

The anterior surface, which is approximately 2 cm posterior to the pubic symphysis, extends from the base to the apex and is connected to the pubic bones by the median puboprostatic ligament and to the arcus tendinous by the lateral puboprostatic ligaments. The urethra emerges from this surface just superior and anterior to the apex of the gland.

The posterior surface is approximately 4 cm from the anus. The two ejaculatory ducts enter through this surface and divide the gland into two portions (Fig. 3.27). The small superior portion which is bounded by the two ejaculatory ducts and the urethra anteriorly forms the me-

dian lobe. The large inferior portion is divided into right and left lobes by a small depression. These lateral lobes form the main mass of the gland and are located posterior to the urethra. The inferior lateral surfaces are prominent areas which are related to the levator ani muscle (Figs. 3.30 to 3.32, 3.36, and 3.39).

The prostate develops as five lobes: anterior, posterior, median (middle), and right and left

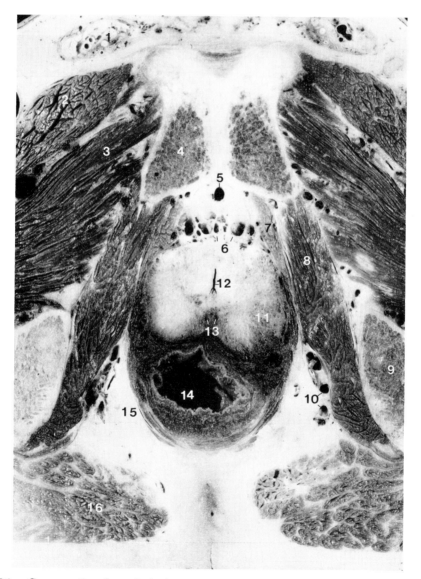

Figure 3.31. Cross-section through the lower portion of the symphysis pubis. *1*, Spermatic cord; *2*, pectineus muscle; *3*, obturator externus muscle; *4*, body of the pubis; *5*, deep dorsal vein of the penis; *6*, prostatic plexus of veins; *7*, pubococcygeus muscle; *8*, obturator internus muscle; *9*, tuberosity of the ischium; *10*, internal pudendal vessels; *11*, lateral lobe of prostate; *12*, prostatic urethra; *13*, ejaculatory ducts; *14*, rectum; *15*, ischiorectal fossa; *16*, gluteus maximus muscle.

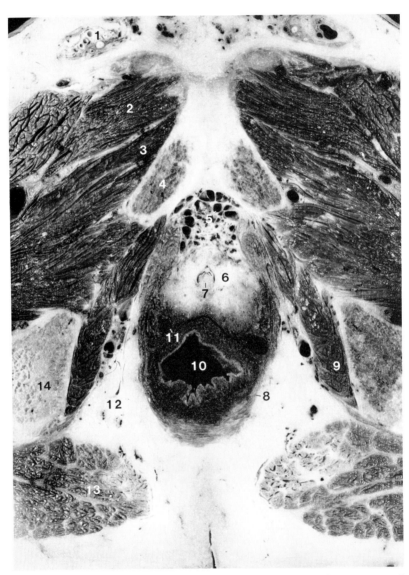

Figure 3.32. Cross-section through the inferior ramus of the pubis. *1*, Spermatic cord; *2*, adductor longus muscle; *3*, obturator externus muscle; *4*, inferior ramus of the pubis; *5*, prostatic venous plexus; *6*, prostatic urethra; *7*, colliculus seminalis; *8*, levator ani muscle; *9*, obturator internus muscle; *10*, rectum; *11*, rectal veins; *12*, ischiorectal fossa; *13*, gluteus maximus muscle; *14*, tuberosity of the ischium.

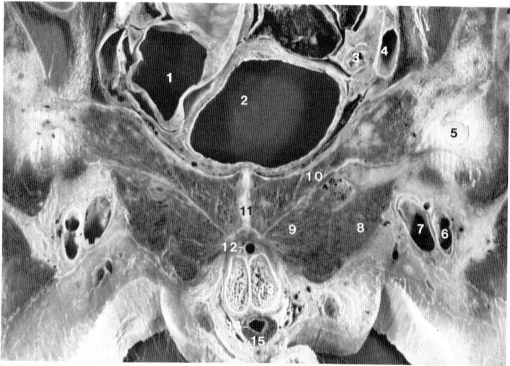

Figure 3.33.   Coronal section through the interpubic disc. *1*, Ileum; *2*, urinary bladder; *3*, sigmoid colon; *4*, external iliac vein; *5*, head of femur; *6*, femoral artery; *7*, femoral vein; *8*, pectineus muscle; *9*, obturator externus muscle; *10*, superior ramus of the pubis; *11*, interpubic disc; *12*, deep dorsal vein of the penis; *13*, corpus cavernosum penis; *14*, penile urethra; *15*, bulbospongiosum penis.

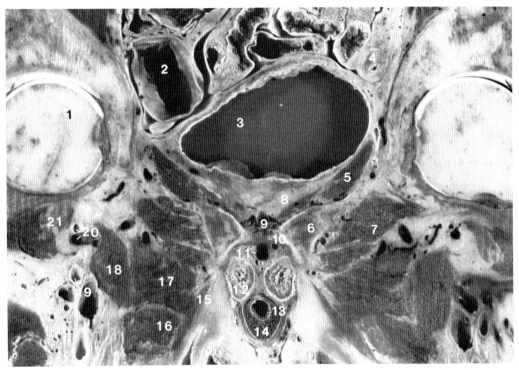

Figure 3.34. Coronal section through the urinary bladder at the level of the head of the femur. *1*, Head of the femur; *2*, ileum; *3*, urinary bladder; *4*, sigmoid colon; *5*, obturator internus muscle; *6*, superior ramus of the pubis; *7*, obturator externus muscle; *8*, prostate; *9*, prostatic venous plexus; *10*, arcuate ligament; *11*, deep dorsal vein of the penis; *12*, corpus cavernosum penis; *13*, penile urethra; *14*, corpus spongiosum penis; *15*, gracilis muscle; *16*, adductor longus muscle; *17*, adductor brevis muscle; *18*, pectineus muscle; *19*, femoral vessels; *20*, medial femoral circumflex vessels; *21*, tendon of iliopsoas muscle.

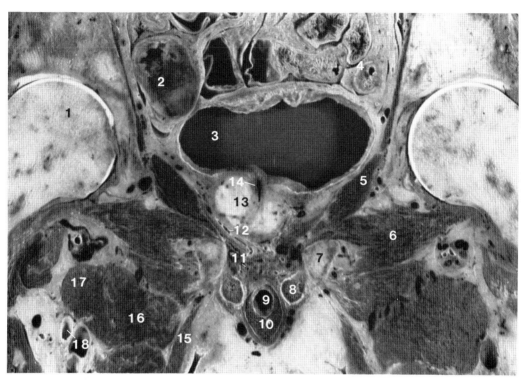

Figure 3.35. Coronal section through the urinary bladder 1 cm posterior to the preceding section. *1*, Head of the femur; *2*, ileum; *3*, urinary bladder; *4*, sigmoid colon; *5*, obturator internus muscle; *6*, obturator externus muscle; *7*, inferior ramus of the pubis; *8*, crura of the penis; *9*, penile urethra; *10*, corpus spongiosum penis; *11*, branches of internal pudendal vessels; *12*, prostatic venous plexus; *13*, prostate; *14*, internal uretheral orifice; *15*, gracilis muscle; *16*, adductor brevis muscle; *17*, pectineus muscle; *18*, femoral vessels.

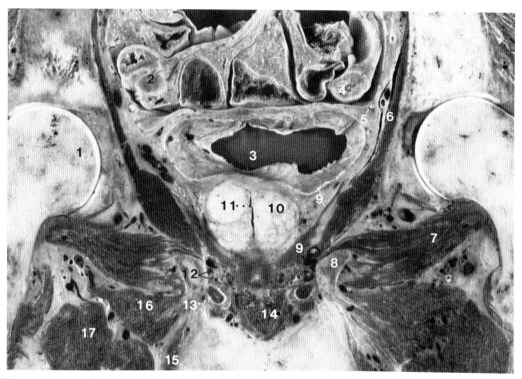

Figure 3.36. Coronal section through the prostate gland. *1*, Head of the femur; *2*, ileum; *3*, urinary bladder; *4*, sigmoid colon; *5*, ureter; *6*, obturator internus muscle; *7*, obturator externus muscle; *8*, inferior ramus of pubis; *9*, levator ani muscle; *10*, prostate; *11*, prostatic urethra; *12*, branches of internal pudendal vessels; *13*, crus of the penis; *14*, bulbospongiosum penis; *15*, gracilis muscle; *16*, adductor magnus muscle; *17*, pectineus muscle.

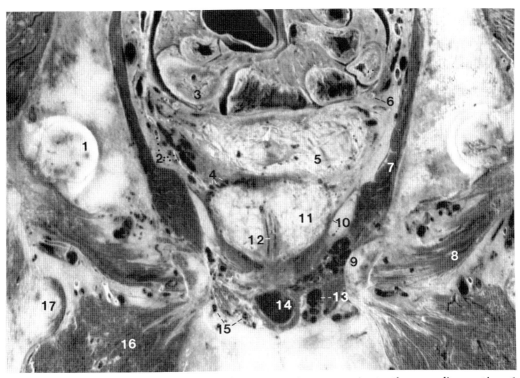

Figure 3.37. Coronal section through the prostate 1 cm posterior to the preceding section. *1,* Head of the femur; *2,* branches of the internal iliac vessels; *3,* ileum; *4,* prostatic venous plexus; *5,* wall of the bladder; *6,* ureter; *7,* obturator internus muscle; *8,* obturator externus muscle; *9,* ramus of the ischium; *10,* levator ani muscle; *11,* prostate; *12,* colliculus seminalis; *13,* crus of the penis; *14,* bulbospongiosum penis; *15,* branches of internal pudendal vessels; *16,* adductor magnus muscle; *17,* lesser trochanter.

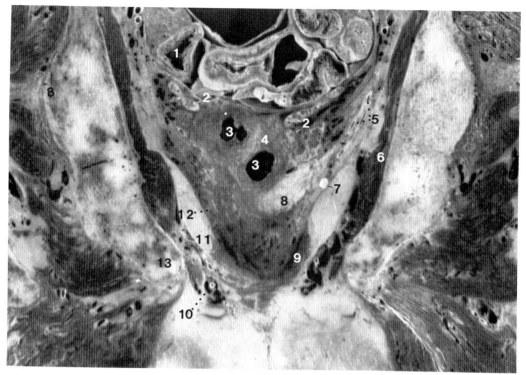

Figure 3.38. Coronal section through the seminal vesicles. *1*, Ileum; *2*, seminal vesicles; *3*, rectum; *4*, wall of the rectum; *5*, branches of the internal iliac artery; *6*, obturator internus muscle; *7*, calcified nodule; *8*, prostate; *9*, external anal sphincter; *10*, pudendal canal; *11*, ischiorectal fossa; *12*, levator ani muscle; *13*, ischium.

lateral. Both the anterior and posterior lobes atrophy, and the other three lobes form the adult gland.

The transverse diameter at the base of the gland is 4 cm, the anterior-posterior diameter is 2 cm, and the distance from the base to the apex is 3 cm.

The prostate gland is traversed vertically by the urethra (Figs. 3.26, 3.27, 3.29 to 3.32, and 3.35 to 3.37). Projecting from the posterior wall of the urethra is the urethral crest, and the prostatic ducts open in the small depressions on each side of the crest. The urethral crest expands into the colliculus seminalis which contains the openings of the prostatic utricle and the ejaculatory ducts (Figs. 3.26, 3.32, and 3.37).

The gland has a distinct capsule on its external surface which is made up of fibrous tissue and smooth muscle. In addition, the prostate has a distinct fibrous sheath which is continuous with the parietal layer of the surrounding fascia. Between the fibrous sheath and the capsule, a plexus of veins surrounds the sides and base of the gland. This prostatic plexus of veins (Figs. 3.30, 3.37, and 3.39) receives the dorsal vein of

the penis (Figs. 3.31, 3.33, and 3.34), communicates with the vesical plexus of veins, and terminates in the internal iliac veins.

The arteries to the prostate arise from the internal pudendal, inferior vesical, and middle rectal arteries.

SEMINAL VESICLES

The seminal vesicles (Figs. 3.25, 3.27 to 3.29, 3.38, and 3.39) are paired sacculated structures which are located posterior to the fundus of the bladder and anterior to the rectum. They are pyramidal in shape, approximately 5 cm long, and directed laterally and superiorly. Each consists of a single tube which is closed at the superior end and is curled upon itself. The lower end of the tube is constricted to form a small narrow duct which joins the termination of the ductus deferens to form the ejaculatory duct. It is separated from the rectum by the fascia of Denonvillier. The median margin of each vesicle is related to the ampulla of the ductus deferens (Fig. 3.25), whereas the lateral margin is related to the prostatic plexus of veins.

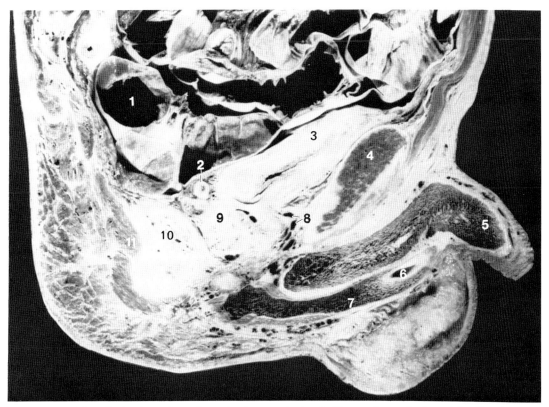

Figure 3.39. Sagittal section through the prostrate. *1*, Ileum; *2*, seminal vesicle; *3*, urinary bladder; *4*, body of the pubis; *5*, corpus cavernosum; *6*, urethra; *7*, corpus spongiosum; *8*, prostatic venus plexus; *9*, prostate; *10*, rectum; *11*, levator ani muscle.

The arteries to the seminal vesicles rise from the inferior vesical and middle rectal arteries.

EJACULATORY DUCTS

The two ejaculatory ducts (Figs. 3.26, 3.27, 3.30, and 3.31) are formed by the union of the lower end of the seminal vesicles and the terminal portion of the ductus deferens. They are approximately 2 cm long and begin at the base of the prostate gland and pass between the median and right and left lateral lobes. The ducts terminate by opening on each side of the prostatic utricle on the colliculus seminalis (Fig. 3.26).

CHAPTER 4

Normal Ultrasonic Anatomy of the Genitourinary System

ROGER C. SANDERS, M.D.

Much detailed information about the kidney, bladder, and prostate is now available with modern ultrasound systems. To assess renal pelvic anatomy adequately, correct examination techniques should be used.

TECHNIQUE

Traditionally, the kidneys were examined in the prone position because the kidneys lie close to the posterior aspect of the body (1) (Fig. 4.1). It soon became apparent that a posterior approach might be unsatisfactory because of overlying ribs. Nowadays, the usual approach to the right kidney is in the supine position (Fig. 4.2). This view utilizes the liver (an excellent acoustic window) to place the right kidney at the optimal focal depth with a medium focus transducer; therefore, one frequently obtains excellent detail

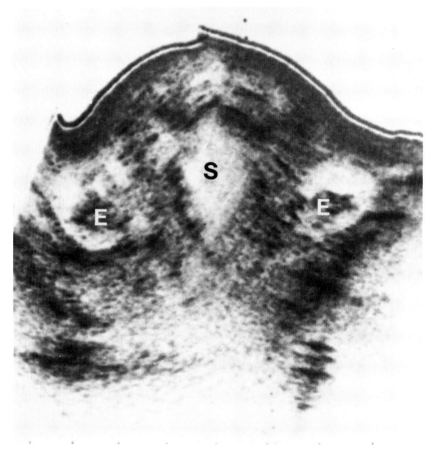

Figure 4.1. Prone transverse section showing both kidneys. Note the anteromedial location of the pelvicalyceal echoes (*E*). *S*, spine.

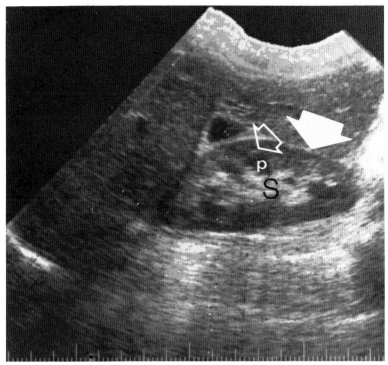

Figure 4.2. Supine longitudinal view of the right kidney. The pyramids (*p*) can be seen within the kidney. The arcuate arteries are visible at the apex of the pyramids (*open arrow*). Note the relatively echogenic sinus echoes (*S*) and the renal capsule (*solid arrow*).

of the intrarenal anatomy on the right side (2).

Techniques for viewing the left kidney are not as satisfactory, and the usual technique adopted is a decubitus or "coronal" view (3, 4) (Fig. 4.3). In this approach the patient is in a decubitus left side up position leaning forward approximately 20 to 40° depending on the angle at which the sinus echoes leave the kidney. The appropriate angle can be established on an initial transverse scan (5). In this position the spleen provides a mediocre acoustic window, but it is better than nothing. The "coronal" view is also of value on the right if the liver is small.

The prone position may be required both on the right and left sides, particularly when the lower poles are inadequately seen through a small liver or spleen. If a prone position is adopted, visualization is improved by placing a compression pillow under the abdomen; the thickness of the soft tissues overlying the kidney is reduced (6), and the kidneys are pushed closer to the transducer. On rare occasions, it may be necessary to examine the patient erect so that the kidneys fall to a low position and are less cloaked by ribs. A sitting position with the administration of 500 to 1,000 ml of degassed water

plus oral fat is an additional technique that has been found helpful (7).

Real-time, particularly a sector scanner, is invaluable in examining the kidneys; a sector scanner can be used between ribs to obtain the ideal axis. Linear array real-time systems are surprisingly effective but are less ideal because ribs may prevent long axis views of the kidneys from being obtained so renal lengths may be underestimated.

To examine the bladder and prostate adequately, the bladder must be full. It may sometimes be necessary to catheterize the bladder to see these structures. The catheter itself forms a visible linear structure within the bladder. The normal bladder wall is well seen as a black line around the bladder (Fig. 4.4). The actual thickness of the wall cannot be measured unless it is hypertrophied or thickened by pathology. The prostate can be seen at the posteroinferior aspect of the bladder as a more or less rounded structure with an echogenic structure at the center representing the urethra (Figs. 4.4 and 4.5). Protruding from the superior aspect of the prostate are the symmetrical mustache-shaped seminal vesicles which vary in size depending

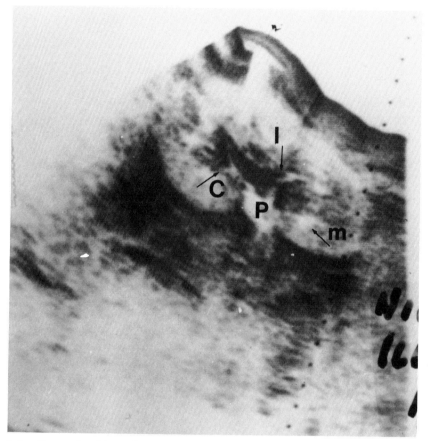

Figure 4.3. Prone decubitus view of the left kidney showing the pelvis (*P*), infundibulum (*I*), calyx (*C*), and renal sinus echoes from collagen tissue and fat. Pyramids (*m*) can be made out within the renal parenchyma.

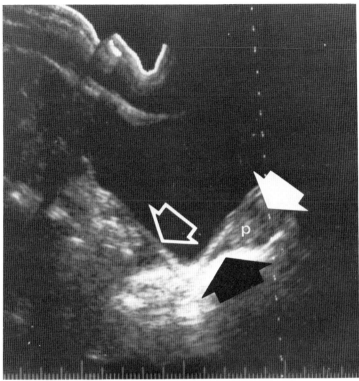

Figure 4.4. Supine longitudinal view of the bladder. The wall of the bladder is normally densely echogenic (*open arrow*). The prostate (*p*) can be seen posterior to the inferior aspect of the bladder. The seminal vesicles are visible (*black arrow*). The prostatic urethra may be an echopenic (*solid arrow*) or echogenic line.

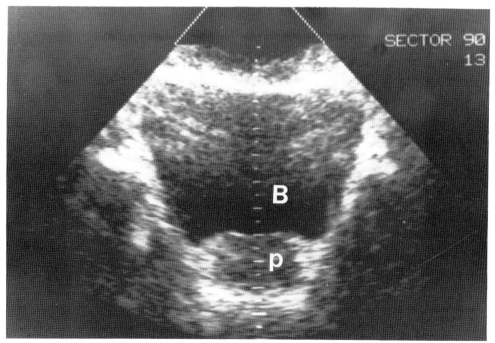

Figure 4.5. Transverse view showing the bladder (*B*) and the prostate (*p*).

upon the amount of spermatozoa present (Figs. 4.4 and 4.6).

ANATOMY

Detailed analysis of renal sonograms has revealed an ultrasonic picture which allows the identification of most of the structures that can be seen on cut section at gross pathology (8). In vitro sonograms have been performed on kidneys injected with a suspension of barium sulfate so that arteries were definitely identified. Subsequent cut sections clearly showed that the pyramids were visible distinct from the cortex (Fig. 4.2) and that the arcuate vessel site could be recognized.

The normal kidney is located so that the major structures that supply the kidneys—the renal artery, the renal vein, and the renal pelvis—exit in an anteromedial direction (Fig. 4.7). For this reason, a desirable ultrasonic view of the kidney is one in which the patient is in a semiprone position and a longitudinal section is obtained along an anteromedial axis; the renal vessels and pelvis are shown. An echogenic line surrounding the kidney, which represents fat in the renal capsule and perinephric fat, connects with the sinus echoes in this axis.

The Sinus

The predominant feature of the normal kidney sonogram is the sinus echoes, otherwise known as the central pelvicalyceal echo complex (Figs. 4.2 and 4.3). This central group of echoes is in continuity with the capsular echoes via a medial insertion. The sinus echo group can be smooth in outline or tentacled. The major component of the echoes within the sinus is the fat which surrounds the pelvis, infundibulum, and calyces. The amount of fat varies; in the neonate there is a relatively small amount of fat, and consequently the sinus echoes are poorly seen (9). In emaciated individuals the sinus and capsular fat can be much reduced (Fig. 4.8). There is a steady increase in sinus echogenicity and fat with age. In old age and in some instances of chronic infection, the amount of sinus fat is increased, and the sinus echoes become more prominent in the normal variant known as fibrolipomatosis (Fig. 4.9, A and B).

Pelvis and Calyces

Incorporated within the sinus echoes are echoes originating from the borders of the pelvis, infundibulum, and calyces. Not too infrequently,

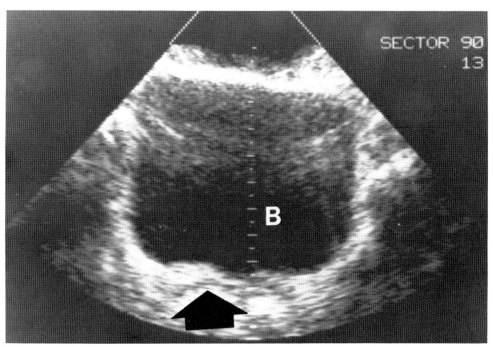

Figure 4.6. Supine transverse view at a higher level showing seminal vesicles (*arrow*). These have a mustache-shaped configuration and vary in size depending on contents. *B*, bladder.

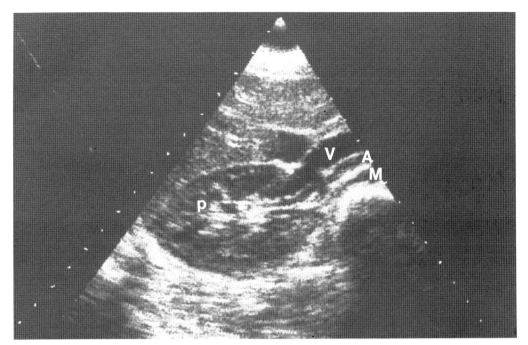

Figure 4.7. Transverse supine view of the right kidney. The pyramids (*p*) can be seen. The renal vein (*V*) can be seen entering centrally anterior to the renal artery (*A*). The crus of the diaphragm is the most posterior of the three structures (*M*).

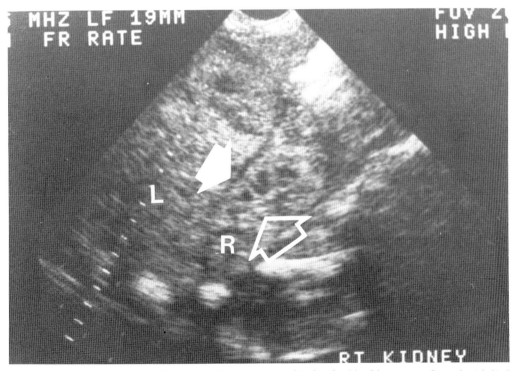

Figure 4.8. Supine longitudinal view. This emaciated individual had been on a 'binge' with little or no food for about 2 months. Sinus echoes are barely visible (*open arrow*). The renal capsule is seen as a sonolucent area because there is no fat (*solid arrow*). There is excess echogenicity in the liver (*L*) and in the renal parenchyma (*R*) due to fat deposition.

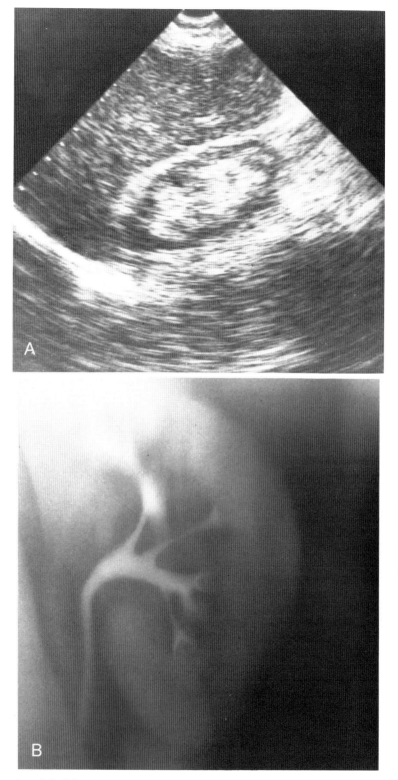

Figure 4.9. *A* and *B*, Fibrolipomatosis. Longitudinal section. There is excess size to the sinus echoes, although the echogenicity is slightly decreased. Note the perirenal fat on the intravenous pyelogram (*B*).

the pelvis shows mild dilatation with urine as a normal variant; sonographically, a cystic lesion is seen at the center of the kidney surrounded by dense echoes (Fig. 4.10). This dilatation may extend into the infundibulum (major calix) and, rarely, may outline a cupped calix. As a rule, normal calyces are not visible. Deliberate attempts to see the pelvis and calyces have been made by either ureteric compression, as for an intravenous pyelogram, or a fluid load accompanied by a diuretic (10). After the injection of 480 ml of water, the collecting system expands and becomes visible in most people. In a particularly confusing variant when hydronephrosis is a possibility, the pelvis may lie in an extrarenal location, becoming more prominent when fluid is administered.

Vascular Structures

Vascular structures can be seen within the sinus echoes. Many renal veins are relatively easy to see as they enter the kidney because they are large structures which lie anterior to the renal artery, pelvis, and ureter (Fig. 4.7).

The left renal vein pursues a long course before it enters the inferior vena cava, passing anterior to the aorta behind the superior mesenteric artery. It is often particularly large before it passes through this narrowed area; the narrow angle between the superior mesenteric artery and aorta can act as a "nutcracker" (Fig. 4.11); catheter studies may show an increased pressure distal to this point. Indeed the left renal vein can become so large that it looks like an aneurysm coming off the aorta; the interface between the left renal vein and the aorta may be very difficult to see.

The renal arteries can also be seen but are much smaller and difficult to visualize (Fig. 4.7). They lie posterior to the renal vein and anterior to the pelvis. The right renal artery passes behind the inferior vena cava; it often forms a bump in the posterior surface of the inferior vena cava (Fig. 4.12). Decubitus views are the best way of showing the renal artery entering the aorta (11). There may be multiple renal arteries (Fig. 4.12)—only the major ones are seen with ultrasound.

The ureter can be traced from the renal pelvis for a short distance in the normal individual. If it can be seen for any distance, this is usually an indication that renal obstruction is present and the obstruction is below the level of the

ureteropelvic junction. Other causes of ureteric dilatation are discussed in Chapter 7.

Cortex and Medulla

Several structures are visible within the renal parenchyma providing a black background is used (12). Abutting on the sinus fat are areas which are slightly more sonolucent than the rest of the parenchyma, known as the pyramids or medulla (Fig. 4.2). These areas are approximately heart shaped with the sharp end of the heart directed toward the renal sinus. At the border with the cortex, an echogenic focus may be seen representing the arcuate vessels. Locating the arcuate arteries and, therefore, the border between the cortex and medulla allows one to assess the cortical width and visualize cortical scarring (8). Visualization of the pyramids and medulla is common in children and thin adults, and it is especially easy on the right where the liver provides an acoustic window. Some segment of the pyramids is visible in most people when a black background and good scanning techique are used.

The cortex surrounds the pyramids and extends to the peripheral margins of the kidney. The cortex is slightly more echogenic than the pyramids but less echogenic than the adjacent liver and spleen except in the neonate. In the neonate it is normal for the cortex to be more echogenic than the liver or spleen; this is thought to be a result of the presence of immature glomeruli (9). Judging the echogenicity of the cortex is best performed in a supine view. One should be cautious about judging the echogenicity of the cortex in the presence of ascites. It can look unduly dense and yet be normal.

Length and Volume Measurements

The normal renal length as seen by ultrasound is less than that seen by x-ray since there is no magnification effect. It is generally considered that a length of between 8 and 14 cm is normal in adults on the right (mean 10.74) and between 7 and 12.5 (mean 11.10) on the left (13). Several tables of renal length are available. Renal length tables have also been developed for children (14). Ultrasound is undoubtedly more accurate than intravenous pyelography in obtaining renal length as long as a diligent effort is made to obtain the longest axis. Intravenous pyelogram lengths always underestimate the true length

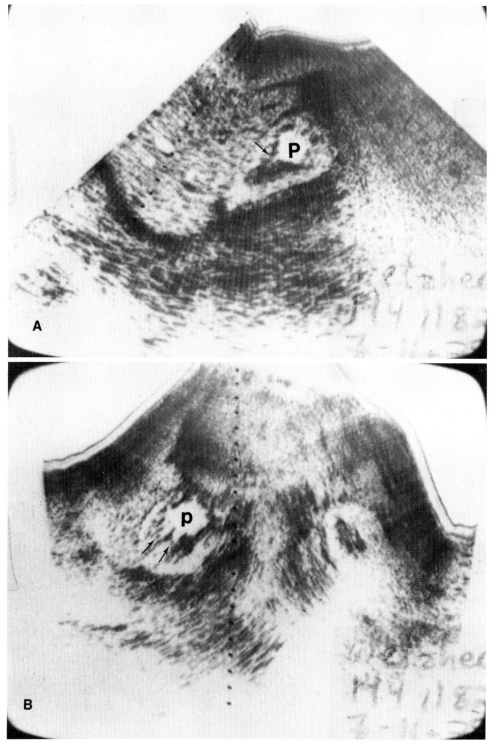

Figure 4.10. *A*, Longitudinal; *B*, transverse. Patient with a prominent extrarenal pelvis (*p*). Infundibula connecting to the pelvis can be seen (*arrows*). The pelvis is fairly large but normal by intravenous pyelography.

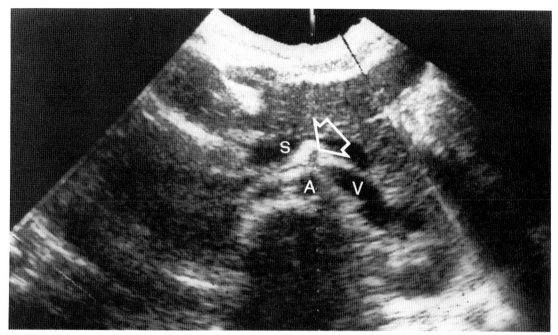

Figure 4.11.   The left renal vein (*V*) is frequently dilated prior to the points where it passes between the superior mesenteric artery (*arrow*) and the aorta (*A*) as a normal variant. *S*, splenic vein.

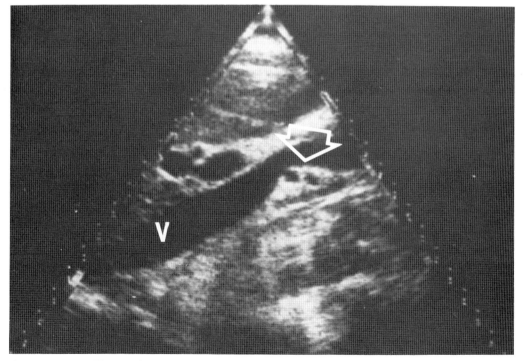

Figure 4.12.   The renal arteries (*arrow*) can be seen as they pass posterior to the inferior vena cava (*V*). In this instance there was a dual renal arterial supply to a neoplasm.

because some degree of anterior tilt to the inferior pole always occurs in normal individuals. Since the amount of tilt is highly variable (between 5 and 64°), a standard correction factor cannot be used (15).

A cruder ultrasonic method of obtaining a normal renal length is to compare the kidney length with the vertebral length. The normal kidney is about four transverse processes in length (16). This technique allows one to deduce whether the kidney is an appropriate length for the patient; this can be used in children or large individuals in whom normal standards would be inappropriate.

Although renal length is the easiest way of assessing the kidney, measurements of renal volume obtained by measuring the renal height, width, and length and using the formula for a prolapse ellipse are more accurate for follow-up (17). Again, tables are available for children (18). A slightly more cumbersome method for obtaining volume which is probably of no greater accuracy is to take serial areas at 1-cm distances in transverse or longitudinal axis above the kidney in a stepwise fashion and add them together to give a renal volume (19, 20). This technique may be technically difficult to perform because breath holding is unpredictable and motion artifacts may occur.

Prostate volume can be calculated by making the assumption it is a sphere and using the following formula

$$\frac{4}{3}\pi^3$$

Normal standards of prostate size are available (21, 22). There is steady enlargement of the prostate with age, but anything over 15 g is considered abnormal.

A number of recognizable normal variant sonographic appearances exist.

PREGNANCY

In pregnancy the collecting system dilates as a normal variant. Maximum dilatation occurs at 28 weeks on the right side. The left side is less affected. Normal standards of renal sinus distension are available (23, 24). The anteroposterior dimension of the renal sinus is measured. If the left renal distension exceeds the right, obstruction can be assumed. An unexpected correlation between a fetus in a breech lie and severe right pyelocaliectasis in pregnancy has been observed (25).

SMALL INFANTS

In small infants the amount of renal sinus fat is limited, and the capsular echoes are barely seen. In addition, there is increased cortical echogenicity due to immature glomeruli morphology (9). As a result of the increased cortical echogenicity, the pyramids are more obvious and the sinus echoes are less obvious. It is not uncommon for a neonatal kidney to be thought to contain multiple cysts by the novice sonographer (26). Fetal lobulation is more pronounced at this age than later when quite marked impressions on the renal border can be seen.

PELVIC KIDNEY

Should either kidney not be found in its usual location, it may well be that there is a pelvic kidney present. Pelvic kidneys will be seen in the pelvis on a supine view, and they have a reniform configuration. Pelvic kidneys are not infrequently mistaken for pelvic masses by gynecologists (27). Sonographic appearances are distinctive, because there will be sinus echoes within the renal mass (Fig. 4.13A). However, pelvic kidneys not infrequently have a dilated renal pelvis (Fig. 4.13B) and/or a malrotated axis, in which case confusion with other pelvic masses, such as an ectopic pregnancy or an ovarian mass, can occur. A variant of a pelvic kidney seen at a slightly higher level on the scan is a "pancake" kidney. Both kidneys are fused into one central kidney with a distorted sinus echo complex (Fig. 4.14). The clue to the sonographic diagnosis of a pelvic kidney or variant is for the examiner to make it a reflex to look into the pelvis whenever a kidney is not seen in its normal location.

MALROTATION

A somewhat confusing normal variant on intravenous pyelogram is malrotation of the kidney. Malrotation of the kidney occurs when the major structures exit from the kidney in an anterior direction rather than an anteromedial direction. When this anomaly is present, one can get the impression on a sonogram that there is a collection in Rutherford Morison's pouch on a supine view, when in reality one is merely seeing a malrotated, slightly dilated extrarenal pelvis (Fig. 4.15). Observation of the axis of the sinus echoes on a transverse view readily gives the diagnosis.

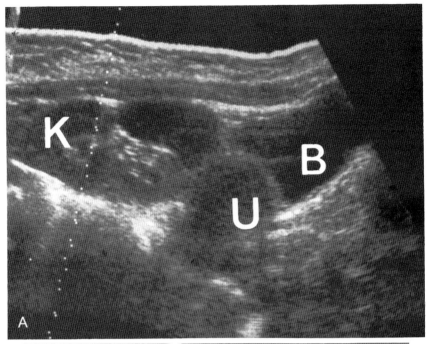

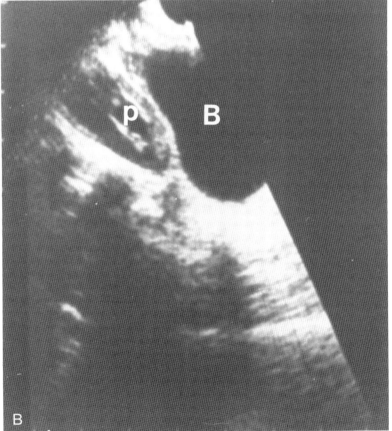

Figure 4.13. *A*, Pelvic kidney. This pelvic kidney was thought to be a gynecological mass prior to the sonogram. The kidney (*K*) lies above the uterus (*U*) and bladder (*B*). *B*, Pelvic kidney. Longitudinal section. This pelvic kidney had a dilated renal pelvis (*p*) and was initially mistaken for an ectopic pregnancy. No left kidney was found in its usual location. *B*, bladder.

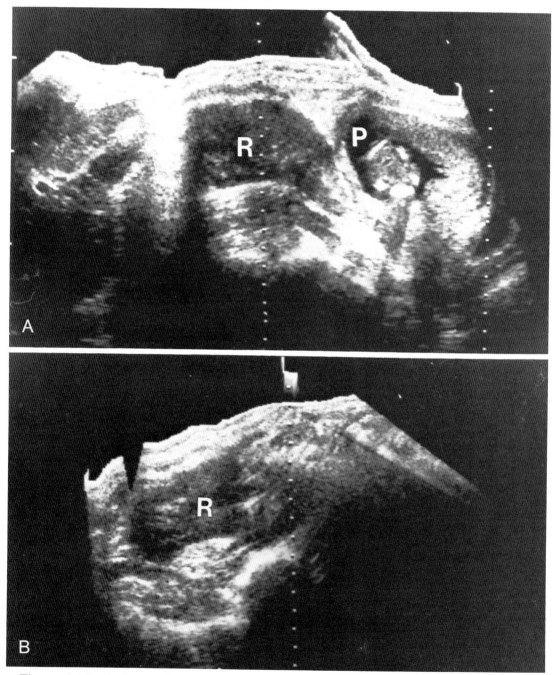

Figure 4.14. *A,* Longitudinal section. Pancake kidney with crossed fused renal ectopia and pregnancy. The fused kidney (*R*) lies above the pregnant uterus (*P*). *B,* Transverse section. The two sinuses of the pancake kidney (*R*) can be seen as echogenic areas.

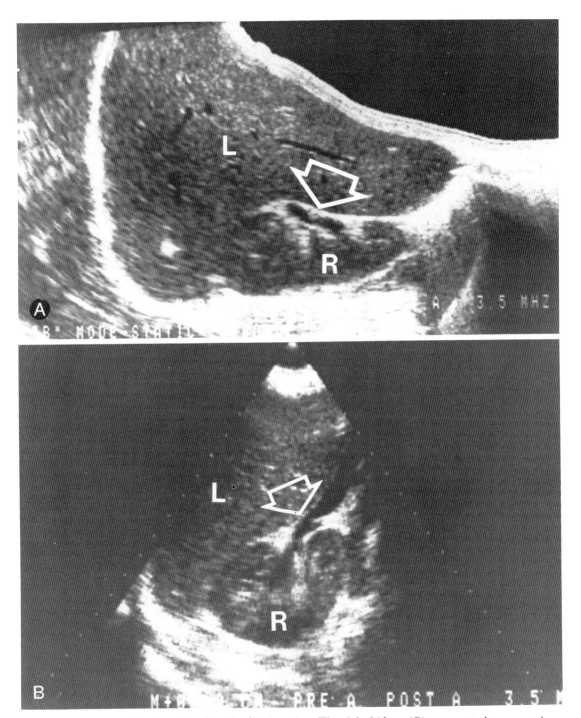

Figure 4.15. *A*, Malrotation. Longitudinal section. The right kidney (*R*) appears to have a cystic space lying anterior to it (*arrow*) which actually represents the renal pelvis. *L*, liver. *B*, A transverse view shows that the major structures enter the kidney (*R*) anteriorly rather than anteromedially. The renal vein (*arrow*) is well seen. The pelvis accounts for the apparent cystic space anterior to the kidney.

CROSSED RENAL ECTOPIA

In this condition both kidneys lie on the same side and are fused. A very long kidney is seen ultrasonically with two separate groups of sinus echoes.

INTRATHORACIC KIDNEY

On occasion, the kidney lies at a high level just below the diaphragm (Fig. 4.16) or even above the diaphragm in an intrathoracic location. The latter variant is usually easily recognized since the kidney lies adjacent to but just above the diaphragm (28). The diaphragm may well show a hump where the kidney is if it is infradiaphragmatic but high.

HORSESHOE KIDNEY

Another normal variant which can be confusing sonographically is a "horseshoe" kidney (29). In this situation, both kidneys lie more medially than usual and are joined by a lower pole "isth-

mus" of renal tissue. The axis of the fused kidney is usually rotated medially. The "isthmic" portion of the kidney can be confused with nodes, fluid-filled gut, or retroperitoneal fibrosis (Fig. 4.17, A and B). It is at too low a level to represent pancreas and has an unusually smooth border for nodes. Careful transverse scanning will show a connection between the two medially placed kidneys. A "horseshoe" kidney isthmus lies in front of the aorta and inferior vena cava. Hydronephrosis and multiple renal vessels are more common in persons with "horseshoe" kidneys than in the rest of the population. A pelvic "horseshoe" kidney has been described (30).

DOUBLE COLLECTING SYSTEM

A relatively commonplace normal variant is a double collecting system or bifid pelvicalyceal system. It is not easy to distinguish between these two situations by ultrasound. In both conditions the sinus echoes are divided into two groups, and in the intervening area the renal

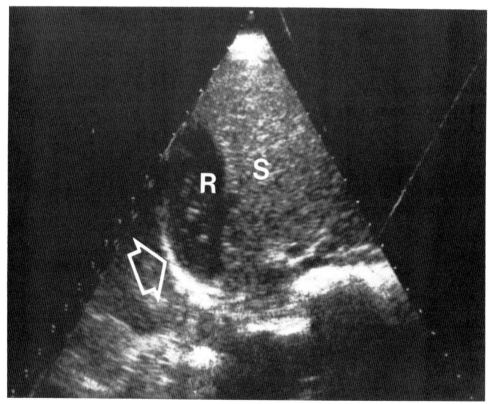

Figure 4.16. High left kidney. The kidney (*R*) lies adjacent to the diaphragm (*arrow*) above the spleen (*S*) and is almost in a thoracic location.

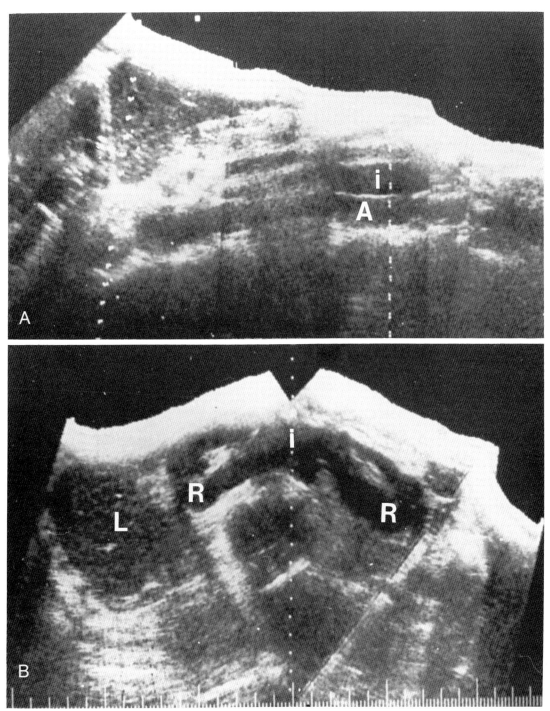

Figure 4.17. *A*, Horseshoe kidney. Longitudinal section. The isthmus (*i*) lies anterior to the aorta (*A*) and could be mistaken for nodes or retroperitoneal fibrosis. *B*, A transverse view shows both kidneys (*R*) lying in a more midline location than usual and connected by the isthmus (*i*). *L*, liver.

texture is normal. In the coronal section that outlines the hiler structures best, one can see that the sinus echoes exit from the kidney in two separate groups (Fig. 4.18). The area of normal renal tissue between the two systems may make one worry about a neoplasm on an intravenous pyelogram; this area is commonly termed a pseudotumor or column of Bertin. Columns of Bertin are seen elsewhere in the kidney as prominent cortical masses between pyramids. A large central area of normal parenchyma with a cortical echogenicity is seen usually at the upper pole. An ultrasonic image akin to that seen with duplication or a bifid pelvicalyceal system can be created if casual scanning techniques are used and rib shadows a segment of the pelvic echoes (31).

DROMEDARY HUMP

A bulge can occur from the lateral border of the kidney, particularly on the left side in which the parenchymal texture is normal but the outline of the kidney is widened (Fig. 4.19). This anomaly is known as a "dromedary hump." If the parenchymal texture is normal, it is practically never worth further investigating by more expensive techniques, such as computed tomography or angiography.

FETAL RENAL LOBULATION

The outline of the kidney can be indented by lobulation related to the embryology of the kidney. One should be certain when observing this anomaly that one is not confusing lobulation with a slight malrotation of the kidney and the entrance of the sinus into the kidney.

NEPHROPTOSIS

The amount of mobility of the kidney can be readily assessed with real-time ultrasound since the patient can be examined sitting, erect, in a

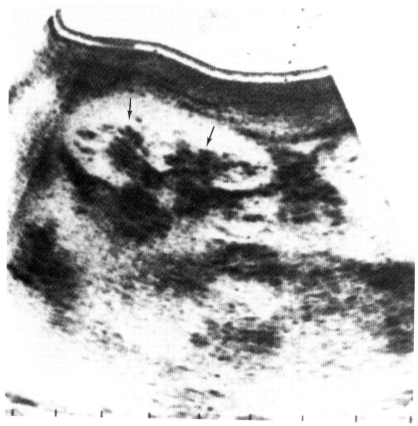

Figure 4.18.   Prone oblique ("coronal") section showing the central echoes entering from the kidneys and splitting into two groups (*arrows*). This is the picture of a bifid pelvicalyceal system.

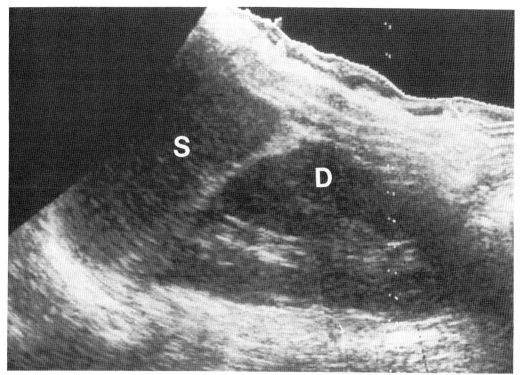

Figure 4.19. Dromedary hump. Longitudinal coronal section. The lateral aspect of the left kidney is more prominent than usual (*D*), but the texture is normal. *S*, spleen.

supine position, or in a decubitus position with the transducer constantly over the patient. Although undue renal mobility is no longer generally thought to be a valid reason for operation, a group of three patients has been described in whom lying on the left side reproduced symptoms. Local tenderness over the right kidney was evident. Two of these patients had been asymptomatic after avoiding the left side down position, and one was cured by nephropexy (32).

AGENESIS

In renal agenesis one kidney is absent. A portion of the splenic flexure of the colon falls into the position where the kidney should lie if the left kidney is absent (the most common anomaly). The splenic flexure adopts a characteristic configuration at barium enema. When the colon is empty, one may have the sonographic impression that the colon is actually a kidney because the mucosa of the colon gives rise to an echogenic appearance and the walls are sonolucent (Fig. 4.20) (33). A colonic pseudokidney can usually be distinguished from a kidney because its walls are less well defined and it may contain a portion of gas with acoustical shadowing. Real-time may show evidence of some peristalsis.

RIGHT KIDNEY AS A MASS

Sometimes the kidney is markedly anteriorly tilted at the inferior pole and can indeed present as a palpable mass (34). The kidney responds to hepatomegaly in various ways. In one response it is pushed inferiorly and tilted anteriorly (Fig. 4.21). When this occurs, it is readily palpable and has been a source of serious clinical confusion.

FIBROLIPOMATOSIS

When excess fat is deposited in the region of the renal sinuses, it appears that two different ultrasonic patterns may occur. As a rule, the sinus echoes are larger and the cortical width is reduced (Fig. 4.9, *A* and *B*). A second pattern may be seen when the sinus echoes, although more diffuse, are relatively echopenic (35).

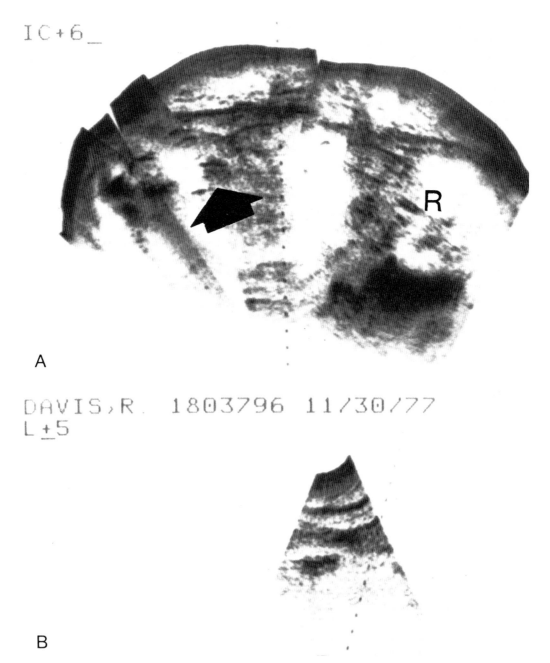

Figure 4.20. *A*, Transverse. A small "kidney" (*arrow*) appears to be present on the left. An enlarged kidney (*R*) is seen on the right. *B*, Longitudinal view. The left "kidney" has an indifferent posterior margin. At surgery no kidney was found. The apparent kidney was a loop of splenic flexure of the colon.

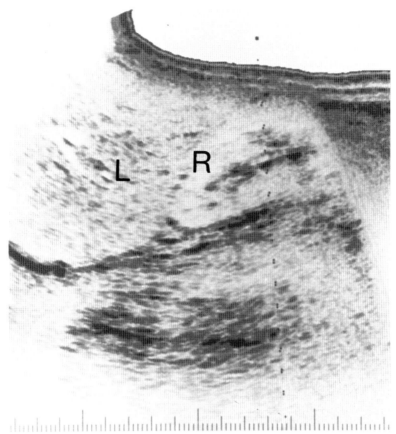

Figure 4.21. Longitudinal section. This anteriorly placed and anteriorly tilted right kidney (*R*) presented as a right upper quadrant mass. It lies within 2 cm of the abdominal wall but is a normal variant. *L*, liver.

Cronan et al. (36) maintain that the echopenic form is actually due to the presence of a number of small peripelvic cysts.

References

1. Sanders RC: Renal ultrasound. *Radiol Clin North Am* 13:417–434, 1975.
2. Rosenfield AT, Taylor KJ, Crade M, De Graaf CS: Anatomy and pathology of the kidney by gray scale ultrasound. *Radiology* 128:737–744, 1978.
3. Albarelli JN, Lawson TL: Renal ultrasonography: advantages of the decubitus position. *J Clin Ultrasound* 6:73–142, 1978.
4. Thompson IM, Kovac A, Geshner J: Coronal renal ultrasound. *Urology* 17:210–213, 1981.
5. Bazzocchi M, Rizzato G: The value of the posterior oblique longitudinal scan in renal ultrasonography. *Urol Radiol* 1:221–225, 1980.
6. Skolnick ML: Enhanced ultrasonic visualization of kidneys via an abdominal compression pillow. *J Clin Ultrasound* 6:377–456, 1978.
7. Rosenberg ER, Clair MR, Bowie JD: The fluid-filled stomach as an acoustic window to the left kidney. *AJR* 138:175–176, 1982.
8. Cook JH, Rosenfield AT, Taylor KJ: Ultrasonic demonstration of intrarenal anatomy. *AJR* 129:831–835, 1977.
9. Hricak H, Slovis TL, Callen CW, et al: Neonatal kidneys: sonographic anatomic correlation. *Radiology* 147:699–702, 1983.
10. Rosenfield AT, Taylor KJ, Dembner AG, et al: Ultrasound of renal sinus: new observations. *AJR* 133:441–448, 1979.
11. Isikoff MB, Hill MC: Sonography of the renal arteries: left lateral decubitus position. *AJR* 134:1177–1179, 1980.
12. Sanders RC: Comparison between black and white backgrounds for ultrasonic images. *J Clin Ultrasound* 8:413–415, 1980.
13. Brandt TD, Neiman HL, Dragowski MJ, Bulawa W, Claykamp G: Ultrasound assessment of normal renal dimensions. *J Ultrasound Med* 1:49–52, 1982.
14. Hangstvedt S, Lundberg J: Kidney size in normal children measured by sonography. *Scand J Urol Nephrol* 14:251–255, 1980.
15. Farrant P, Meire HB: Ultrasonic measurement of renal inclination; its importance in measurement of renal length. *Br J Radiol* 51:628–630, 1978.

16. Lewis E, Ritchie WG: A simple ultrasonic method for assessing renal size. *J Clin Ultrasound* 8:417–420, 1980.
17. Jones TB, Riddick LR, Harpen MD, et al: Ultrasonographic determination of renal mass and renal volume. *J Ultrasound Med* 2:151–154, 1983.
18. Holloway H, Jones TB, Robinson AE, et al: Sonographic determination of renal volumes in normal neonates. *Pediatr Radiol* 13:212–214, 1983.
19. Rasmussen SN, Haase L, Kjeldsen H, Hancke S: Determination of renal volume by ultrasound scanning. *J Clin Ultrasound* 6:143–214, 1978.
20. Moskowitz PS, Carroll BA, McCoy JM: Ultrasonic renal volumetry in children. *Radiology* 134:61–64, 1980.
21. Henneberry M, Carter MF, Neiman HL: Estimation of prostatic size by suprapubic ultrasonography. *J Urol* 121:615–616, 1978.
22. Abu-Yousef MM, Narayana AS: Transabdominal ultrasound in the evaluation of prostate size. *J Clin Ultrasound* 10:275–278, 1982.
23. Peake SL, Roxburgh HB, Langlos S: Ultrasonic assessment of hydronephrosis of pregnancy. *Radiology* 146:167–170, 1983.
24. Erickson LM, Nicholson SF, Lewal DB, Frischke L: Ultrasound evaluation of hydronephrosis of pregnancy. *J Clin Ultrasound* 7:128–132, 1979.
25. Finberg H: Renal ultrasound: anatomy and technique. *Semin Ultrasound* 2:1, 7–20, 1981.
26. Scheible W, Leopold GR: High-resolution real-time ultrasonography of neonatal kidneys. *J Ultrasound Med* 1:133–138, 1982.
27. Granat M, Gordon T, Issaq E, Shabtai M: Accidental puncture of pelvic kidney: a rare complication of culdocentesis. *Am J Obstet Gynecol* 138:233, 1980.
28. Sumner TE, Volberg FM, Smolen PM: Intrathoracic kidney—diagnosis by ultrasound. *Pediatr Radiol* 12:78–80, 1982.
29. Mindell HJ, Kupic EA: Horseshoe kidney: ultrasonic demonstration. *AJR* 129:527, 1977.
30. Trackler RT, Resnick ML, Leopold GR: Pelvic horseshow kidney: ultrasound findings and case report. *J Clin Ultrasound* 6:1–72, 1978.
31. Haller JO, Friedman AP, Lebensart DP: Pseudoduplication: a scanning artifact of renal ultrasonography. *Urol Radiol* 1:187, 1980.
32. Patel AS, Barber-Riley WP: Symptomatic medial nephroptosis—an ultrasonic diagnosis. *Br J Radiol* 55:244–246, 1982.
33. Teele RL, Rosenfield AT, Freedman GS: The anatomic splenic flexure: an ultrasonic renal impostor. *AJR* 128:115–120, 1977.
34. Bree RL: Anterior position of the lower pole of the right kidney: potential confusion with right upper quadrant mass. *J Clin Ultrasound* 4:283–285, 1977.
35. Yeh HC, Mitty HA, Wolf BS: Ultrasonography of renal sinus lipomatosis. *Radiology* 124:799–801, 1977.
36. Cronan JJ, Amis ES, Yoder IC, Kopans DB, Simeone JF, Pfister R: Peripelvic cysts: an impostor of sonographic hydronephrosis. *J Ultrasound Med* 1:229–236, 1982.

CHAPTER 5

Renal Cystic Disease: Fluid-filled Lesions in the Kidney Parenchyma

ROGER C. SANDERS, M.D.

Ultrasonic accuracy in defining whether a mass found within the kidney is a fluid-filled "cyst" or a solid lesion is reported between 98 and 100% accurate (1) using gray-scale and real-time. With further improvement in real-time instrumentation, results of this quality should be commonplace. Errors mostly relate to solid homogeneous mass lesions miscalled "cysts" or vice versa because the ultrasonic criteria for a cyst were not strictly followed.

To avoid misdiagnosis, technique should be optimal. The time gain compensation settings for the kidney should be set so that at the same depth within the body as the cyst lies other normal fluid-filled organs, such as the gallbladder and bladder, do not contain internal echoes. There should be low level echoes present within the adjoining renal parenchyma. The fluid-filled mass will stand out as an essentially echo-free structure (Fig. 5.1), although low level echoes will be seen from reverberations (Fig. 5.2) or the partial volume effect. A simple cyst will show "good transonicity": there will be high level echoes distal to the cyst and not in the surrounding renal parenchyma. If the mass is a solid homogeneous mass, there will only be low level

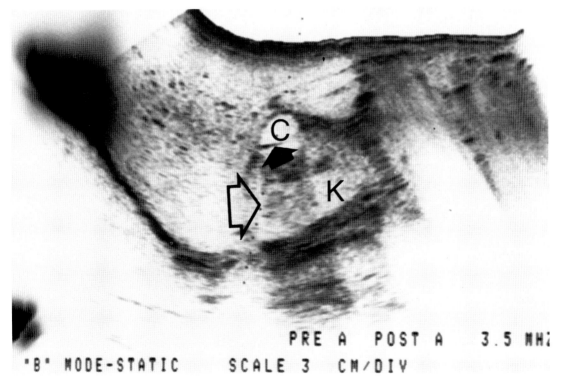

PRE A   POST A   3.5 MH?
"B" MODE-STATIC   SCALE 3   CM/DIV

Figure 5.1. Longitudinal section. Cyst (*C*) at the anterior aspect of the right kidney (*K*) with a partially seen septum within (*solid arrow*). The acoustic enhancement effect is well seen posterior to the cyst (*open arrow*).

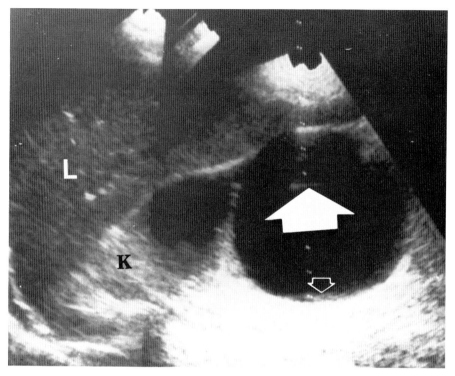

Figure 5.2. Longitudinal view. Two cysts arise from the inferior pole of the right kidney (*K*). Reverberations (*solid arrow*) can be seen on the near side of the cyst to the transducer, and echoes from the slice thickness effect (*open arrow*) can be seen on the far side of the cyst from the transducer. *L*, liver.

echoes distal to the lesion. It may be of help to use a transducer of higher frequency to emphasize the "enhanced transonicity" sign. In comparison with the adjacent renal parenchyma, there will be few or no echoes within a cyst, although, if the "cyst" contains fluid with a high protein content (such as an abscess), there may be some echoes within a fluid-filled lesion (2). It is preferable to decide whether the mass is a cyst without the presence of overlying ribs. A possible cyst of the right kidney is best examined with the patient supine looking through the liver (Fig. 5.1). Lesions of the left kidney are best looked at with the patient in the right decubitus (left coronal) position so that the spleen lies just superior to the kidney forming another acoustic window and one can look at the kidney without the presence of too many overlying ribs.

SINGLE FLUID-FILLED LESIONS

Simple Renal Cyst

Simple cysts of the kidney, if benign, are of no clinical significance unless they cause distor-tion of adjacent calyces with local hydronephrosis or mechanically induced pain. They may be located anywhere in the kidney and, if found in the region of the pelvis, are known as peripelvic. If located outside the renal capsule but in the region of the pelvis, they are termed parapelvic. Simple cysts contain yellow fluid and become more common as patients get older. Some 40 to 50% of patients over the age of 60 are reputed to have renal cysts (3). Their etiology is uncertain, but they develop commonly in patients with impaired renal function, particularly those on dialysis.

The usual simple renal cyst at echography is smooth walled, echo free, and spherically indents the pelvicalyceal echo system or protrudes exophytically from the kidney (Figs. 5.1 and 5.2) (4). The walls of such a cyst can show changes which may be confusing. If the cyst is multilocular, distinct septa may be seen (Figs. 5.1 and 5.3) provided the transducer is placed at sufficient different angles to the cyst and septum. Such septa are easier to see by ultrasound than computed tomography (CT) (5). Sometimes a septa may provoke echoes but be at an angle

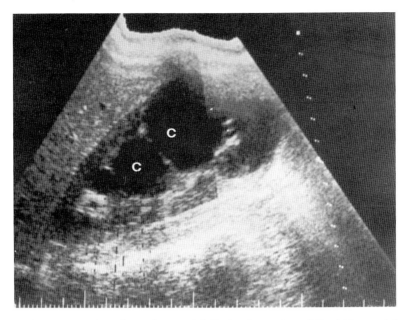

Figure 5.3. Coronal section. Several cysts (*c*) lie in the center of the kidney, giving an initial impression of hydronephrosis. However, septa are present between the cysts, and a portion of the renal sinus echoes can be seen at the upper pole of the kidney.

difficult to visualize ultrasonically because the transducer cannot be placed at right angles to the acoustic interface. The resultant echo may not be linear and may suggest the presence of a neoplasm in the wall. Sometimes the apparent irregularities of the wall seen on sonography represent minor infoldings of the cyst wall. Parapelvic cysts frequently have an irregular wall and can be confused with hydronephrosis (Fig. 5.3) (6). Nearly all cysts show some reverberation echoes in the cyst on the near side to the transducer (Fig. 5.2) (7), but some cysts show further echoes on the distal aspect of the cyst thought to be due to the width of the beam (about 0.5 cm wide) partially showing cystic fluid and partially showing wall (Fig. 5.2). These echoes are termed the slice thickness artifacts and are akin to the "partial volume effect" seen on CT scanning (8). Linear side lobe artifacts also cause echoes at the periphery of a cyst (9). A linear horizontal echo, more or less parallel to the borders of a cyst, is termed a grating artifact and is seen particularly with linear arrays (10). However, occasionally cysts may show a definite fluid level due to debris within the cyst; in such cases the fluid level persists when the patient's position changes. Calcification in a cyst wall confuses the ultrasonic appearance (Fig. 5.4). Calcification will prevent through transmission;

therefore, a reliable assessment of whether there is fluid in a cyst cannot be made.

Simple cysts may occur in childhood (11–13); their ultrasonic appearance and management are the same as in adults. Cysts become very common with old age (3), and it is our practice not to intervene on asymptomatic cysts in elderly patients (see Chapter 16).

Although the vast majority of single cystic lesions in the kidney represent simple cysts, other lesions should be considered.

Cystic Neoplasms

Neoplasms within cysts are exceedingly rare. Such neoplasms generally cause such symptoms as hematuria or pain. In our limited experience (eight cases) they appear to have a typical sonographic appearance. Very few lesions have been reported examined with gray-scale (14). There are irregularities of the wall of the cyst associated with echoes within the lumen (Fig. 5.5). Numerous septum may be present (15). However a few septa may occur in benign cysts. In my view, sonographic cyst wall irregularities represent a strong indication for the performance of a cyst puncture with a subsequent cystogram. A cystic lesion with wall irregularities has been reported with malakoplakia (16). Indications for puncture are considered in Chapter 16.

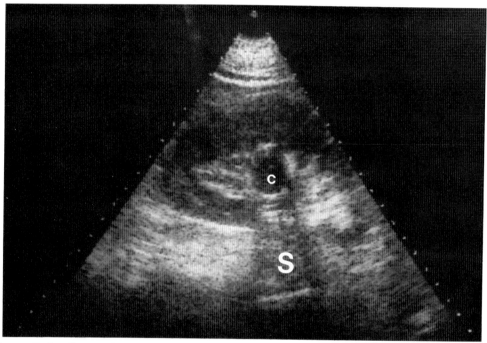

Figure 5.4. Cyst with a calcified wall (c). Instead of acoustical enhancement beyond the cyst, one can see an area of relative shadowing (S). Note the echogenic walls of the cyst.

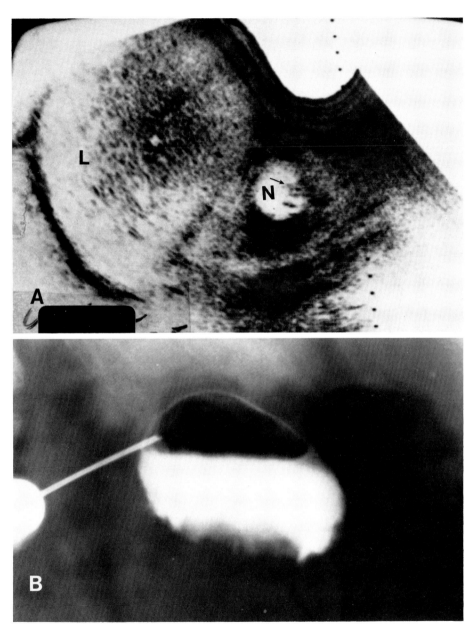

Figure 5.5. *A,* Supine longitudinal view through the liver of the right kidney. A large cystic neoplasm (*N*) is present in the anterior aspect. Echoes and an irregular border due to the neoplasm can be seen within the cyst (*arrow*). *L,* liver. *B,* Double contrast cystogram shows irregular border to the inferior aspect of the cyst.

Tumors are seen with necrotic fluid-filled centers. Necrotic centers are particularly common in the later evolution of Wilms' tumors (Fig. 5.6). Unlike simple cysts or cysts with a neoplasm in the wall, an abnormal area of decreased echoes surrounds the sonolucent area. Fluid-filled necrotic areas are almost unknown with other renal tumors apart from the occasional cystic hypernephroma (Fig. 5.7).

Lymphoma can appear like a sonolucent cyst. It may be very hard to distinguish between a cyst and lymphoma because the amount of through transmission is critical in making this distinction and the homogeneous lymphomatous mass conducts sound well (Fig. 5.8) (17). Renal lymphoma can be seen either as focal deposits within the kidney or as a generalized process causing an alteration in the renal texture.

Hemorrhagic Cyst

Hemorrhagic cysts are a serious problem for the ultrasonographer because the ultrasonic appearance can be indistinguishable from those of a cystic neoplasm (Fig. 5.9, A and B). Such cysts are thought to be the result of old trauma and contain altered blood. They are usually treated as neoplasms (18). Of the five cases seen with gray-scale, one looked like a simple cyst. In three others the walls were irregular and there were low level central echoes (Fig. 5.9, A and B), but the acoustic transmission was greater than would be expected with a neoplasm. In a fifth, a mass protruded into the cyst. On puncture, old blood was obtained from all five cysts. Clot can have a variable appearance depending on its composition (19, 20). Arteriography shows displacement of adjacent vessels but no evidence of neovascularity. CT scanning has been helpful in the noninvasive diagnosis of such cysts because it shows a density number compatible with hemorrhage different from that seen in a simple cyst.

Mimics of Renal Cysts

PYRAMIDS

With the exceptional resolution available with current equipment it is possible to visualize the renal pyramids in about 80% of adults (see Chapter 4) (21); they have a different acoustic density from the surrounding renal cortex. Occasionally, particularly in neonates (22), the pyramids stand out so well that it is possible to confuse them with a cystic lesion of the kidney (see Chapter 4) (Fig. 5.10). The echogenicity of the cortex is as great or greater than the liver up to about age 6 months so the pyramids look more obvious. However, it will be noticed that they are arranged symmetrically in the medul-

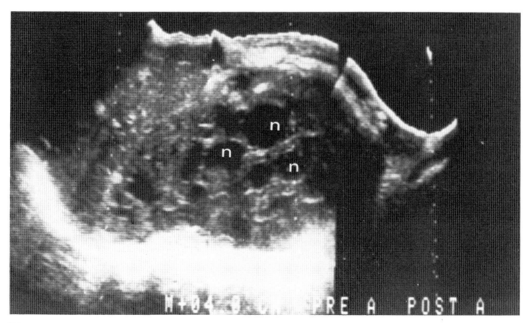

Figure 5.6. Wilms' tumor with numerous areas of necrosis (*n*). These cystic structures are fluid filled but are surrounded by a kidney neoplasm.

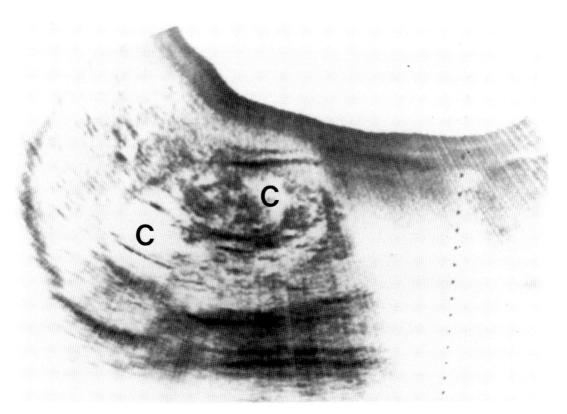

Figure 5.7. Cystic hypernephroma. This unusual lesion contains a number of cysts (C) in addition to echogenic material.

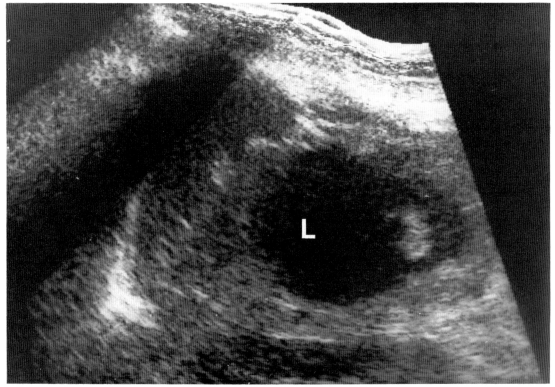

Figure 5.8. Lymphomatous mass in kidney. At first glance this large lymphomatous deposit (*L*) mimics the appearance of hydronephrosis, but notice the absence of through transmission.

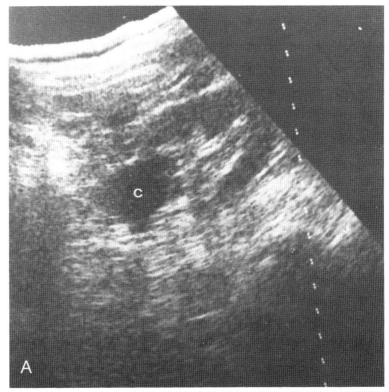

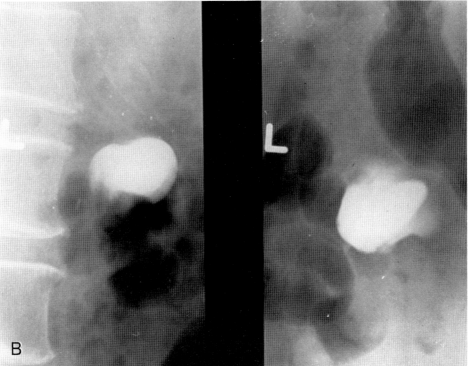

Figure 5.9. *A*, Hemorrhagic cyst. Note the irregular borders and the internal echoes within this cystic lesion (*c*). The cyst was punctured, and old blood was obtained. *B*, Same case. Cystogram showing the internal margins of the hemorrhagic cyst. The cyst has been unchanged on conservative treatment over the last 2 years.

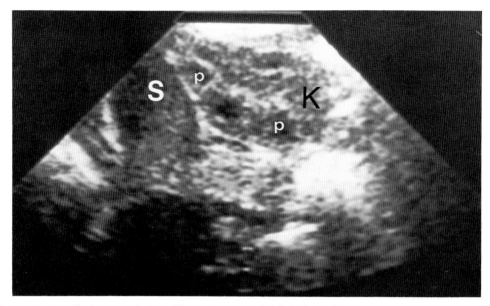

Figure 5.10. Left coronal view. Normal neonatal left kidney. Note the increased echogenicity of the kidney (K) in comparison with the spleen (S). The pyramids (p) stand out and can, at this age, be mistaken for cysts.

lary zone, that more than one "lesion" can be seen, and that all the "lesions" are approximately the same size.

RENAL SINUS LIPOMATOSIS

Renal sinus lipomatosis has variable acoustic features. These have been summarized by Yeh et al. (23) and Becker et al. (24). Although in most instances sinus lipomatosis gives rise to an echogenic center to the kidney, in others the fat provokes a zone of decreased echoes that can at first mimic a cystic lesion (Fig. 5.11). However, if the examination is performed with proper gain settings, it will be apparent that there are low level echoes within the apparently cystic area of about the same number as in the surrounding renal parenchyma outside the pelvicalyceal system. Some of the sonolucent areas previously thought to represent fat have been shown to be parapelvic cysts (25).

RENAL ABSCESS

The ultrasonic appearance of renal abscess is variable depending on whether (a) the pus is liquified in a form ready for drainage or (b) there are multiple tiny abscesses and inflammation. Ultrasonically, there may be a parenchymal cystic area surrounded by a zone of altered echoes (Fig. 5.12) (26, 27), or there may be an area

which differs from the remainder of the renal parenchyma in having fewer echoes but which is not frankly cystic. Generally, the clinical features allow the distinction of an abscess from a tumor, but the acoustic patterns may be the same. Infection may be superimposed on a simple cyst, producing some extra echoes (28).

RENAL HEMATOMA

Renal hematomas vary in acoustic appearances markedly. The natural history of a hematoma is such that the sonographic findings vary from day to day. In the first instance, the blood is liquid and presents a typical cystic appearance, but as clot develops, groups of internal echoes occur (19, 20, 29, 30). Eventually the hematoma may liquefy and develop into a seroma with a cystic appearance, or it may become organized and develop low level echoes. Neither a hematoma nor an abscess has a smooth wall.

HYDRONEPHROTIC UPPER COLLECTING SYSTEM

When a "cyst" is located at the upper pole of either kidney, the possibility of a second dilated upper collecting system should be considered and the excretory urogram (EVC) should be examined with this in mind. If the lesion does

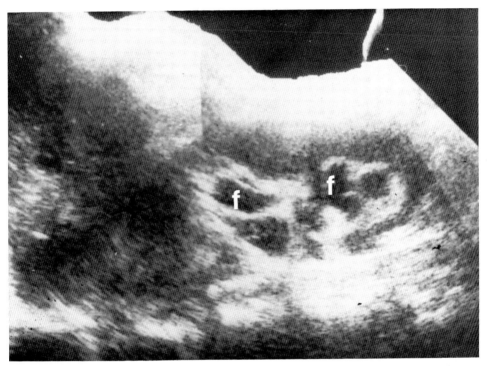

Figure 5.11. Sinus lipomatosis. The sonolucent areas (*f*) at the center of the kidney were initially mistaken for hydronephrosis, but a subsequent CT scan showed them to have fat density. This is one of the variant appearances that fat can assume.

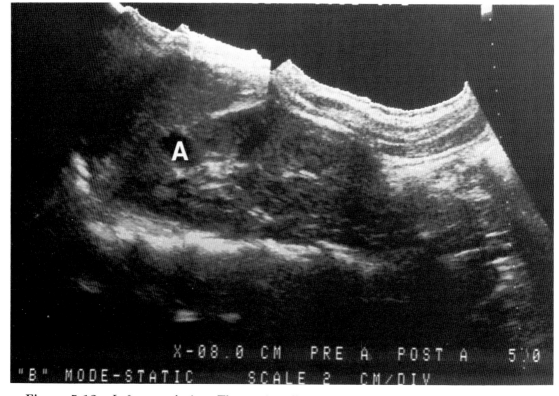

X-08.0 CM   PRE A   POST A   5:0
"B" MODE-STATIC   SCALE 2   CM/DIV

Figure 5.12. Left coronal view. The cystic collection at the upper pole of the kidney (*A*) represents an abscess. A subsequent sonogram 2 weeks later showed disappearance on antibiotic therapy.

represent a hydronephrotic upper collecting system, a tubular echo-free structure may be seen (31) passing medial to the normal lower collecting system representing the dilated ureter. If more than one calyx formed the upper collecting system before it became hydronephrotic, septa will be seen within the system. However, a hydronephrotic upper collecting system can mimic the appearance of a simple cyst if only a single calyx is involved (Fig. 5.13). The bladder should be examined in such a case to be certain a ureterocele is not present (31–33).

PYLOGENIC CYST

A pylogenic cyst is a calyceal diverticulum which communicates with the pelvicalyceal system and fills with contrast. The sonographic appearance is usually indistinguishable from a simple cyst, but the diagnosis can be made by correlation with the intravenous pyelogram (34).

RENAL ARTERY ANEURYSM

Large noncalcified renal artery aneurysms resemble cysts since they are usually small spherical structures in the renal hilum (35, 36). A large arteriovenous fistula has been reported resembling a hydronephrotic kidney (37). A large renal vein draining the aneurysm may be seen. Doppler is an aid in showing that the lesion is vascular. In some systems the Doppler beam can be directed along the same axis as the B-scan or real-time ultrasonic beam. If there is evidence of arterial flow from the suspect area, one can conclude that the lesion is not a cyst or other liquid nonvascular structure; however, the lesion still can be either normal renal parenchyma or tumor.

MULTIPLE FLUID-FILLED LESIONS

Multiple Simple Cysts

Particularly in elderly patients, numerous simple renal cysts may occur in one or both kidneys. Several ultrasonic features allow simple cysts to be distinguished from other types of renal cystic diseases. As already stated, simple cysts are smooth walled, although they may

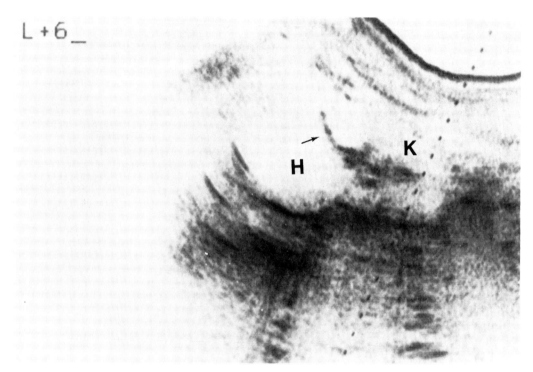

Figure 5.13.   Prone longitudinal view. Hydronephrotic second collecting system (*H*)—a cystic area with septa (*arrow*). Note normal kidney inferiorly (*K*).

demonstrate septa if multilocular. With simple cysts a distinct renal pelvicalyceal echo is present which may be spherically distorted by a cyst or cysts. Simple cysts are relatively few in number, and so far the most that I have seen in a single kidney is eight (Fig. 5.14).

Multiple cysts develop in patients on long-term chronic dialysis. These cysts may be especially confusing because they occur in kidneys that are small and distorted by pyelonephritis (38–41).

HYDRONEPHROSIS

Some forms of hydronephrosis may be confused with cystic disease (42). In one variant, pressure dilatation of the pelvicalyceal system occurs almost exclusively in the calyces, which balloon out to form several loculated, almost equal-sized cavities sonographically reminiscent of multiple simple cysts in the kidney (Fig. 5.15). However, no pelvicalyceal echo complex can be seen, and the "cysts" are all approximately the

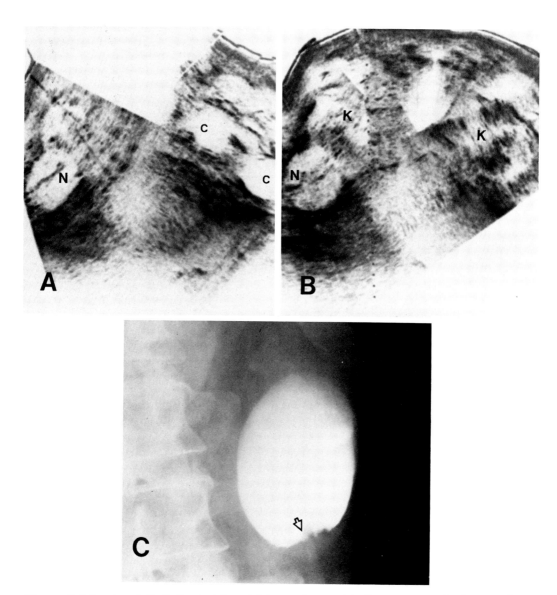

Figure 5.14. *A* and *B*, Patient with multiple renal cysts (*c*). One cyst contained a prominent irregular septum and a number of internal echoes (*N*). This was, therefore, the cyst selected for puncture. *K*, kidney. *C*, Contrast inserted in the cyst shows an irregular inferior wall (*arrow*) which at operation proved to be the site of a neoplasm.

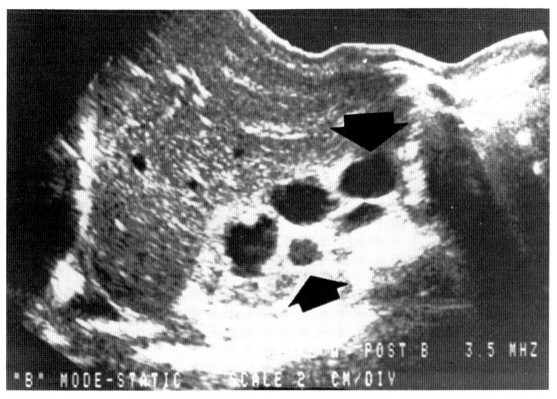

Figure 5.15. Longitudinal section. View of hydronephrosis obtained with a B-scanner. Several dilated calyces (*arrows*) resembling cysts are seen. They all connected when real-time views were obtained.

same size. There is a relative absence of renal parenchyma. Often this form of dilatation is associated with a large extrarenal pelvis, i.e., one large, medially located cyst surrounded and communicating with several laterally placed, equal-sized, smaller cysts. Another common form of hydronephrosis is represented by dilatation of the renal pelvis along with effacement of the calyces (Fig. 5.16). In this type of hydronephrosis, only a single cystic mass may be seen replacing the normal kidney. Usually it has a slightly lobulated lateral border. Should this be all that can be seen where the kidney is normally placed, the first diagnosis should be hydronephrosis. However, in the neonate, confusion can occur with multicystic kidney which can also present as a single large cyst, the smaller associated cysts being below the ultrasonic threshold.

A difficult situation occurs if the patient has hydronephrosis and one or two simple cysts. The clue, again, is the absence of a normal pelvicalyceal echo complex. Sometimes a dilated ureter may be seen. Focal dilatation of a few calyces, as with infundibular stenosis, can be confusing. Although the dilated calyces are separated by a dense linear echo, they have an appearance strongly reminiscent of several adjacent, similar-sized renal cysts.

A simple peripelvic cyst sitting centrally in the pelvicalyceal system is hard to separate from hydronephrosis (25). This false positive type of hydronephrosis is not of much clinical significance because the subsequent retrograde or intravenous pyelogram shows absence of obstruction and demonstrates the presence of the peripelvic cyst.

MULTICYSTIC (DYSPLASTIC) KIDNEY

In most series this condition represents the commonest cause in the neonate of a mass in the abdomen, yet it is still rare. These kidneys have little or no blood supply and are connected to an atretic ureter. They lack any significant quantity of functioning renal nephrons. The characteristic appearances are of a group of cysts of variable size and shape occupying the renal bed and responsible for the palpable mass (43, 44) (Fig. 5.17). The cysts are sometimes separated by small echogenic areas presumably representing tiny cysts too small to resolve by ultrasound, but no normal renal parenchyma or pelvicalyceal echo pattern can be seen. Since these infants are very small, technique is all important. The use of a low frequency transducer and the wrong time gain conversion factors (TGC) can give confusing appearances, because the first few centimeters are poorly visualized. The details of the more superficial aspects of the cyst can easily be eliminated if a 5-

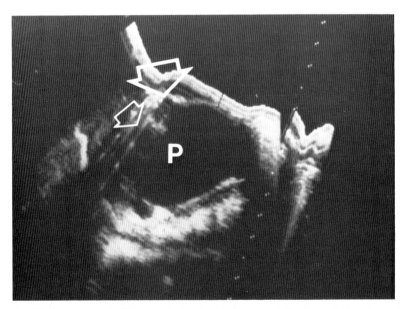

Figure 5.16.   Hydronephrosis. The pelvis (*P*) is the dominant fluid-filled structure. A few almost effaced calyces (*arrows*) can be seen at the superior margin.

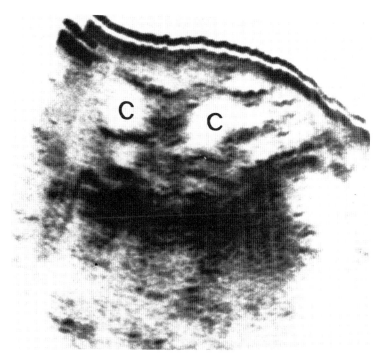

Figure 5.17. Multicystic kidney. Several cysts (C) of differing sizes are present within this neonatal kidney. The intervening echogenic areas represent even smaller cysts that are, however, large enough to cause echoes.

MHz transducer is not used. Real-time views are essential in patients who are squirming.

In two recent reviews of multicystic kidneys in which a comparison was made with hydronephrosis (43, 44) the following features were found to be of help: In multicystic kidney the cysts were eccentrically located away from the renal pelvis, did not communicate, and were often very large. Multiple cysts were seen. A rim of apparent renal parenchyma around the kidney was most unusual, although echogenic areas within the kidney representing very small cysts were present. A single large cyst can be seen in a multicystic kidney indistinguishable from a hydronephrotic kidney. In another form, the hydronephrotic pelvis with budding calyces coming off of it is seen without renal parenchyma. This "hydronephrotic" type of multicystic kidney is, however, associated with atretic ureter and hypoplastic renal artery. In still another form, numerous cysts are present too small to be seen as cysts on sonography yet large enough to cause echoes; the resulting mass may resemble a tumor.

Although most cases of multicystic kidney are discovered in the neonate, some present later in childhood and can be confused with adult polycystic kidney. Occasional cases of adult polycystic kidney are seen in which the condition is much more severe on one side than the other (45) (Fig. 5.23).

Multicystic kidney has been diagnosed in utero. A multilocular cystic lesion is seen in the trunk of the fetus. Several examples have been seen of a fetal syndrome consisting of urethral atresia and bilateral multicystic kidney (46). The sonographic appearances consisted of multiple cystic lesions in the areas of the fetal kidney with one large single cystic lesion representing the bladder in the pelvis.

A focal abnormality of the kidney may be seen due to multicystic or dysplastic renal disease. This is presumed to be the result of obstruction of an infundibulum. The appearances are identical to diffuse disease, although focal.

ADULT MULTICYSTIC KIDNEY

If the multicystic kidney is left in situ and not surgically removed, renal growth does not occur in the affected kidney. The cystic lesion remains the same size, whereas the rest of the abdominal trunk enlarges. Should a patient with multicystic kidney be encountered as an adult, the cysts are usually calcified and the kidney is small without a renal pelvis (47) (Fig. 5.18). Calcification of the border of the cyst may be sufficiently dense to cast an acoustic shadow and is certainly sufficient to prevent a distinction between a cystic lesion and a solid homogeneous mass.

Calcification in a cyst wall is always confusing ultrasonically. Examination of the EVU before a report is issued on a sonographic examination of the kidney will avoid errors such as the confusion of a cystic mass with calcified border with a solid homogeneous lesion.

ADULT POLYCYSTIC DISEASE

In adult polycystic kidney, a dominant inherited condition, cysts may arise from any portion of a collecting system whether glomerulus or tubule. This condition is quite common in adults (1 in 1,000), but it can be present in children and has even been recognized in infancy (48). Patients present with hypertension and its consequences, berry aneurysms or hematuria. By the time the patient is 30 to 50, renal failure has usually supervened. Diagnosis is important from a prognostic point of view.

The ease with which a diagnosis of adult polycystic disease can be made by sonography varies with the severity of the condition. When the cysts are small, i.e., around 1 mm in size, they are not visible, but once they reach a few millimeters in size, although they may not be visible as distinct cysts, they may produce echoes and the acoustic texture of the parenchyma changes. The kidneys are enlarged and dotted throughout with incresed echoes (Fig. 5.19). There may well be one or two cysts which are larger than the remainder and become visible as distinct small cysts at a stage when no other changes are seen.

Once the cysts reach a size at which they are ultrasonically visible, a typical sonographic appearance is seen (Figs. 5.20 and 5.21). The cysts are variable in shape and size and bordered by rather irregular walls. These walls are jagged and irregularly lobulated. The usual central pelvicalyceal echoes are almost always seen, although they may well be severely distorted and displaced by the cysts. There is enlargement of the kidney, but it usually retains its reniform configuration even though there are lobular pro-

trusions from the margin. In 30 to 40% of cases there will also be cysts in the liver (49). In up to 10% there will be cysts in the pancreas, and 5% are alleged to show cysts in the spleen.

The sensitivity of ultrasound in the detection of adult polycystic kidney has been compared with EVU in the investigation of families at risk for polycystic kidney (50–55). It is slightly more sensitive than the excretion urogram and is diagnostic even when the patient has renal failure and cannot be examined by contrast techniques. In a family study of 39 individuals, two 14-year-olds were shown by sonography to have the disease (50).

Coincidental hydronephrosis creates confusion because of a loss of the pelvicalyceal echo complex; an apparent further cyst centrally located within the pelvicalyceal echo complex will be seen. Generally, the borders of the pelvis will be thicker, and its outline will be smoother than those of a polycystic cyst.

Localized infection in a cyst may be a diagnostic problem. The presence of internal echoes within a cyst is suggestive of concomitant infection (see Chapter 16); however, bleeding into cysts is common and may also cause such echoes.

A pattern which may be confused with adult polycystic kidney is seen in patients with severe hydronephrosis superimposed on chronic pyelonephritis (Fig. 5.22). Scarring causes the dilated calyces to adopt unusual configurations. A number of cystic structures will be seen with irregular shapes and sizes. The clue to the diagnosis of hydronephrosis as opposed to polycystic kidney lies in the configuration of the cortex changes in chronic pyelonephritis which will be seen to communicate and often to have a longitudinal configuration (56). Polycystic cysts have a more lobulated appearance.

Adult polycystic kidney may present as a mainly unilateral condition (45, 57); correlation with the intravenous pyelogram is helpful in avoiding confusion with a renal mass; otherwise, hydronephrosis may be mistaken for cysts or vice versa (Fig. 5.23).

A variant exists with similar pathology to polycystic kidney in which cysts are mixed with masses due to tuberosclerosis.

INFANTILE POLYCYSTIC KIDNEY

This rare condition has a quite different ultrasonic appearance from adult polycystic kidney. In this form of tubular ectasia, the tubules

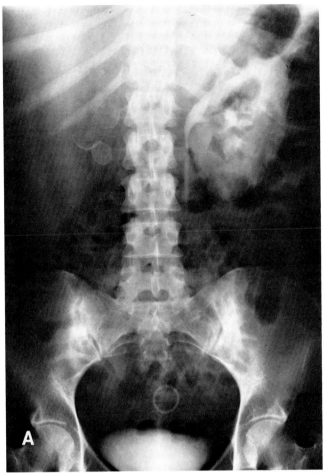

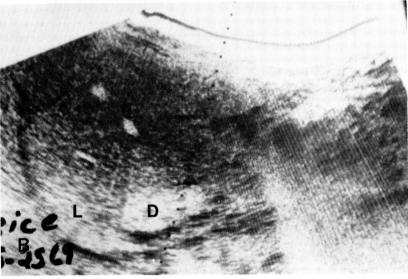

Figure 5.18. *A*, Intravenous pyelogram in a 25-year-old female showing an enlarged left kidney due to compensatory hypertrophy and several small calcified circular rings just to the right of the spine at L1 and L2 level which represent a multicystic kidney. *B*, Supine longitudinal view through the region of the calcified rings shows a mass (*D*) which has few or no internal echoes but shows poor through transonicity. It is the remnant of the multicystic kidney that was present in infancy. *L*, liver.

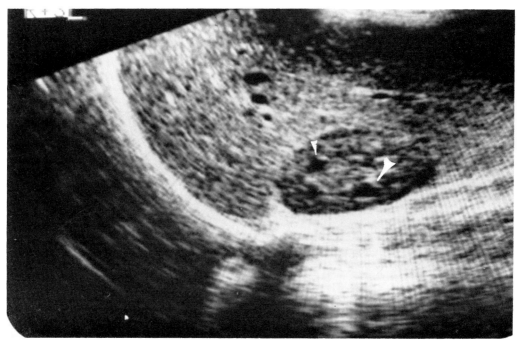

Figure 5.19. Supine longitudinal view. The patient was a 10-year-old boy with a strong family history of adult polycystic disease. Note several small cysts in kidney (*arrows*) representing the first evidence of adult polycystic disease.

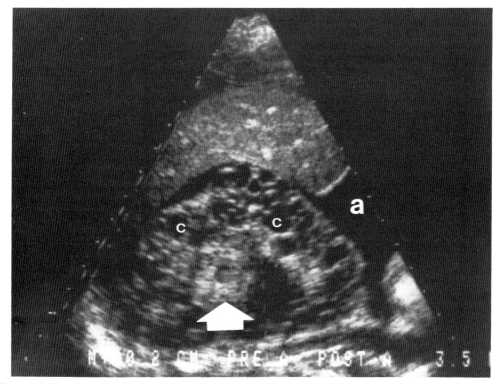

Figure 5.20. Longitudinal section of a patient with severe adult polycystic disease. Numerous cysts (*c*) of differing sizes are present within the kidney. The renal sinus echo complex can still be seen (*arrow*), and some ascites (*a*) is present. Note the overall increase in parenchymal echogenicity.

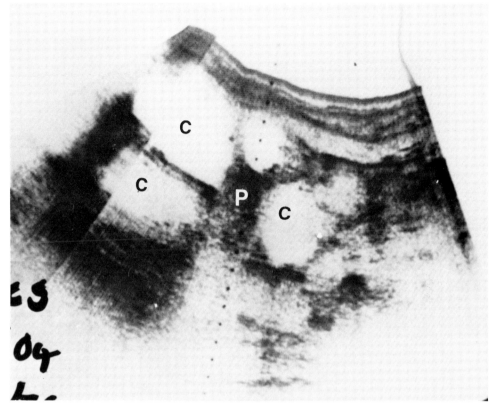

Figure 5.21. Prone longitudinal view. Advanced adult polycystic disease. The pelvicalyceal system is present, although distorted (*P*). Note the large size of the cysts (*C*) in this patient. The cysts show marked irregularity and lobulation.

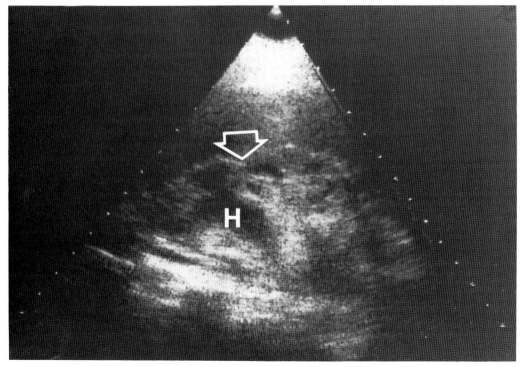

Figure 5.22. Chronic pyelonephritic kidney with superimposed hydronephrosis. Note the dilated calix (*H*). The outline of the kidney is irregular due to scarring (*arrow*).

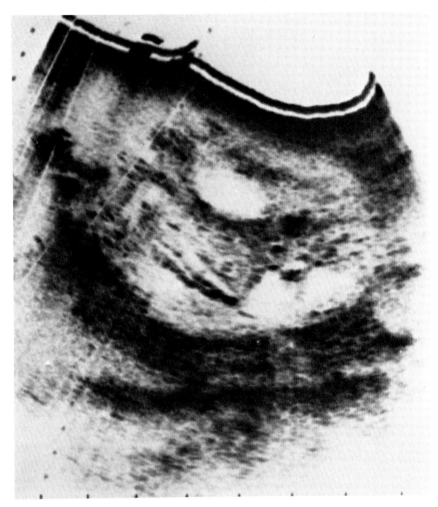

Figure 5.23. Prone longitudinal section of a child with adult polycystic disease presenting as a unilateral renal mass. At ultrasonic examination, the cystic areas were believed, without comparison with the intravenous pyelogram, to represent hydronephrotic calyces. The parenchyma was noticed to be markedly variable in texture, and the mass was considered likely to be a Wilms' tumor. It was removed surgically and at pathology was found to be a polycystic kidney. The contralateral kidney appeared quite normal.

in the distal collecting systems dilate to form cystic structures with a largest size of 2 to 3 cm.

Pathologically, infantile polycystic kidney is divided into four types. In type I, which presents in newborn babies, about 90% of the tubules are involved and the disease is rapidly fatal. In type II, some 60% of the tubules are affected; these infants are also uremic but survive somewhat longer. In type III, occurring in young children, about 25% of the renal tubules are affected. These children may have no renal symptoms and present with hypertension and chronic renal failure. They may have hepatic fibrosis. An even milder variant exists in which the predominant clinical features relate to hepatic fibrosis with portal hypertension and hepatomegaly. In the milder types there may be relatively large cysts which are predominantly located in the medulla, but some are seen in the cortex (58).

In the severe cases (types I and II), most cysts are too small to be seen ultrasonically as fluid-filled structures but are large enough to cause echoes; the predominant ultrasonic pattern is the development of prominent medullary echoes (Fig. 5.24) (59). There are also increased echoes in the cortex, although to a lesser extent. Both

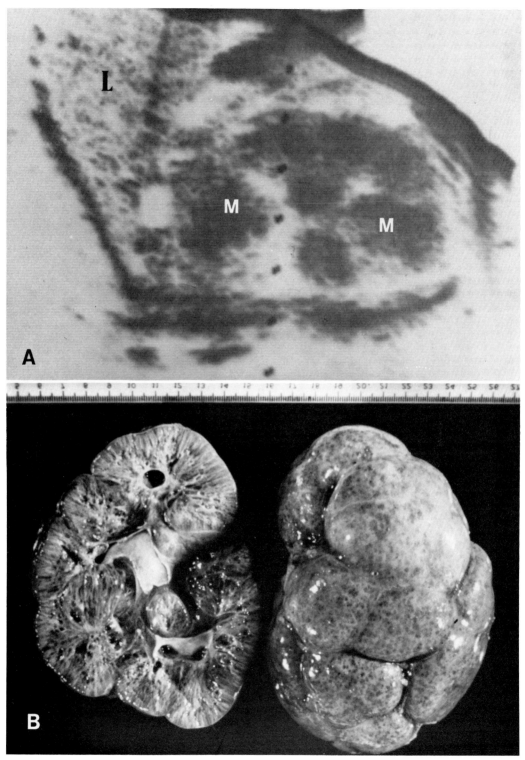

Figure 5.24. *A*, Infantile polycystic kidney. Note the echogenic areas (*M*) in the region of the medulla due to infantile polycystic kidney. *B*, Pathological specimen showing cystic dilatations with the largest dilation located within the medulla. (Courtesy of W. Scott, M.D.)

kidneys become greatly enlarged. Whereas in the normal there is a relatively echo-free area in the region of the papilla, a reversed pattern is seen with the infantile polycystic kidney. Within the densely echogenic medullary areas, one may see small cysts. The sinus echoes cannot be distinguished from the medulla (60, 61). The cortex is relatively spared (62). Patients with infantile polycystic kidney that present in childhood rather than in infancy have less marked changes, although the cysts may reach a larger size (Fig. 5.25). More echoes are seen in the cortex, and the pyramidal echoes are not so densely echogenic in this variant. It is said that liver changes may occur (48). The hepatic parenchyma is said to become more echogenic, and the portal collaterals become more prominent.

A normal variant that can easily be confused with infantile polycystic kidney is seen in the neonate. The pyramids show a transient increase in size and a decrease in echoes as a normal variant (63).

MEDULLARY CYSTIC DISEASE OR JUVENILE NEPHRONOPTHOSIS

This rare condition causes renal failure in children and young adults (64). The kidneys are small and filled with cysts millimeters in size often not visible by gross pathology; their presence is indicated by enlargement of the pelvicalyceal system and some echoes in the parenchyma (Fig. 5.26). Fibrosis also occurs and may contribute to the enlargement of the pelvicalyceal system echoes. Individual cysts may become up to 2 cm in size and ultrasonically visible.

Congenital Nephrosis

Congenital nephrosis of the Finnish type is a cause of nephrotic syndrome in infancy. In this rare condition, the kidneys show dilatation of the proximal tubules and widening of Bowman's spaces. The condition is sometimes termed microcystic disease of the kidney. Sonographically,

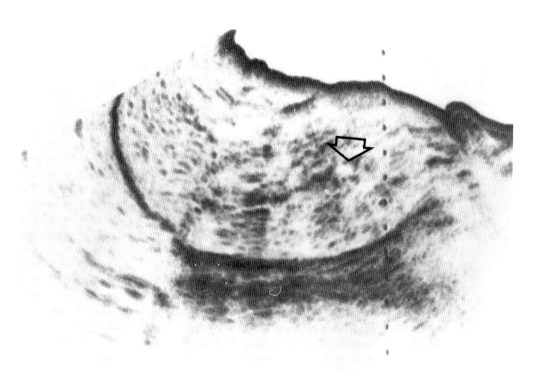

Figure 5.25. Longitudinal section. Infantile polycystic disease presenting at age 3. The kidney (*K*) is very large. The sinus echoes can still be seen. There are dense echoes in the regions where the pyramids should normally lie, but some increased echoes are also seen in the cortex where there are additional cysts. A few small cysts can be seen.

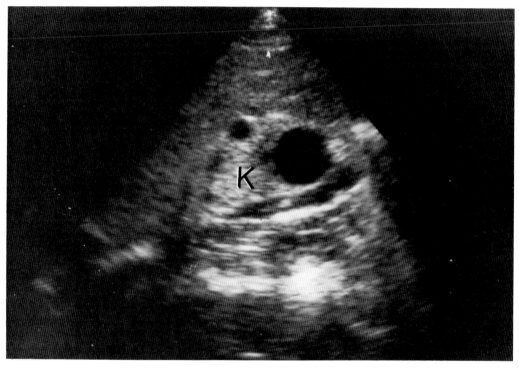

Figure 5.26. Medullary cystic disease (juvenile nephronopthosis). These densely echogenic small kidneys (*K*) contain many tiny and a few visible cysts. One cyst achieved a 3 cm size. The condition is bilateral.

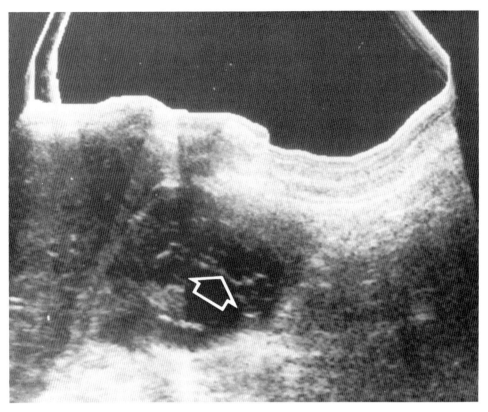

Figure 5.27. Multilocular cystic nephroma. This cystic mass which contains septum (*arrow*) with relatively thick borders is a benign condition with malignant potential.

the kidneys are enlarged and densely echogenic, presumably because the cysts are large enough to reflect sound (65).

Multilocular Cystic Nephroma

This rare condition, otherwise known as benign multilocular cyst, usually occurs in middle-aged women or in small infants (66). A "cyst" is present which contains a number of septa and some structure (Fig. 5.27). The appearances are usually sonographically distinct (67), although there can be confusion with a neoplasm (68). In all five examples seen at Johns Hopkins Hospital, a number of septa with frond-like protrusions were present. All had been considered to be simple cysts on angiography and on intravenous pyelography. Occasionally, cases have been seen in which calcification occur. It is important to recognize benign multilocular cyst because it may be preneoplastic (69, 70). Both CT and ultrasound show a complex series of septa, but ultrasound is a little better than CT at showing septa (5).

Papillary Necrosis

The sonographic findings in papillary necrosis have recently been described (71). Although the sinus echoes are intact, a series of cystic lesions representing shelled-out calyces may be seen around the sinus echoes. One may see the same appearance with pyelonephritis with blunting of the calyces.

References

1. Pollack HM, Banner MP, Arger PH, Peters J, Mulhern C, Coleman BG: The accuracy of gray-scale renal ultrasonography in differentiating cystic neoplasms from benign cysts. *Radiology* 143:741–745, 1982.
2. Cunningham JJ, Wooten W, Cunningham MA: Gray scale echography of soluble protein and protein aggregate fluid collections (in vitro study). *J Clin Ultrasound* 4:417, 1975.
3. Laucks SP, McLachlan MS: Aging and simple cysts of the kidney. *Br J Radiol* 54:12–14, 1981.
4. Bree RL, Silver TM: Differential diagnosis of hypoechoic and anechoic masses with gray scale sonography: new observations. *J Clin Ultrasound* 7:249–254, 1979.
5. Araki T, Ohtomo K, Yuji I, Ilo M: Demonstration

of septa in cystic lesions: comparison study by computed tomography and ultrasound. *Clin Radiol* 33:325–329, 1982.

6. Hidalgo H, Dunnick NR, Rosenberg ER, et al: Parapelvic cysts: appearance on CT and sonography. *AJR* 138:667–671, 1982.

7. Sommer G, Taylor KJW: Differential of acoustic shadowing due to calculi and gas collections. *Radiology* 135:399–403, 1980.

8. Goldstein A, Madrazo BL: Slice-thickness artifacts in gray-scale ultrasound. *J Clin Ultrasound* 9:365–375, 1981.

9. Laing RC, Kurtz AB: The importance of ultrasonic side-lobe artifacts. *Radiology* 145:763–768, 1982.

10. Jaffe CC: Rosenfield AT, Sommer G, et al: Technical factors influencing the imaging of small anechoic cysts by B-scan ultrasound. *Radiology* 135:429–433, 1980.

11. Ravden MI, Zuckerman HL, Kay CJ, Rosenfeld AT, Ablow RC, Rosenfeld N: Evaluation of solitary simple renal cysts in children. *J Urol* 124:904–906, 1980.

12. Gordon RL, Pollack HM, Popky GL, Duckett JW: Simple serous cysts of the kidney in children. *Radiology* 131:357–361, 1979.

13. Bartholomew TH, Slovis TL, Kroovand L, et al: The sonographic evaluation and management of simple renal cysts in children. *J Urol* 123:732–736, 1980.

14. Merritt CR, Bluth EI: Sonography of the day. *AJR* 138:783–788, 1982.

15. Lewis RH, Clark MA, Dobson CL, et al: Multilocular cystic renal adenocarcinoma arising in a solitary kidney. *J Urol* 127:314–316, 1982.

16. Charboneau JW, Hattery RR, Ernst EC III, James EM, Williamson B, Hartman GW: Spectrum of sonographic findings in 125 renal masses other than benign simple cyst. *AJR* 140:87–94, 1983.

17. Callen PW, Marks WM: Lymphomatous masses simulating cysts by ultrasonography. *J Assoc Can Radiol* 30:244–246, 1979.

18. Jackman RJ, Stevens GM: Benign hemorrhagic renal cyst. *Radiology* 110:7–13, 1974.

19. Coelho JCU, Sigel B, Ryva JC, et al: B-mode sonography of blood clots. *J Clin Ultrasound* 10:323–327, 1982.

20. Sigel B, Coelho JCU, Schade SG, et al: Effect of plasma proteins and temperature on echogenicity of blood. *Invest Radiol* 17:29–33, 1982.

21. Cook JH III, Rosenfield AT, Taylor KJW: Ultrasonic demonstration of intrarenal anatomy. *AJR* 129:831, 1977.

22. Haller JO, Berdon WE, Friedman AP: Increased renal cortical echogenicity: a normal finding in neonates and infants. *Radiology* 142:173–174, 1982.

23. Yeh HC, Mitty HA, Wolfe BS: Ultrasonography of renal sinus lipomatosis. *Radiology* 124:799, 1977.

24. Becker JA, Schneider M, Staiano S, Cromb E: Renal pelvic lipomatosis: a sonographic evaluation. *J Clin Ultrasound* 2:299, 1976.

25. Cronan JJ, Amis ES, Yoder IC, et al: Peripelvic cysts: an impostor of sonographic hydronephrosis. *J Ultrasound Med* 1:229–236, 1982.

26. Fallon B, Gershon C: Renal carbuncle: diagnosis

and management. *Urology* 17:303–309, 1981.

27. Plainfosse MC, Mercier-Pageyral B, Bacques O, et al: Apport de l'echographic dans le diagnostic des abces du rein. A propos de treize observations. *Ann Radiol* 23:7–13, 1980.

28. Schneider M, Becker JA, Staiano S, et al: Sonographic-radiographic correlation of renal and perirenal infections. *AJR* 127:1007, 1976.

29. Hill M, Sanders RC: Gray scale characteristics of intraabdominal cystic masses. *J Clin Ultrasound* 6:217, 1978.

30. Kaplan G, Sanders RC: The use of ultrasound in post-operative haematoma. *J Clin Ultrasound* 1:5–13, 1973.

31. Mascatello VJ, Smith EH, Carrera GF: Ultrasonic evaluation of the obstructed duplex kidney. *AJR* 129:113–120, 1977.

32. Sumner TE, Crowe JE, Resnick MI: Diagnosis of ectopic ureterocele using ultrasound. *Urology* 15:82, 1980.

33. Rose JS, McCathy J, Yeh HC: Ultrasound diagnosis of ectopic ureterocele. *Pediatr Radiol* 8:17–20, 1979.

34. Medani CR, Dunn MG: The ultrasonic appearance of pyelogenic cysts: a report of two cases. *J Clin Ultrasound,* in press.

35. Hantsman SS, Barie JJ, Glendening TB, et al: Giant renal artery aneurysm mimicking a simple cyst on ultrasound. *J Clin Ultrasound* 10:136–139, 1982.

36. Raja Rao AK, Kimball WR: Ultrasonic appearance of an arteriovenous fistula of the kidney. *J Clin Ultrasound* 6:295–382, 1978.

37. Tepper JP, Udoff EJ, Minkin SD, et al: Renal arteriovenous fistula—angiographic and sonographic correlation. *J Urol* 127:106–108, 1982.

38. Mirahmadi MK, Vaziri J: Cystic transformation of end-stage kidneys in patients undergoing hemodialysis. *Artif Organs* 3:267–270, 1980.

39. Krempien B, Ritz E: Acquired cystic transformation of the kidneys of haemodialysed patients. *Virchows Arch* 386:189–200, 1980.

40. Hughson MD, Hennigar GR, McManus JPA: Atypical cysts, acquired renal cystic disease and renal cell tumors in end stage dialysis kidneys. *Lab Invest* 42:475–480, 1980.

41. Feiner HD, Katz LA, Gallo GR: Acquired cystic disease of kidney in chronic dialysis patients. *Urology* 17:260–264, 1981.

42. Ralls PW, Esensten KL, Boger D, et al: Severe hydronephrosis and severe renal cystic disease: ultrasonic differentiation. *AJR* 134:473–475, 1980.

43. Stuck KJ, Koff SA, Silver TM: Ultrasonic features of multicystic dysplastic kidney: expanded diagnostic criteria. *Radiology* 143:217–221, 1982.

44. Sanders R, Hartman D: Ability of ultrasound to separate multicystic kidney from hydronephrosis. *Radiology,* accepted for publication.

45. Lee JKT, McClennan BL, Kissane JM: Unilateral polycystic kidney disease. *AJR* 130:1165–1167, 1978.

46. Bartley JA, Golbus MS, Filly RA, et al: Prenatal diagnosis of dysplastic kidney disease. *Clin Genet* 11:375, 1977.

47. Marsidi PJ, Lin WI, Pilloff B: Congenital multicystic dysplastic kidney in the adult. *Urology* 16:511–514, 1980.

48. Garel L, Montagne JPh, Faure C: Rare pediatric conditions: contribution of grey-scale ultrasonography. *Pediatr Radiol* 8:237–245, 1979.

49. Bartolozzi C. Carlesi G, Ciatti S, et al: Ultrasonographic examination of the kidney, liver and pancreas in the polycystic disease. In *Current Concepts on Ultrasound*, Proceedings of the 2nd Italo-Yugoslavian US Meeting, 1980.

50. Wolf B, Rosenfield AT, Taylor KJW, et al: Presymptomatic diagnosis of adult onset polycystic kidney disease by ultrasonography. *Clin Genet* 14:1, 1978.

51. Lufkin EG, Alfrey AC, Trucksess ME: Polycystic kidney disease: earlier diagnosis using ultrasound. *Urology* 4:5, 1974.

52. Denney JD, Marty R, Milutinovich J, Fialkow P, Phillips LA, Rdd TG, Lowe-Davis MC, Aufleger MA: Polycystic kidney disease: early detection by gray scale echography. *Ultrasound Med* 4:197, 1977.

53. Kelsey JA, Bowie JD: Gray-scale ultrasonography in the diagnosis of polycystic kidney disease. *Radiology* 122:791, 1977.

54. Weitzel D, Bahlmann J, Otto P: Die Wertigkeir der Sonographie fur die Diagnostik von Zystennieren. *Dtsch Med Wochenschr* 31:1, 1974.

55. Rosenfield AT, Lipson MH, Wolf B, et al: Ultrasonography and nephrotomography in the presymptomatic diagnosis of dominantly inherited (adult-onset) polycystic kidney disease. *Radiology* 135:423–427, 1980.

56. Sanders RC, Conrad MR: The ultrasonic characteristics of the renal pelvicalyceal echo complex. *J Clin Ultrasound* 5·373, 1977.

57. Hantman SS: Unilateral adult polycystic kidney. *J Ultrasound Med* 1:371–374, 1982.

58. Blythe H, Ochenden BJ: Infantile polycystic kidney clinical features. *J Med Genet* 8:257, 1971.

59. Sanders RC, Scott W, Conrad MR, et al: The sonographic pattern of infantile polycystic disease. *Ultrasound Med* 4:251, 1977.

60. Boal DK, Teele RL: Sonography of infantile polycystic kidney disease. *AJR* 135:575–580, 1980.

61. Metreweli C, Garel L: The echographic diagnosis of infantile renal polycystic disease. *Ann Radiol* 23:103–107, 1980.

62. Melson GL, Shackelford GD, McClennan BL, et al: Infantile polycystic kidney disease: new sonographic observations with radiographic, clinical and pathological correlations. Presented at the Society of Uroradiologists, Palm Beach, FL, 1982.

63. Stepleton FB, Hilton S, Wilcox J, et al: Transient nephromegaly simulating infantile polycystic disease of the kidneys. *Pediatrics* 67:554–559, 1980.

64. Rosenfield AT, Siegel NJ, Kappelman NB, Taylor KJW: Gray scale ultrasonography in medullary cystic disease of the kidney and congenital hepatic fibrosis with tubular ectasia: new observations. *AJR* 129:297, 1977.

65. Graif M, Lison M, Strauss S, Manor A, Itzchak Y, Sack J: Congenital nephrosis: ultrasonographic features. *Pediatr Radiol* 12:154–155, 1982.

66. Madewell JE, Goldman SM, Davis CJ, Hartman, DS, Feigin DS, Lichtenstein J: Multilocular cystic nephroma: a radiographic-pathologic correlation of 58 patients. *Radiology* 146:309–321, 1983.

67. Slasky BS, Wolfe PW: Cross-sectional imaging of multilocular cystic nephroma. *J Urol* 128:128–131, 1982.

68. Javadpour N, Dellon AL, Kumpe A: Multilocular cystic disease in adults: imitator of renal cell carcinoma. *Urology* 1:596, 1973.

69. Feldberg MA, van Waes PF: Multilocular cystic renal cell carcinoma. *AJR* 138:953–955, 1982.

70. Sadlowski RW, Smey P, Williams J, et al: Adenocarcinoma in multilocular renal cyst. *Urology* 14:511–512, 1979.

71. Hoffman JC, Schnur MJ, Koenigsberg M: Demonstration of renal papillary necrosis by sonography. *Radiology* 145:785–787, 1982.

CHAPTER 6

Renal Neoplasms

BEVERLY G. COLEMAN, M.D.
PETER H. ARGER, M.D.

Ultrasound is now well established as an accurate, noninvasive means of evaluating patients with a suspected renal neoplasm. Most authorities concede that sonography is optimally utilized as a complement to other imaging modalities. It should clearly not be relied upon as an initial screening procedure to diagnose renal masses. Simple cysts and other predominantly fluid-filled lesions are likely to be readily apparent. But neoplasms, particularly small lesions that do not distort the renal contours or pelvicalyceal system, could be easily missed. A high degree of accuracy should result if patients are referred only for further characterization of a true renal mass previously documented by standard uroradiological or radionuclide studies. One notable rare exception is pregnancy with complications suggestive of a renal neoplasm. Because of the lack of ionizing radiation, ultrasound should virtually always be the first diagnostic tool to investigate genitourinary complaints in obstetrical cases.

In view of the survey scanning applications of real-time sonography, serendipitous presentation of renal neoplasms is frequent, in which patients are actually being examined for nonurological problems. A less common occurrence is the discovery of renal neoplasms in patients having sonography as the initial study because of compromised renal function, severe iodine allergy, or suspected perinephric disease.

Clinical manifestations of renal neoplasms are quite variable, ranging from a total lack of symptoms to complete debilitation at diagnosis. Clearly, the laboratory and physical findings are not always clues to the final pathology. The systemic effects of fever, anemia, weight loss, etc. are nonspecific and may be seen in countless disorders. Local effects that supposedly herald an adenocarcinoma can also be seen with other neoplasms. The classic triad of a renal malignancy includes flank pain, mass, and gross hematuria [1–3]. These features actually occur in only 10 to 15% of carcinomas and, unfortu-nately, indicate far-advanced disease as evidenced by the finding of metastases in a high percentage of cases at presentation [4]. Endocrine effects are rather unusual phenomena that may divert medical attention away from the genitourinary tract. The spectrum of endocrinopathies that can signal a malignancy includes hypercalcemia, erythrocytosis, and hypertension [5].

TECHNIQUE

No specific patient preparation is required for renal mass studies. In those occasional situations which require ultrasound-guided aspiration biopsy at the initial setting, patients are often apprehensive and may benefit from low dose sedation. Oral intake, especially good hydration, should be maintained unless specific restrictions are indicated for medical reasons. It is preferable that sonography be scheduled prior to fluoroscopy in order to minimize interference from air-containing bowel. Perhaps the ideal situation is to scan patients prior to the post-evacuation views that routinely accompany the intravenous urogram. In this manner, both studies would be performed under identical physiological conditions, enhancing their comparability.

The principles and techniques of ultrasound scanning have been continuously altered as ongoing technological advancements occurred. Prone scanning was once the standard means of investigating renal masses for diagnosis and biopsy purposes. Compound and sector scanning were usually required with this approach. Compound scans consist of multiple transducer passes over the same area at different angles or positions. Sector scans are created by pivoting the transducer so that the sound beam is rotated about the transducer face [6]. These techniques were needed to overcome rib artifacts that often obscured the internal architecture of the kidney. Less compound and sector scanning are now required because of smaller transducer probes that are capable of scanning between ribs. Very high gain settings were sometimes required to penetrate the subcutaneous connective tissues and thick muscles of the back. This increased gain consequently produced more background noise. Additionally, the mapping process was rather time consuming.

Soon after gray-scale ultrasound equipment appeared, an anterior approach to renal scanning was introduced (7). Higher frequency focused transducers and better signal processing made it possible for sonographers to perform this new technique. The right kidney was examined in a supine position, utilizing the liver as an acoustic window. Single pass transverse and longitudinal scans were done with the transducer aimed under the costal margin. As a result, excellent views of normal intrahepatic and intrarenal structures were produced. The left kidney, however, could rarely be seen in a supine position because of overlying gastrointestinal air that reflected the sound waves. It was found to be seen best with scans done in a right lateral decubitus position using the spleen as a window.

The standard static B-mode technique consists of a grid pattern approach with serial transverse and longitudinal scans at 1-cm intervals over the renal fossae. Similarly, the real-time examination should proceed in an orderly fashion to cover the kidneys completely in both planes. Detailed supplementary views can then be made of the region of interest, as previously determined by the urogram or radionuclide scans. Before the examination is completed, a thorough comparison must be made between the sonogram and the earlier screening procedure to ensure that the mass being investigated actually corresponds in size and location between the two studies.

Real-time units have added a critical new dimension to ultrasound because of the improved resolution and more versatile scanning. The kidneys can now be quickly examined from an anterior approach, which has sharply reduced the time constraints of the scanning process. The ease and speed of this technique have made ultrasound more accessible to many patients, particularly those with very acute or prolonged illnesses. Patient cooperation is no longer an issue since prone scans in suspended respiration are not required.

Patient body habitus is the single factor that determines transducer selection. As a rule, the highest frequency transducer which permits adequate penetration should be used. Most static

and real-time units now have probes with 3.5 mHz and 5.0 mHz focused transducers. Rarely, 2.25 mHz transducers are needed for morbidly obese patients. The transducers should be swept in a smooth, continuous arc with varying degrees of angulation as needed. The sound beam should be kept perpendicular to the area being examined. Alterations in the time-gain curve or overall output may be needed during a study, but the normal renal parenchyma should always contain evenly distributed low and medium level echoes.

A routine renal sonogram might consist of anterior scans done with the patient in right and left posterior oblique positions. Additional supine, erect, and decubitus views could be obtained as needed, depending on the location of a neoplasm and the information desired. For example, the renal hilum is best demonstrated by decubitus scans. Moreover, transverse scans in this position provide an exceptional view of the renal pedicle. In cases where a malignancy is strongly suspected, survey views of the liver, lymphatic pathways, blood vessels, and the contralateral kidney can be quickly obtained with real-time scans. This serves as a useful, albeit less accurate, staging procedure than computed tomography. Chiba-needle aspiration biopsy with ultrasound guidance is a proven method of obtaining histopathological confirmation in nonsurgical candidates.

The task of evaluating the renal vascular structures poses many problems. The left renal vein is probably the easiest vessel to demonstrate with sonography due to its long course between the aorta and superior mesenteric artery. In contrast, the right renal vein is more difficult to visualize because it follows a very short path to the inferior vena cava. The renal arteries that lie posterior to the veins can only be demonstrated with certainty if their junction with the aorta is seen. The diaphragmatic crura, often prominent and asymmetrical, also run transversely. They lie just posterior to the renal arteries and should not be mistaken for vascular structures since the characteristic pulsation of vessels is now evident with real-time. The renal veins are the earliest and most frequently involved vessels by a neoplastic process because of their very thin walls which lack strong supporting connective tissues. Some venous changes that result from a neoplastic process include complete or partial thrombosis, venous lakes, and arteriovenous fistulae producing premature opacification of veins. Renal arterial involvement that can occur in neoplastic and inflammatory disorders includes microaneurysms, amputation, encasement, and displacement. Since peripheral-pulsed Doppler has been useful in defining the vascular flow patterns in the carotid system, the advent of deep abdominal Doppler may permit an appraisal of the major renal vessels as well as the internal vascularity of neoplasms without instrumentation or contrast injection of the patient.

GENERAL DIAGNOSTIC PRINCIPLES

There are three broad sonographic categories of renal masses—cystic, complex, and solid. A mass that fulfills the strict sonic criteria for a cyst should be echo free, smooth, regularly shaped with thin, sharply marginated walls, and demonstrate excellent through sound transmission. This type image is produced by fluid-filled masses, the majority being simple renal cysts. Localized collections of urine or blood, such as a calyceal diverticulum, seroma, arteriovenous fistula, etc., may exhibit a similar appearance. However, these entities are quite rare in comparison to the frequency of benign cysts in a general hospital population. There have been unusual documented cases of mural tumor nodules or microscopic evidence of malignant cells within simple or multilobular cysts; however, these lesions do not appear purely cystic on scans (8). A solid ultrasound pattern is characterized by the presence of internal echos and acoustic impedance of the sonic beam. These masses are often variable in shape, without smooth, well-defined borders. With some static scanners that have A-mode capability, it is still possible to quantitate sound attenuation by comparing the intensity of the near and far wall echoes. Sound absorption by a solid mass is evident as less echo amplitude originating from the far wall. This type of analysis cannot be performed with real-time scans, in which case estimation of the degree of sound attenuation is more subjective. The observer then compares the intensity of the posterior echoes beyond the mass with those beyond the uninvolved portions of the kidney. The majority of renal neoplasms, regardless of histological type, are solid on sonograms. By definition, complex renal masses are mixed, containing cystic and solid components. This type of pattern may result from necrotic or hemorrhagic neoplasms, complicated renal cysts, and inflammatory disorders.

The limit of resolution of solid renal masses with ultrasound is approximately 2 cm. Contin-

ued improvements in gray-scale and new real-time equipment have made it possible to diagnose precisely some cystic and complex masses less than 1.0 cm in size (9). This has permitted the detection and characterization of masses often unrecognizable with urography or nephrotomography. Consequently, some authorities have stressed the validity of still performing ultrasound in the face of a normal urogram, as in a case of unexplained hematuria (10). Nevertheless, the potential resolution of solid masses has probably changed little over the past few years, most likely because the echogenicities of a very small neoplasm and the normal renal cortex are similar. Recording renal scans on a black background enhances subtle textural differences and renders excellent scans of intrarenal anatomy (11). This type of display can be helpful in evaluating small neoplasms that may have only slightly different echo characteristics from the uninvolved parenchyma.

The ability to resolve a mass clearly is in part dependent upon its location. Since the liver provides an excellent acoustic window, right renal masses are more easily demonstrated. The polar regions of both kidneys are the most difficult to visualize, left greater than right. Ribs pose technical problems with the examination of upper pole masses, and intestinal bowel gas may occasionally obscure the lower pole. There are also pitfalls in investigating peripelvic masses in the mid-portion of the kidney because of juxtaposition to renal sinus structures. The adjacent fat and fibrous tissues may impart an irregular, thick-walled appearance to the margins of a mass and interfere with sound transmission as well. A single multilocular cyst or multiple contiguous cysts may become insinuated between the infundibuli and calyces. Internal echoes within these masses may result from septations. Anterior surface renal masses are often easier to evaluate than deep posterior ones. The more superficial anterior masses are readily penetrated by the sonic beam, but near-field reverberation echoes appear. Beam divergence is responsible for spurious echoes that may appear in posterior masses. Both types of artifacts are most obvious with higher frequency transducers. An important point of differentiation is that true echoes, generated from dissimilar tissue interfaces within a solid mass, are more apt to persist at varied gain settings and in different scan planes.

Perhaps the single most important contribution of ultrasound toward the diagnosis of genitourinary disease involves the differentiation of cystic and solid masses. Since its inception, a high accuracy rate of between 90 and 95% has been reported for ultrasound in this regard (9–11). Early on, many patients were often subjected to cyst puncture because of a false positive rate of approximately 5%. The detailed intrarenal anatomy now affordable with high resolution gray-scale technology has not only increased the detection but also the overall accuracy of diagnosing benign renal cysts. Experienced radiologists using state-of-the art equipment have recently reported a 98% accuracy in the sonographic diagnosis of an unequivocal cyst. The 2% inaccuracy was due to complicated cysts, hematomas, etc. and not to poorly echoproductive neoplasms (12).

MALIGNANT RENAL NEOPLASMS

Renal Adenocarcinoma

Renal adenocarcinomas are common, accounting for more than 90% of all malignancies of the kidney (13). These primary epithelial neoplasms of the renal parenchyma are known to originate from the proximal convoluted tubule. However, it is not yet entirely clear whether lesions arise de novo from the renal tubular cell or evolve through adenomatous hyperplasia or renal cortical adenomas (14–16). The exact etiology of this neoplasm remains obscure despite exhaustive investigation of physical, chemical, and viral carcinogens.

Renal adenocarcinoma is a disease predominantly of adults, with fewer than 100 cases ever documented in children (17). It most frequently afflicts patients over 40 years of age with peak occurrence among males in the sixth and seventh decades of life (18, 19). The familial frequency of this neoplasm is very low except in association with von Hippel-Lindau disease (polycystic kidneys, cerebral and retinal angiomas).

There is a vast array of gross and microscopic findings in renal adenocarcinomas which relate to such factors as overall size, vascular supply, and degree of differentiation. These tumors exhibit a spectrum of gray-scale sonographic characteristics that reflects the various histopathological appearances. In characterizing these tumors with ultrasound, the important features to examine include echo intensity, number and distribution of internal echoes, type of external margin, size, and through sound transmission. The overall echogenicity (number and intensity

of echoes) may be more, less, or equal to that of the uninvolved renal cortex (Fig. 6.1). Echoes within solid tumors were once thought to derive from blood vessels and other connective tissues. But it has now been clearly shown that there is no direct correlation between the number of internal echoes and the vascularity of these tumors (20).

Small neoplasms that are still localized to the kidney are typically spherical, cortical-based masses without a true capsule (21). Light microscopy reveals homogeneous stroma with solid sheets of cells that exhibit various growth patterns. On ultrasound, these tumors tend to be moderately echogenic (Fig. 6.2). The interface between normal and abnormal renal parenchyma was earlier believed to be imperceptible. But it now appears that distinct margins can result from a pseudocapsule of compressed renal parenchyma. In some cases it is even difficult to demonstrate the site of origin of exophytic neoplasms from the kidney. Occasionally, upper pole lesions may seem to arise from the adrenals, and lower pole tumors may simulate bowel lesions. More invasive carcinomas may infiltrate the kidney to the extent that no normal cortex is identifiable. Classically, these masses have irregular shapes with ill-defined borders (Fig. 6.3). Necrosis and hemorrhage may occur in tumors that have outgrown their blood supply. In such cases the sonogram shows central, anechoic areas within a solid mass (Fig. 6.4). Localized hydronephrosis and blood pooling within vascular lakes are other sonolucent regions that can now be seen on scans (Fig. 6.5). Calcifications and fibro-fatty deposits appear as focal, intense echoes that may demonstrate acoustic shadowing (Fig. 6.6).

The growth pattern of renal carcinomas ranges from indolence to rapid progression. Long-standing neoplasms may attain massive proportions with dissemination locally by direct extension and distantly via the lymphatic and venous systems. Within the abdomen, the single most frequently involved organ in metastatic renal carcinoma is the liver. Neoplasms of the right kidney, particularly those arising in the upper pole, tend to invade the liver locally. Such an occurrence is always a diagnostic possibility unless a distinct fascial plane is seen between the kidney and liver (Fig. 6.7). The adrenals, diaphragm, colon, and spleen may also be affected by local tumor extension. The most common pathway of dissemination is venous, with neoplastic invasion and thrombosis present in approximately 30% of surgical specimens (22,

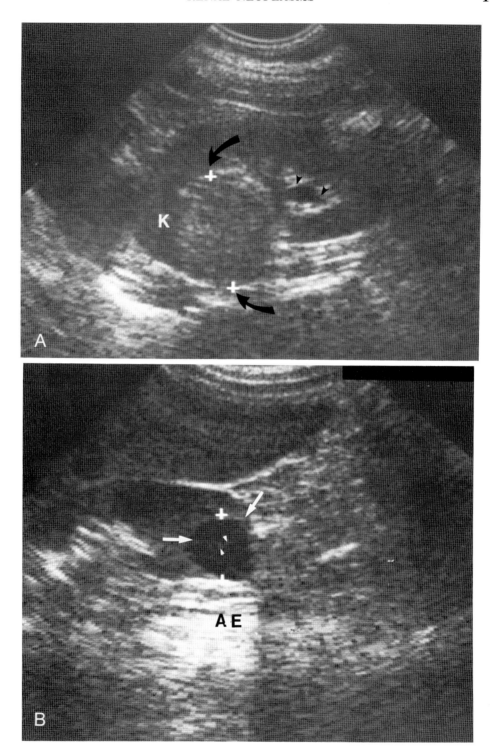

Figure 6.1. Highly echogenic adenocarcinoma. *A*, Longitudinal decubitus scan of left upper pole carcinoma (*curved arrows*) which is clearly more echogenic than the adjacent renal parenchyma (*K*). The mass is compressing the collecting system causing localized hydronephrosis (*arrowheads*). *B*, Longitudinal oblique scan of the contralateral kidney showing irregularly shaped lower pole mass (*arrows*) demonstrating some acoustic enhancement (*AE*) and low level internal echoes (*arrowheads*). Ultrasound-guided aspiration performed prior to left radical nephrectomy revealed a simple cyst.

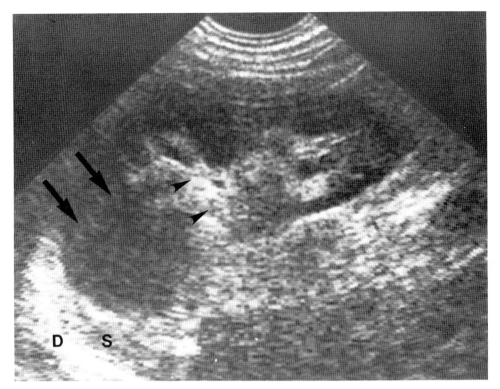

Figure 6.2. Moderately echogenic adenocarcinoma. Longitudinal oblique scan of the left kidney demonstrates a moderately echogenic adenocarcinoma (*arrows*) of the upper pole. The mass borders on the renal sinus (*arrowheads*) in this obese patient with sinus lipomatosis. *S*, spleen; *D*, diaphragm.

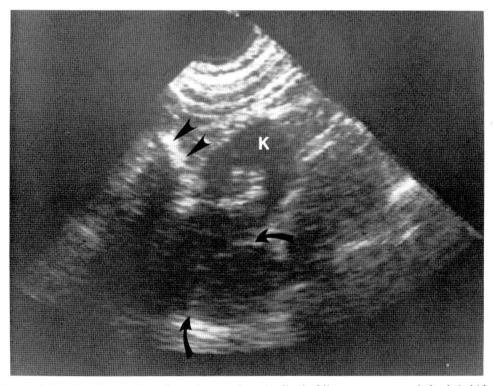

Figure 6.3. Poorly marginated carcinoma. Longitudinal oblique sonogram of the left kidney demonstrates a large, lobular upper pole mass (*arrows*) similar in echogenicity to the uninvolved portions of the kidney (*K*). This position afforded better renal images because of interference from air-containing gastrointestinal structures (*arrowheads*).

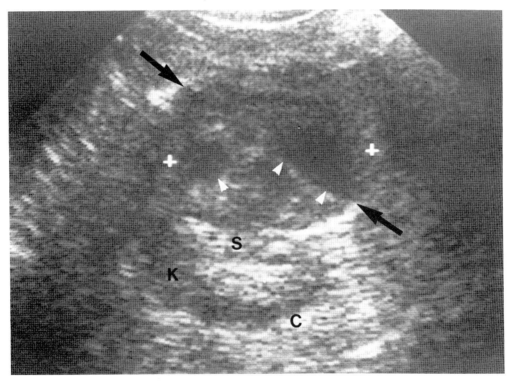

Figure 6.4. Necrotic carcinoma. Transverse supine sonogram of a large, necrotic carcinoma (*arrows*) of the right kidney. At least two echo-free areas (*arrowheads*) can be identified. *S*, sinus; *C*, capsule; *K*, normal cortex.

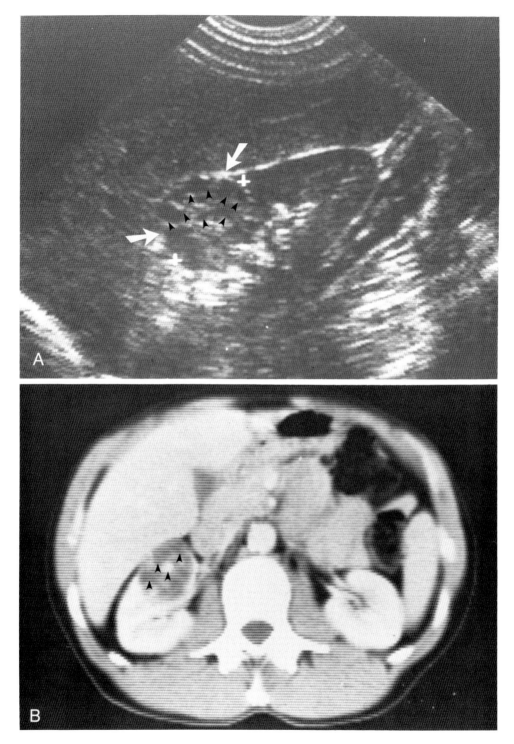

Figure 6.5.   Multilocular carcinoma. *A*, Longitudinal supine scan of the right kidney in a potential renal transplant donor demonstrates a round, sharply marginated carcinoma (*arrows*) with multiple discrete anechoic areas (*arrowheads*). *B*, Corresponding CT scan reveals both low and high density areas (*arrowheads*) secondary to cystic degeneration and contrast puddling within vascular lakes.

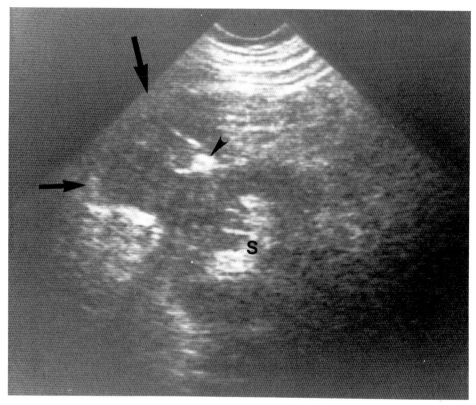

Figure 6.6. Exophytic carcinoma. Transverse supine scan of the right kidney demonstrates an irregular, exophytic carcinoma (*arrows*) with dense calcification (*arrowhead*) that demonstrates acoustic shadowing. The mass indents the renal sinus (*S*) at the mid-pole of the kidney and has an overall echogenicity similar to the uninvolved cortex.

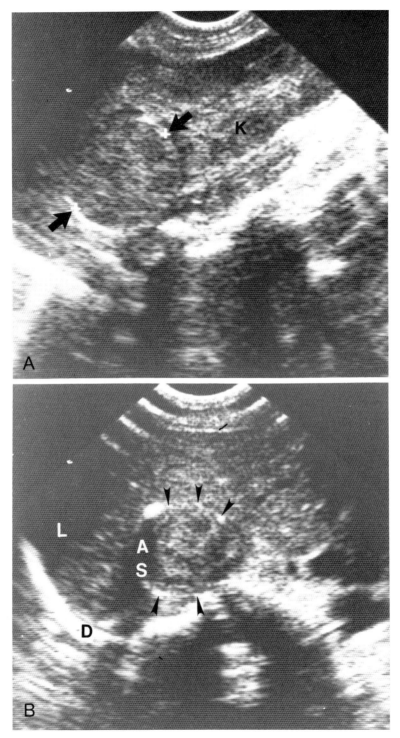

Figure 6.7.   Calcified adenocarcinoma. *A*, Longitudinal supine scan of the right kidney demonstrates a round, well-circumscribed mass (*arrows*) involving the upper pole of the kidney (*K*) which is not clearly separate from the adjacent liver. *B*, Transverse supine scan reveals circumferential mural densities (*arrowheads*) which clearly demarcate the mass from the adjacent liver (*L*). *AS*, acoustic shadowing; *D*, diaphragm.

23) (Fig. 6.8). Malignant cells within the major renal veins may take one or more alternate routes: (*a*) directly antegrade up the inferior vena cava and through the right heart to the lungs; (*b*) from the lung via pulmonary arterial channels to very remote sites, such as the brain, thyroid, and skin: (*c*) retrograde through the left spermatic or ovarian vein to the pelvis; and (*d*) along the axial skeleton via Batson's plexus of paravertebral veins (24) (Fig. 6.9).

Radical nephrectomy is the mainstay of therapeutic management of renal adenocarcinoma and the accepted, definitive treatment for all stages of the disease except distant metastases and local invasion of organs other than the adrenals (25–27). Since no curative standard exists for patients with very advanced disease, some authors advocate more aggressive therapy for solitary metastases as well as surgical removal of the involved portion of adjacent organs (1, 5, 28). Ultrasound staging of renal adenocarcinoma should include scans of the entire retroperitoneum, abdomen, and pelvis. This procedure has been clearly shown to be less accurate than computerized tomography (CT) (29–31). Nevertheless, ultrasound can be quite valuable if CT is not readily available. In cases where

widespread disease is evident on the sonogram, the morbidity and expense of unnecessary radical surgery can be avoided. In surgical candidates, the sonographic findings of contralateral renal masses, renal hilar adenopathy, and venous thrombi can aid clinicians in preoperative planning.

Papillary Cystadenocarcinoma

Papillary cystadenocarcinoma is a relatively uncommon variant of renal malignancies which has distinctive histological features. These are typically well-differentiated, encapsulated, and poorly vascularized tumors, which renders angiography of limited value in the diagnostic process. The natural history of a papillary tumor is one of slow growth and late or infrequent metastasis. A study correlating the sonographic and pathological findings suggested that there is a statistically significant difference in the echogenicity of papillary and nonpapillary renal carcinomas (32). Papillary tumors are characteristically hypoechoic due to extensive ischemic necrosis and hemorrhage. There is usually some degree of acoustic enhancement demonstrated on the sonogram because of their higher fluid

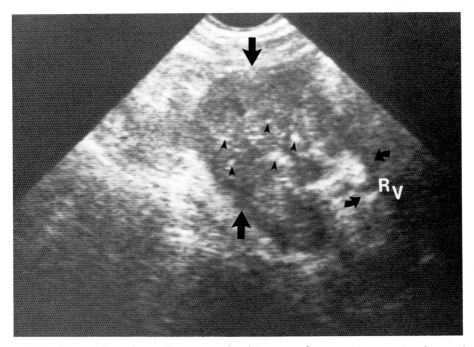

Figure 6.8. Venous thrombosis. Transverse decubitus scan demonstrates an extensive carcinoma (*arrows*) with scattered internal microcalcifications (*arrowheads*) and extension into the renal vein (*RV*).

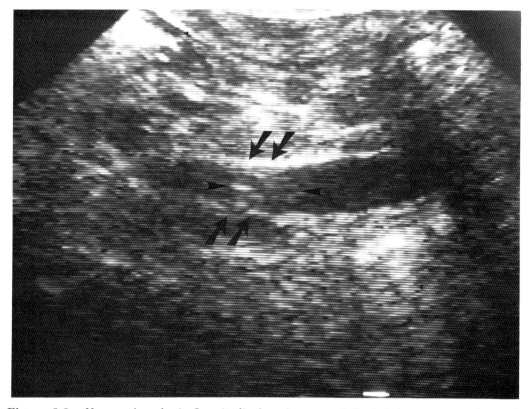

Figure 6.9. Venous thrombosis. Longitudinal supine scan of the inferior vena cava (*arrows*) reveals solid tumor thrombus (*arrowheads*) secondary to extensive renal adenocarcinoma.

contents (Fig. 6.10). Meticulous scanning is crucial in evaluating these minimally echogenic neoplasms to avoid the erroneous diagnosis of a benign simple cyst. The end point in the diagnostic investigation of all tumor must be based upon a correlative approach utilizing the clinical, urographic, sonographic, and angiographic data. This is particularly true in a case of suspected papillary cystadenocarcinoma. Any disparities among confirmatory studies necessitate percutaneous aspiration or exploratory laparotomy. Fine needle aspiration biopsy is a well-estalished technique that can be used to obtain a cytological diagnosis in equivocal cases.

Urothelial Carcinoma

The majority of infiltrating urothelial neoplasms are transitional cell carcinomas, with the remainder being squamous cell carcinomas. They are derived from the epithelial lining of the renal pelvis, calyces, ureter, and bladder. Histologically, transitional cell carcinomas are similar regardless of the site of origin. Patients usually present for intravenous urography relatively early because of hematuria. The appearance of these tumors is quite variable depending on the extent of disease at diagnosis. There may be one or more filling defects within the pelvicalyceal system, localized hydronephrosis, or a large mass infiltrating the renal parenchyma. Extrapelvic extension of transitional cell carcinomas to involve the renal parenchyma is a sign of advanced disease that portends a poor prognosis. These bulky tumors may be impossible to distinguish from an invasive renal adenocarcinoma, except at final pathology.

In a straightforward case of irregular renal pelvic filling defects, retrograde pyelography with brush biopsy is the generally accepted procedure to follow the screening urogram. Ultrasound may be valuable when smooth, round lesions are present. This urographic appearance can occur with early urothelial tumors, benign papillomas, radiolucent calculi, or blood clot. A definitive diagnosis of calculus disease can be made only if acoustic shadowing is evident on scans. Calculi are very dense and highly reflec-

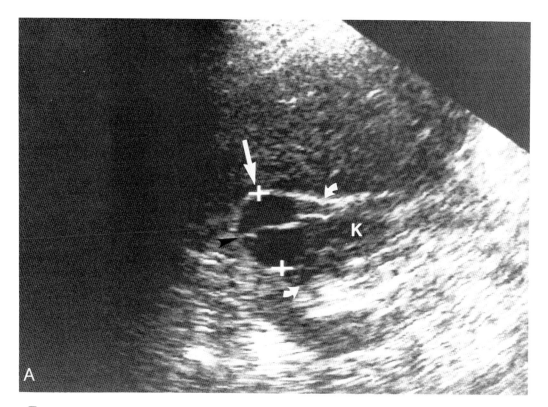

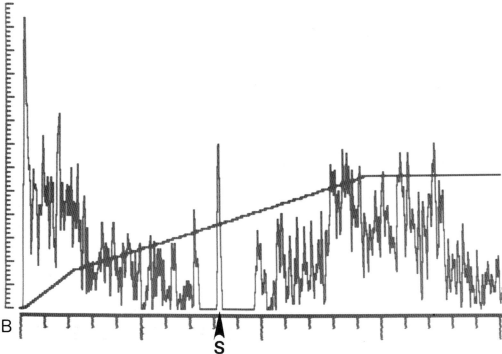

Figure 6.10. Papillary cystadenocarcinoma. *A*, Transverse supine scan of the right kidney demonstrates a single septum (*arrowhead*) within a fluid-filled mass (*arrow*). The anterior superior wall (*curved arrows*) of this carcinoma blends imperceptibly with the renal cortex (*K*). *B*, A-mode tracing demonstrates high intensity far-wall echoes indicative of acoustic enhancement. No internal echoes could be identified other than the single septum (*S*).

tive of the ultrasound beam; therefore, shadowing should occur regardless of the chemical composition or the presence of calcium. Blood clot can only be diagnosed with certainty when serial sonograms demonstrate retraction or total resorption.

Since ultrasound is seldom required to diagnose urothelial neoplasms, their sonographic characteristics have not been clearly elucidated. Limited, early reports have described transitional cell malignancies as anechoic or poorly echogenic with low amplitude echoes (33, 34). Small tumors situated within a calyx may be impossible to visualize on scans. Localized hydronephrosis may be apparent with obstructing tumors in the absence of a distinct mass (35). It is quite likely that with gray-scale technology, the echogenicity of these tumors is actually more variable than previously appreciated (Fig. 6.11).

Lymphoma

Extranodal renal involvement is common in patients with different types of lymphomas, more so in non-Hodgkin's disease. In most cases,

renal lymphoma is a manifestation of long-standing disease. The findings of reduced renal function, flank pain, palpable flank mass, and hematuria or lymphocyturia in lymphoma patients may signal the onset of renal disease (36). Lesions of the kidney are rarely due to primary lymphoma, but rather to local extension from adjacent perinephric nodal masses or distant hematogenous metastases (37).

Lymphomatous masses are apt to be minimally echogenic or totally echo free on sonograms because of their uniform cellularity. Acoustic enhancement may even result from the lack of reflecting tissue interfaces within these masses. In the early era of ultrasound, lymphomatous tissues were frequently mistaken for fluid-filled bowel or simple cysts because of this appearance. It is now apparent, however, that the degree of through sound transmission of lymphomas is less than that of cystic masses. Solitary lymphomas tend to exhibit a more solid sonographic pattern and may mimic other renal tumors, such as adenocarcinoma (Fig. 6.12). Ultimately, the ultrasonic image is a result of numerous factors: (*a*) the pathways of spread to

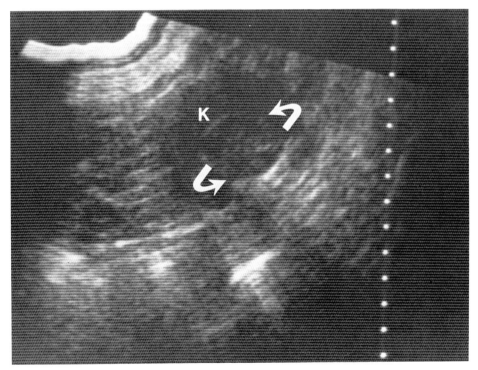

Figure 6.11. Transitional cell carcinoma. Transverse decubitus scan of the upper pole of the left kidney demonstrates a round, moderately echogenic carcinoma (*arrows*) within the pelvicalyceal system. At low gain settings, the mass contains more echoes than the renal cortex (*K*).

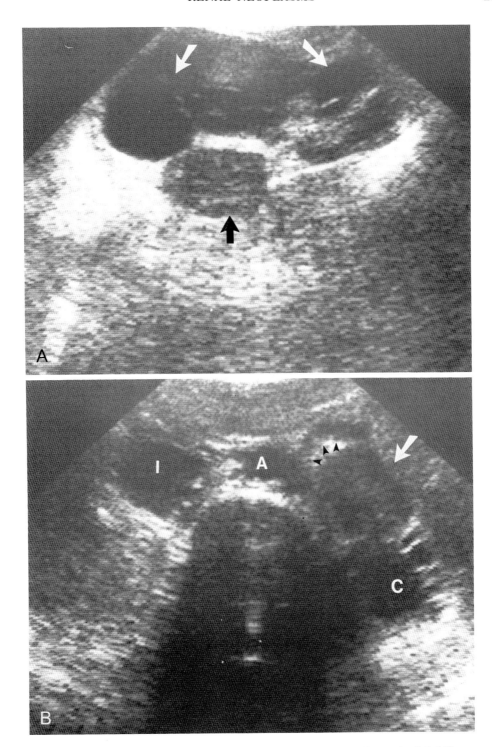

Figure 6.12. Mixed lymphoma. *A,* Longitudinal decubitus scan of the native left kidney reveals cystic degeneration (*white arrows*) secondary to end-stage interstitial nephritis. There is a solitary echogenic mass (*black arrow*) involving the upper pole. *B,* Transverse supine scan reveals lymphadenopathy (*arrow*) displacing the left renal artery (*arrowheads*). *A,* aorta; *I,* inferior vena cava; *C,* renal cysts.

the kidney; (b) the mechanism of intrarenal growth; (c) the extent of extrarenal involvement; and (d) the size, number, and distribution of renal lesions (38). In considering these variables and the diverse behavior patterns of different lymphomas, a wide range of ultrasound appearances is to be expected. Some of the previously described abnormalities include single or multiple cortical masses; retroperitoneal lymphadenopathy and perirenal masses displacing, obstructing, and/or invading the kidney; and infiltration of the renal parenchyma secondary to progressive multifocal disease (Fig. 6.13). Once a diagnosis of lymphoma has been established, ultrasound is an excellent means of following patient response to therapy, especially in cases of decreased or absent renal function.

Metastatic Neoplasms

Metastatic renal disease may occur secondary to practically any end-stage neoplastic process. Autopsy series of malignancies report a high incidence of renal metastases. The usual route

of these tumor deposits is hematogenous, which makes lung, breast, and melanoma common offenders (Fig. 6.14). The ultrasonic features of metastatic renal disease have not been well documented. A few isolated cases reported earlier in conjunction with other solid renal tumors describe metastatic foci as less echogenic than the normal renal parenchyma. However, the ultrasonic appearance of metastases is more likely a reflection of the primary neoplasm. Hypovascular tumor with homogeneous cell types and tumors that undergo cystic degeneration, necrosis, or hemorrhage should logically be poorly echo productive. Likewise, heterogeneous tumors should appear more echogenic. Therefore, metastatic tumors, particularly when solitary, may closely resemble primary renal carcinomas (Fig. 6.15). Multiple unilateral or bilateral renal masses associated with adrenal metastases or retroperitoneal lymphadenopathy make metastatic disease seem probable (39). It should always be borne in mind that a diagnosis of renal metastasis is feasible only in the face of a known primary neoplasm.

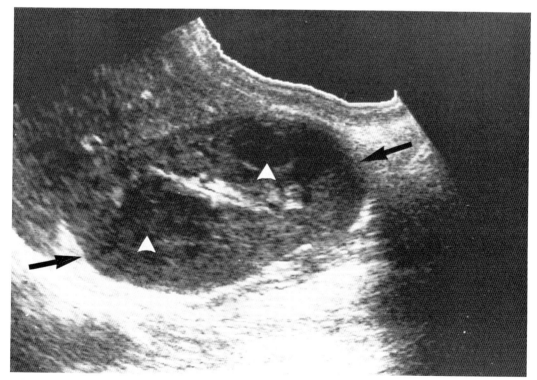

Figure 6.13. Multifocal lymphoma. Longitudinal supine scan in an 11-year-old male demonstrates a massively enlarged right kidney (*arrows*). There is gross distortion of the intrarenal anatomy with multiple poorly echo-productive areas (*arrowheads*) identified secondary to progressive multifocal lymphoma.

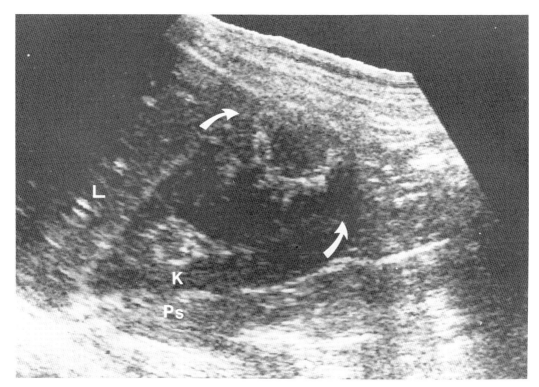

Figure 6.14. Metastatic melanoma. Longitudinal supine scan demonstrates a right lower pole renal mass (*arrows*) which is much less echogenic than the normal renal parenchyma (*K*). *L*, liver; *Ps*, psoas muscle.

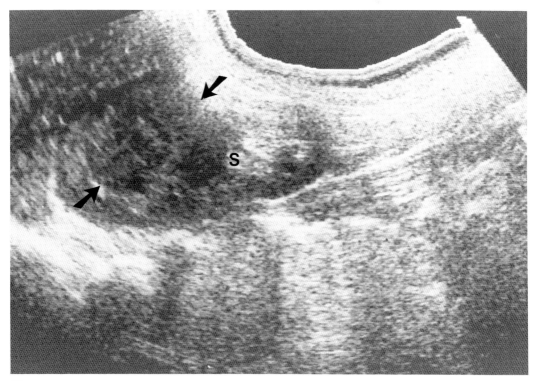

Figure 6.15. Metastatic carcinoid. Longitudinal supine scan of the right kidney reveals a large upper pole metastatic deposit (*arrows*) which is distorting the renal sinus (*S*).

Sarcomas

Sarcomas are rare malignant neoplasms that originate from the mesenchyma or connective tissue elements of the kidney. Most commonly, they arise from the capsular surface of the kidney. There have been isolated case reports of different histological types, i.e., rhabdomyosarcoma, liposarcoma, leiomyosarcoma, fibrosarcoma, and hemangiopericytoma. The clinical symptomatology, physical findings, and ultrasonic features of renal sarcomas are not distinctive from other malignancies. Retroperitoneal sarcomas may invade the adjacent kidney; hence, it is often not possible to determine the site of origin in extensive cases.

BENIGN NEOPLASMS

Angiomyolipomas

These are classically rare, benign mesodermal tumors composed of muscle, blood vessels, and fat in varying proportions. A significant percentage of angiomyolipomas, usually multiple lesions involving both kidneys, occur in association with tuberous sclerosis. Unilateral, solitary tumors in otherwise normal middle-aged females may be a "forme fruste" of the disorder. The clinical presentation, physical findings, and roentgen images of angiomyolipomas are not distinctive. Consequently, problems have been encountered in discriminating these benign neoplasms from renal malignancies. Masses are often richly vascular with microaneurysms on arteriograms resembling the tumor neovascularity of renal carcinomas (40). The diagnosis may be suggested when there is sufficient fat content to produce radiolucency on plain films. Fortunately, these tumors have more characteristic ultrasound features. They tend to be highly echogenic without total reflection of the sound beam. The very dense internal echoes of angiomyolipomas persist even at low gain settings and are believed due to a high fat content (41). Since these tumors are histologically mixed, there is a spectrum of sonographic findings depending on the proportions of the different tissue components. Some tumors may actually appear complex and others even poorly echogenic (42). The exact site of origin may not be apparent in those neoplasms that primarily extend into the retroperitoneum with compression and displacement of the kidney (Fig. 6.16).

Oncocytomas

Oncocytomas are benign renal adenomas that have been alternately referred to as granular cell adenomas or eosinophilic adenomas. This entity remains a subject of great debate, and controversy even surrounds its very existence. Some authorities consider these adenomas as localized renal adenocarcinomas because of many clinical, pathological, and radiological similarities. Oncocytomas are usually solitary, well-encapsulated tumors. Different pathological classifications have been devised based on cell type (i.e., tubular, papillary, alveolar), staining characteristics (i.e., eosinophilic, basophilic), and site of origin (i.e., proximal or distal convoluted tubules, collecting duct) (43). Their cells impart a granular appearance on light microscopy because of an abundant eosinophilic-staining cytoplasm. Despite the large dimensions some adenomas may reach, no incidence of metastasis has ever been documented (44). These tumors are even rarer than angiomyolipomas, so there is little available information on their sonographic features. A small series reported homogeneously solid masses of moderate echogenicity, and some later cases have confirmed these earlier observations (Fig. 6.17). Presently, it is just not possible to distinguish these adenomas from carcinomas with ultrasound. Furthermore, conventional urograms, computed tomograms, and radioisotope studies have not been helpful in this regard. An oncocytoma can be suspected on arteriography if a solitary mass exhibits a stellate vascular pattern, rim vessels, and a uniform tumor blush without neovascularity (43). Although a preoperative diagnosis seems improbable, it would appear to have merit in any cases where there is a need to preserve renal cortical tissue.

Other Types of Benign Tumors

Some of the other histological types of benign renal tumors include hemangiomas, lipomas, fibromas, and leiomyomas. The actual incidence of these lesions may vary with the hospital population, but all are very unusual. They tend to be small and rarely produce symptoms. Yet, they are now being recognized with increasing frequency (45) because of high resolution screening modalities like ultrasound and computed tomography. Their significance lies in differentiating them from renal malignancies with a high degree

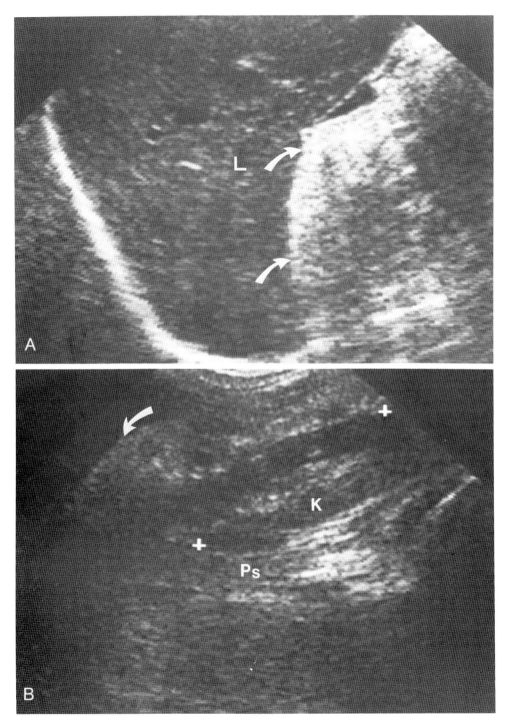

Figure 6.16. Angiomyolipoma. *B,* Longitudinal supine scan reveals many highly reflective echoes (*arrows*) inferior to the liver (*L*) secondary to an exophytic angiomyolipoma arising from the upper pole of the right kidney. *B,* At low gain, this longitudinal supine scan reveals the kidney (*K*), enveloped by this angiomyolipoma (*arrow*) which arose from the upper pole and was adherent to the psoas muscle (*Ps*).

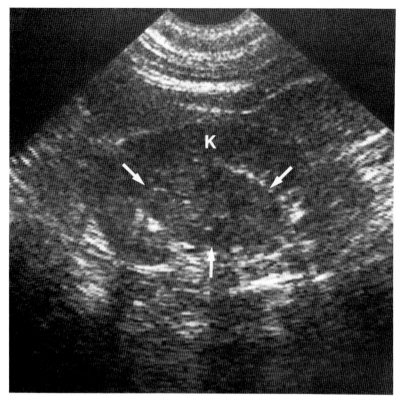

Figure 6.17. Oncocytoma. Longitudinal supine scan in a 61-year-old male with hematuria reveals a moderately echogenic mass (*arrows*) with echoes similar to the noninvolved portions of the kidney (*K*). Final pathology revealed a proximal tubular adenoma with uniform cellularity and no mitoses.

of confidence and at minimum risk and cost to the patient. Aspiration biopsy is an acceptable alternative means of establishing a histopathological diagnosis. Small bore cutting needles can now be used to obtain adequate tissue samples for typing.

RENAL PSEUDOTUMORS

Normal Variants

A renal pseudotumor has been defined as a real or simulated mass resembling neoplasm but composed of pathologically normal renal tissue (46). Persistent fetal lobation is a result of incomplete fusion of fetal renal lobes, which normally disappear by the fourth or fifth year of life (47). The distribution of these lobes corresponds to the anterior calyces, creating a multinodular renal outline with cortical indentations between the calyceal groups. Although fetal lobations may involve either kidney, the dro-

medary hump is a rather unique feature of the left kidney. This is believed due to pressure on the developing fetal kidney by the contiguous spleen. Medial contour deformities may occur just above, below, or at the level of the renal hilum. These have been termed renal uncus, hilar lips, and hilar bulges. There may be compression or splaying of adjacent pelvicalyceal structures by these redundant folds of renal cortex. This pseudotumor most frequently involves the suprahilar region of the left kidney (48).

The hypertrophied column of Bertin is a prominent invagination of the renal cortex to varying depths within the medullary substance of the kidney. The internal renal substance is affected rather than the cortical margins. It has been postulated that this lesions results from the fusion of two septa into a single column of twice the normal thickness (48). These islands of cortical tissue tend to be most exggerated in complete or partial duplications. Acquired pseudotumors result from hyperplasia, hypertrophy and regeneration of renal tissue in response to some preceding disease process. They represent nodules of functioning parenchyma dispersed among scarred, damaged renal segments. Chronic inflammatory disorders, infarction, and trauma are common causes of acquired pseudotumors (46).

Radionuclide imaging is the optimal means of confirming the diagnosis of renal pseudotumor. There are numerous radiopharmaceuticals that are preferentially concentrated and retained by functioning nephrons (49). Renal tumors lack normal parenchyma and apppear as cold defects on nuclear scans. It was once believed that pseudotumors could be accurately diagnosed with ultrasound because true neoplasms were thought to be either more or less echo producing than the normal parenchyma (33). But homogeneous, well-differentiated carcinomas can have the same echo characteristics as the normal cortex. Pseudotumors are usually first detected on intravenous urography but may be inadvertently noted with ultrasound. In such cases, a focal accumulation of echoes very similar to the cortical echoes is identified (Fig. 6.18). Typically, there is associated distortion of the renal contour or the pelvicalyceal system. Since pseudotumors cannot be reliably predicted on the basis of the sonogram, radionuclide scans should be used to confirm the diagnosis.

Extrarenal Lesions

Occasionally, nonrenal structures may simulate the appearance of a primary neoplasm of the kidney. This type of pseudotumor usually involves the left kidney. Splenic masses, enlargement, malposition or contour variations, and a fluid-filled gastric fundus were once very common sources of error (50). The flexibility of scanning at different angles and in multiple positions now allows the detection of a distinct fascial plane between the normal spleen and kidney with ultrasound. Gastric peristalsis is now readily identifiable with real-time, so the location of the stomach in relation to the upper pole of the left kidney should be obvious. Splenomegaly and focal splenic masses may compress or displace the kidney such that it is sometimes difficult to demonstrate a sharp interface between the neighboring organs. Retroperitoneal masses, particularly adrenal in origin, can mimic a primary renal neoplasm (Fig. 6.19). Extensive tumors that have secondarily infiltrated the kidney may be impossible to distinguish from an invasive renal carcinoma.

Atypical Renal Cysts

Atypical renal cysts may have a solid or complex ultrasound pattern due to complications of infection, hemorrhage, or, rarely, neoplastic infiltration. A wide range of ultrasonic features may be demonstrable in such cases. These cysts can appear smooth with distinct borders and good through sound transmission, yet internal echoes are seen because of viscous particulate matter, purulent debris, or hemorrhagic contents (Fig. 6.20). Occasionally, fluid debris levels are identified. Rather than being round or ovoid, atypical cysts are apt to have nongeometric shapes (Fig. 6.21). Cysts that have been subjected to previous aspiration attempts and contrast cystography may possess all of the characteristics of a carcinoma (Fig. 6.22). In exceedingly rare cases, some benign serous cysts may mimic tumors for no apparent reason (Fig. 6.23).

There is a constellation of mural findings in atypical cysts. Their walls may be thickened circumferentially or segmentally. The demarcation between renal parenchyma and cyst wall is often imperceptible. In the unusual incidence of a neoplasm occurring within a cyst, the wall may appear irregular with one or more nodular excrescences. Bilocular and multilocular are terms that have been used to describe one or more noncommunicating cysts. These cysts are thought to have a distinctive sonographic appearance (Fig. 6.24). The fluid-filled locules are separated by highly echogenic fibrous septa which are often calcified (51). There are at least two other types of calcifications associated with benign serous cysts. "Egg-shell" mural calcification may occur in a small percentage of simple cysts, many of which give evidence of previous inflammation or bleeding. Densely calcified cysts are even more unusual (52). Any calcified renal lesion can be difficult to assess with ultrasound because of the reflection of the sonic beam that results from the calcium deposits. They are probably best evaluated by other imaging modalities, such as computed tomography.

Vascular Disorders

Unusual renal lesions secondary to vascular disorders can sometimes produce a parenchymal mass resembling neoplasm. Although a cystic sonic pattern is more typical of arteriovenous

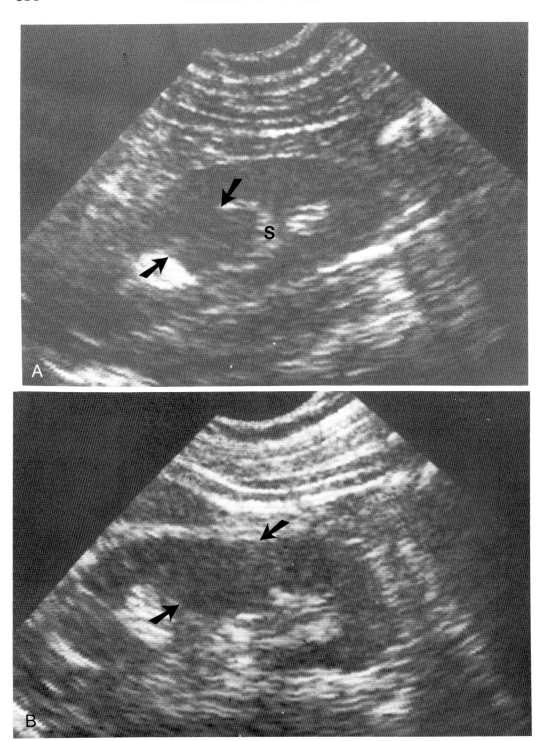

Figure 6.18. Hypertrophied column of Bertin. *A*, Longitudinal supine scan of the right kidney reveals focal distortion of the renal sinus (*S*) by a mid-pole defect (*arrows*) secondary to a hypertrophied column of Bertin. *B*, Longitudinal supine view of the left kidney shows a much less prominent defect (*arrows*).

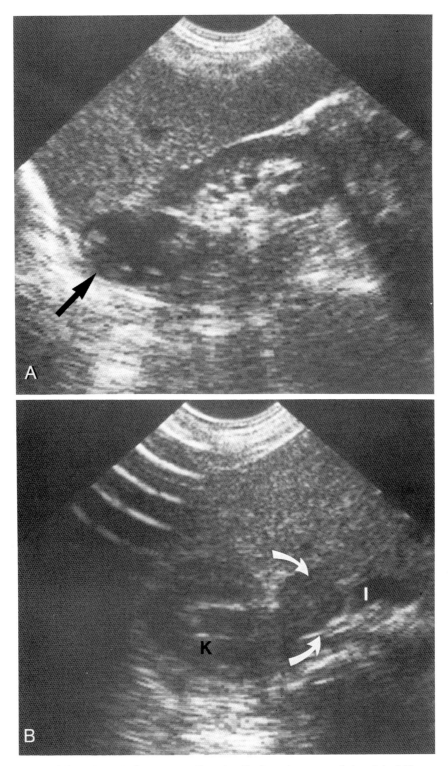

Figure 6.19. Adrenal cortical tumor. *A*, Longitudinal supine scan of the right kidney reveals a poorly echo-productive mass (*arrow*) possibly arising from the right kidney. *B*, Transverse supine scan shows a moderately echogenic mass (*arrows*) between the kidney (*K*) and the inferior vena cava (*I*) which was thought to be a lymph node. Final pathology revealed an encapsulated adrenal cortical neoplasm without renal involvement.

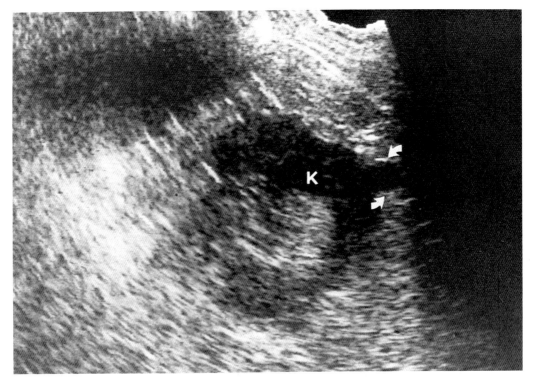

Figure 6.20. Atypical renal cyst. Transverse decubitus scan of the left kidney shows one of multiple small masses (*arrows*) with overall echogenicity similar to the renal cortex (*K*). These simple cysts appeared dense on CT and contained debris at surgery.

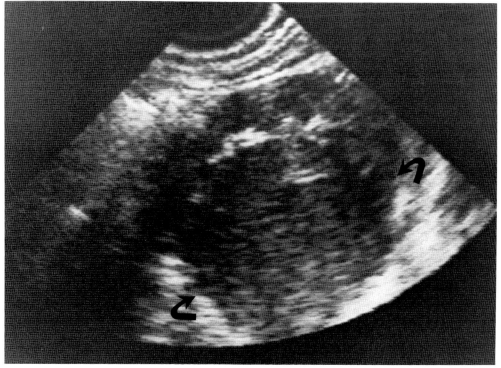

Figure 6.21. Atypical renal cyst. Longitudinal decubitus scan in an 8-year-old with sudden onset of hematuria and a history of trauma 6 weeks earlier. A large, irregularly shaped mass (*arrows*) simulating a Wilms' tumor was identified. A simple renal cyst filled with pink-tinged fluid was found at surgery.

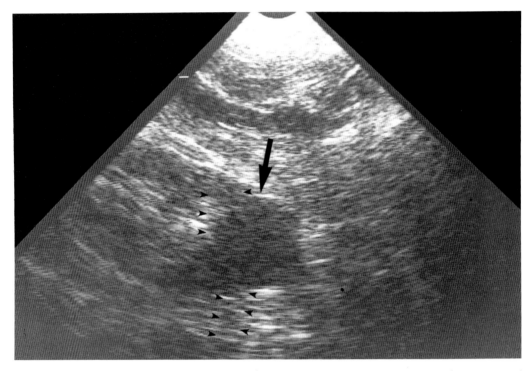

Figure 6.22. Atypical renal cyst. Longitudinal prone real-time examination during second aspiration of this right lower pole mass (*arrow*) reveals shadowing from the needle track (*arrowheads*). Class I reddish fluid was removed, and postaspiration films showed no mural abnormalities.

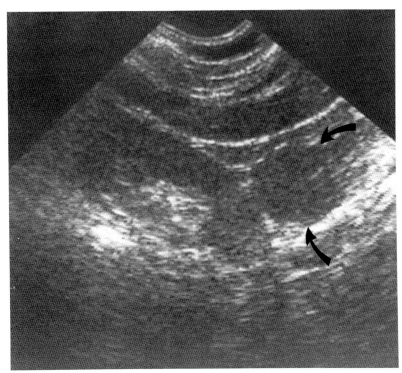

Figure 6.23.   Atypical renal cyst. Longitudinal decubitus scan reveals exophytic lower pole mass (*arrows*) moderately echogenic in nature and without acoustic enhancement. Final pathology revealed a simple serous cyst.

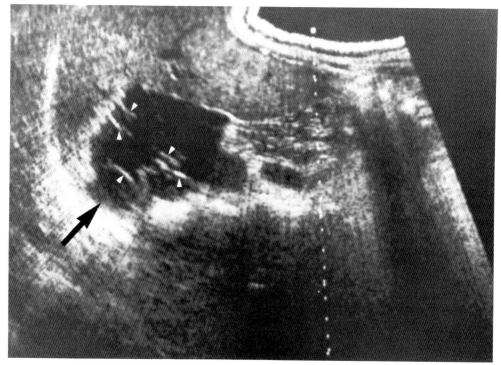

Figure 6.24. Multilocular renal cyst. Longitudinal supine scan of the right kidney shows an irregularly shaped mass (*arrow*) which is predominately fluid filled. There are numerous highly echogenic fibrous septa (*arrowheads*) noted.

malformations, renal artery aneurysm, and hematomas, solid or complex patterns are known to occur. Aneurysms of the main renal artery are located in the parapelvic area. Large, calcified aneurysms that abut the renal sinus can be a diagnostic dilemma unless arterial pulsations are identified. Arteriovenous malformations composed of cirsoid, tortuous vessels contain few internal echoes but seldom conform to the strict criteria for simple cysts (Fig. 6.25). Trauma, excessive anticoagulation, and blood dyscrasias may cause focal renal defects due to hemorrhage. Intrarenal hematomas are extremely diverse sonographically, depending on their organization, presence of calcification, and the time interval between initiation and detection of the hemorrhage. Seromas may be completely cystic, whereas masses of clotted blood tend to be complex with increasing echogenicity as clot fragmentation occurs (53).

Inflammatory Pseudotumors

Inflammatory renal masses can occur in acute and chronic pyelonephritis, pyonephrosis, xanthogranulomatous pyelonephritis, and renal tuberculosis. Acute bacterial pyelonephritis usually causes interstitial edema, which on scans produces generalized renal enlargement and decreased echogenicity. Acute focal bacterial nephritis is a descriptive term that refers to a localized form of inflammation of the renal parenchyma, whose predominant feature is focal swelling or mass. The ultrasound appearance is that of a poorly defined solid mass of slightly less intensity than the normal cortex. This is a medically treatable entity that seldom requires interventional measures. Without adequate therapy, mature abscesses are believed to evolve from this process (54). Frank abscesses can produce an array of ultrasonic images depending on the degree of liquefaction of their contents (Fig. 6.26). They can rarely be totally anechoic and mimic simple cysts. More likely, irregular margins, low level internal echoes, and sound attenuation result from the presence of a purulent exudate and loculations (55). Emphysematous infections may occur from gas-forming organisms such as *Escherichia coli* and *Proteus vulgaris*. Diabetes and obstructive uropathy are fre-

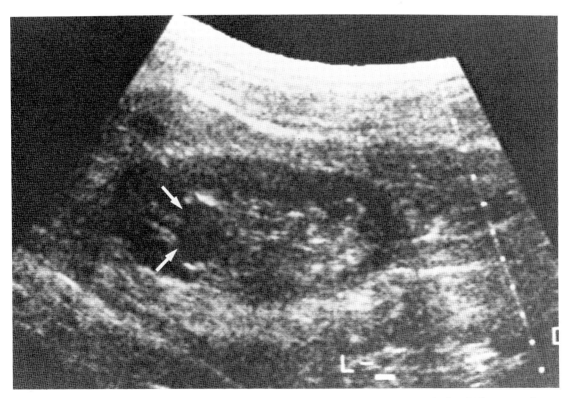

Figure 6.25.   Arteriovenous malformation. Longitudinal decubitus scan of the left kidney reveals an ovoid, poorly echogenic mass (*arrows*) due to an arteriovenous malformation.

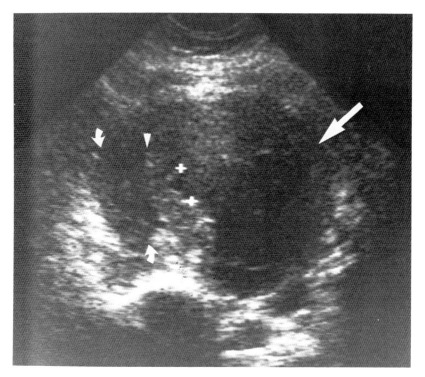

Figure 6.26. Renal abscess. Transverse decubitus scan of the right kidney reveals total disruption of the renal architecture by a large, minimally echogenic abscess (*arrow*) with perinephric extension (*curved arrows*) outside the renal capsule (*arrowhead*).

quently associated with this type of inflammation. Highly echogenic masses can result. In pyonephrosis, it may be possible to localize the air to the collecting system and to demonstrate the mobility of dense echoes with acoustic shadowing (56). Xanthogranulomatous pyelonephritis is a severe form of chronic inflammation usually associated with calculus disease. It is possible to confuse the diffuse type with an infiltrative carcinoma since both conditions may be sufficiently extensive to cause a functionless kidney. A solid parenchymal mass due to the focal variant can simulate a localized carcinoma. It has been encountered at least twice as frequently as the diffuse type (57). Tuberculous involvement of the kidney can occasionally produce a bulky mass secondary to a tuberculoma, pyonephrosis, or abscess (58). Clearly, a close resemblance exists between a number of renal inflammatory and neoplastic processes. To minimize errors, renal mass lesions should always be carefully scrutinized with ultrasound. The final proposed differential diagnosis must always be correlated with the clinical symptoms, physical findings, and available laboratory data.

References

1. Skinner DG, Colvin RB, Vermillion DC, Pfister RC, Lebeader WF: Diagnosis and management of renal cell carcinoma. *Cancer* 28:1165, 1977.
2. Holland JM: Cancer of the kidney—natural history and staging. *Cancer* 32:1030, 1973.
3. Grabstald H: Renal cell tumors. *Surg Clin North Am:* 49:337, 1969.
4. Murphy GP, Schirmer HKA: The diagnosis and treatment of hypernephroma. *Geriatrics* 18:354, 1963.
5. DeKernion JB, Berry D: The diagnosis and treatment of renal cell carcinoma. *Cancer* 45:1947, 1980.
6. Bennington JL, Beckwith JB: Tumors of the kidney, renal pelvis, and ureter. In *Atlas of Tumor Pathology*, fascicle 12. Washington, DC, Air Force Institute of Pathology, 1975, p 93.
7. Taylor KJW, Hill CR: Scanning techniques in gray-scale ultrasonography. *Br J Radiol* 48:918, 1975.
8. Feldberg MAM, van Waes PFGM: Multilocular cystic renal cell carcinoma. *AJR* 138:953, 1982.
9. Scheible W. Talner LB: Gray scale ultrasound and the genitourinary tract: a review of clinical applications. *Radiol Clin North Am* 17:281, 1979.
10. Gleeson MH, Bloom SR, Polak JM, Henry K, Dowling RH: An endocrine tumor in kidney affecting small bowel structure, motility and function. *Gut* 11:1060, 1970.

11. Rosenfield AT, Taylor KJW, Crade M, DeGraaf CS: Anatomy and pathology of the kidney by gray scale ultrasound. *Radiology* 128:737, 1978.
12. Pollack HM, Banner MP, Arger PH, Peters J, Mulhern CB, Coleman BG: The accuracy of gray-scale renal ultrasonography in differentiating cystic neoplasms from benign cysts. *Radiology* 143:741, 1982.
13. Newman HR, Schulman ML: Renal cortical tumors: a 40-year statistical survey. *Urol Surv* 19:2, 1969.
14. Sun CN, Bissada NK, White HJ, Redman JF: The spectrum of ultrastructural patterns of renal cell adenocarcinoma. *Urology* 9:195, 1977.
15. Cooper PH, Waisman J: Tubular differentiation and basement membrane production in a renal adenoma: ultrastructural features. *J Pathol* 109:113, 1971.
16. Pinals RA, Krane SM: Medical aspects of renal carcinoma. *Postgrad Med J* 38:507, 1962.
17. Pratt-Thomas HR, Spicer SS, Upshur JK, Greene WB: Carcinoma of the kidney in a 15-year-old boy—unusual histologic features with formation of microvilli. *Cancer* 31:719, 1973.
18. Holland JF, Frei E III: *Cancer Medicine.* Philadelphia, Lea and Febiger, 1973, p 1655.
19. Ochsner MG, Brannan W, Pond HS III, Goodier EH: Renal cell carcinoma: review of 26 years of experience at the Ochsner Clinic. *J Urol* 110:643, 1973.
20. Coleman BG, Arger PH, Mulhern CB, Pollack HM, Banner MP, Arenson RL: Gray-scale sonographic spectrum of hypernephromas. *Radiology* 137:757, 1980.
21. Bennington JL: Cancer of the Kidney—etiology, epidemiology, and pathology. *Cancer* 32:1017, 1973.
22. Middleton RG: Surgery for metastatic renal cell carcinoma. *J Urol* 97:973, 1967.
23. Mims MM, Christensen B, Schulmberger FL, Goodwin WE: A 10-year evaluation of nephrectomy for renal cell carcinoma. *J Urol* 95:10, 1966.
24. Merrin CE: Renal neoplasms. In Javadpour N: *Principles and Management of Urologic Cancer.* Baltimore, Williams & Wilkins, 1979.
25. Robson CJ, Churchill BM, Anderson W: The results of radical nephrectomy for renal cell carcinoma. *Trans Am Assoc Genitourin Surg* 60:122, 1968.
26. Patel NP, Lavengood RW: Renal cell carcinoma. Natural history and results of treatment. *J Urol* 119:722, 1978.
27. Schafft P, Novick AC, Straffon RA, Stewart BH: Surgery for renal cell carcinoma extending into the inferior vena cava. *J Urol* 120:28, 1978.
28. DeKernion JB, Ramming KP, Smith RB: Natural history of metastatic renal cell carcinoma: computer analysis. *J Urol* 120:148, 1978.
29. Levine E, Lee KR, Weigel J: Preoperative determination of abdominal extent of renal cell carcinoma by computed tomography. *Radiology* 132:395, 1979.
30. Love L, Churchill R, Reynes C, Schuster GA, Moncada R, Berkow A: Computed tomography of renal carcinoma *Urol Radiol* 1:3, 1979.
31. Probst P, Hoogewaud HM, Haertel M, Zingg E, Fuchs WA: Computerized tomography versus angiography in the staging of malignant renal neoplasm. *Br J Pathol* 54:744, 1981.
32. Blei CL, Hartman DS, Friedman AC, Davis CJ: Papillary renal cell carcinoma: ultrasonic/pathologic correlation. *J Clin Ultrasound* 10:429–434, 1982.
33. Maklad NF, Chuang VP, Doust BD, Cho JK, Curran JE: Ultrasonic characterization of solid renal lesions: echographic, angiographic and pathologic correlation. *Radiology* 123:733, 1977.
34. Green WM, King DL, Casarella WJ: A reappraisal of sonolucent renal masses. *Radiology* 121:163, 1976.
35. Sanders RC, Bearman SB: B-scan ultrasound in the diagnosis of hydronephrosis. *Radiology* 108:375, 1973.
36. Lalli AF: Lymphoma and the urinary tract. *Radiology* 93:1051, 1969.
37. Kaude JV, Lacy GD: Ultrasonography in renal lymphoma. *J Clin Ultrasound* 6:321, 1978.
38. Hartman DS, Davis CJ, Goldman SM, Friedman AC, Fritzsche P: Renal lymphoma: radiologic-pathologic correlation of 21 cases. *Radiology* 144:759, 1982.
39. McDonald DG: The complete sonographic evaluation of solid renal masses. *J Clin Ultrasound* 6:402, 1978.
40. Barrilero AE: Renal angiomyolipoma: a study of 13 cases. *J Urol* 117:547, 1977.
41. Lee TG, Henderson SC, Freeny PC, Raskin MM, Benson EP, Harper DP: Ultrasound findings of renal angiomyolipoma. *J Clin Ultrasound* 6:143, 1978.
42. Hartman DS, Goldman SM, Friedman AC, Davis CJ, Madewell JE, Sherman JJ: Angiomyolipoma: ultrasonic-pathologic correlation. *Radiology* 139:451, 1981.
43. Bonavita JA, Pollack HM, Banner MP: Renal oncocytoma: further observations and literature review. *Urol Radiol* 2:229, 1981.
44. Morales A, Wasan S, Bryniak S: Renal oncocytomas: clinical, radiological and histologic features. *J Urol* 123:261, 1980.
45. Lang EK: Roentgenographic assessment of renal lesions. An analysis of the confidence level established by sequential roentgenographic investigation. *Radiology* 109:257, 1973.
46. Felson B, Moskowitz M: Renal pseudotumors: the regenerated nodule and other lumps, bumps, and dromedary humps. *AJR* 107:720, 1969.
47. Effman EL, Ablow RC, Siegel NJ: Renal growth. *Radiol Clin North Am* 15:3, 1977.
48. Hodson J: The lobar structure of the kidney. *Br J Urol* 44:246, 1972.
49. Prichert JH, Wisnton MA: Detection and diagnosis of renal masses with modern radioisotope and ultrasonic techniques. *CRC Crit Rev Clin Radiol Nucl Med* 5:423, 1974.
50. Cunningham JJ: Renal tumors and pseudotumors. In Resnik MI, Saunders RC: *Ultrasound in Urology.* Baltimore, Williams & Wilkins, 1979.
51. Banner MP, Pollack HM, Chatten J, Witzleben C: Multilocular renal cysts: radiologic-pathologic correlation. *AJR* 136:239, 1981.
52. Pollack HM, Banner MP, Arger PH, Goldberg

BB, Mulhern CB: Comparison of computed tomography and ultrasound in the diagnosis of renal masses. In Rosenfield AT: *Genitourinary Ultrasonography.* New York, Churchill Livingstone, 1979.

53. Wicks JD, Silver TM, Bree RL: Gray scale features of hematomas: ultrasonic spectrum. *AJR* 131:977, 1978.

54. Lee JKT, McClennan BL, Melson GL, Stanley RJ: Acute focal bacterial nephritis: emphasis on gray scale sonography and computed tomography. *AJR* 135:87, 1980.

55. Schneider M, Becker JA, Staino S, Campos E: Sonographic, radiographic correlation of renal and perirenal infections. *AJR* 127:1007, 1976.

56. Coleman BG, Arger PH, Mulhern CB, Pollack HM, Banner MP: Pyonephrosis: sonography in the diagnosis and management. *AJR* 137:939, 1981.

57. Malek RS, Elder JS: Xanthogranulomatous pyelonephritis: a critical analysis of 26 cases and of the literature. *J Urol* 119:589, 1978.

58. Tonkin AK, Written DM: Genitourinary tuberculosis. *Semin Roentgenol* 14:305, 1979.

CHAPTER 7

Ultrasonography in Patients with Acute Renal Failure

BARRY H. GROSS, M.D.
HEDVIG HRICAK, M.D.
ROY A. FILLY, M.D.

Despite advances in dialysis and renal transplantation, acute renal failure (ARF) remains a cause of significant morbidity and mortality (1). Prompt diagnosis of surgically correctable causes of ARF is essential (2). In the past, nephrotomography following the intravenous administration of high doses of urographic contrast media was the radiographic examination of choice in such patients (1, 3). Current clinical observations discourage the use of high doses of contrast media in patients with impaired renal function (4).

Over the past 15 years, ultrasonography has assumed an increasingly important role in the evaluation of various urinary tract abnormalities (5). Early studies (6, 7) showed that ultrasound could accurately detect pelvicalyceal dilatation and, therefore, should be emphasized as a primary screening modality in the search for surgically correctable causes of ARF (2, 4, 8, 9). Sonographic and clinical aspects of ARF will be reviewed with emphasis on sonographic technique, diagnosis, and intervention. Special consideration is given to ARF in infants and children and in patients with only one kidney. ARF of the transplanted kidney is considered elsewhere in the text.

CLINICAL ASPECTS OF ACUTE RENAL FAILURE

Renal failure is defined as the degree of renal insufficiency that results in a substantial alteration in plasma biochemistry. It is considered acute if it develops over days to weeks and chronic if it develops over months to years. Acute renal failure may be superimposed upon previously stable chronic renal failure (1).

ARF is categorized as prerenal, renal, or postrenal in etiology. Prerenal ARF results from renal hypoperfusion (10), which in turn can be caused by a variety of extrarenal abnormalities (1). Prerenal ARF can be distinguished from the other two categories by clinical and laboratory data alone (10).

ARF resulting from medical renal disease cannot be readily distinguished from postrenal ARF, caused by outflow obstruction on clinical and laboratory grounds alone. Although obstruction accounts for only 5% of patients with ARF (1), its distinction from renal medical disorders is crucial. Postrenal ARF is potentially correctable (10). Furthermore, prompt diagnosis and intervention are necessary to prevent secondary renal parenchymal loss (11). Obstruction must usually be bilateral to cause acute renal failure. Unilateral obstruction as a cause of ARF should be considered in association with renal agenesis, contralateral nephrectomy, or severe contralateral renal parenchymal diminution (10). Similarly, in patients with stable chronic renal failure, unilateral obstruction may tip the balance against the patient resulting in biochemical evidence of acute deterioration.

Postrenal ARF most often occurs in patients with malignant pelvic neoplasms of the bladder, prostate gland, uterus, ovaries, or rectum (1). Retroperitoneal fibrosis, para-aortic lymph node metastases, primary retroperitoneal neoplasms, renal calculi, and sloughed papillae are less common etiologies of postrenal ARF.

Renal medical disease is far and away the leading cause of ARF and usually results from acute tubular necrosis (ATN) (1, 12). The many entities that cause ATN can be divided into two etiologic categories, ischemic and nephrotoxic injury (13). Uncomplicated ATN is usually reversible, with patients recovering up to 80% of normal renal function (1), but death occurs in approximately 50% of affected patients (14). Other renal medical disorders are less frequently responsible for ARF. These include abnormalities of glomeruli, interstitium, small renal vessels, or, less commonly, major blood vessels (10). Renal artery occlusion is a rare cause of ARF because it is nearly always unilateral. However, complete traumatic avulsion of a renal pedicle may result in ATN of the contralateral kidney (1). By contrast, renal vein thrombosis is often bilateral and may be associated with ARF (15). Renal medical diseases that cause ARF are listed in Table 7.1.

SONOGRAPHIC TECHNIQUE

The technique for examination of the patient in ARF does not differ significantly from examination of the kidney for other indications. However, a few points are worth mentioning. First, such patients are often critically ill and cannot be transported to the ultrasound scanning room. Thus, high resolution portable real-time scanners are mandatory in hospitals which commonly treat such patients.

Although supine or prone longitudinal and transverse scans are useful (Fig. 7.1A), coronal images display the renal pelvis and calyces in continuity (Fig. 7.1B), allowing optimal evalu-

ation for urinary tract dilatation (2, 10, 16–18). Posterior oblique longitudinal scanning, producing images between the coronal and sagittal planes, has been advocated as another method of displaying the pelvicalyceal system (19). In either event, real-time sector scanning not only provides portability but facilitates identification of the appropriate scanning plane and results in the rapid acquisition of images without any loss of diagnostic accuracy (17, 20).

If bilateral dilatation is detected, the scanning procedure should be continued to determine level and etiology of the obstructing lesion, if possible. A dilated proximal ureter can virtually always be demonstrated in the same scanning plane which best displays the pelvicalyceal system in continuity (Fig. 7.1B). Scanning of the pelvis with the urinary bladder distended (retrogradely if necessary) is required to identify obstructing masses of any origin (Fig. 7.2). It is also mandatory to examine the pelvis for an ectopically positioned kidney if none is found in the flank (Fig. 7.3).

SONOGRAPHY OF ACUTE RENAL FAILURE

The Dilated Collecting System

Sonographic depiction of the kidney has reached a level of detail which is to be admired by all physicians interested in noninvasive imaging of renal pathology (21–25). The parenchyma can be seen with sufficient detail to distinguish the more echogenic cortex and column of Bertin from the hypoechoic medullary pyramids (Fig. 7.4). High amplitude punctate echoes reflected from the arcuate arteries and veins help to further discriminate the corticomedullary junction. The renal parenchyma is normally equally or less echogenic than the liver at a comparable distance from the transducer except in neonates, in whom the kidney may be more echogenic than liver in normal patients (23–25). Children differ from adults in two additional aspects: the medullary zones are proportionately larger, and there is comparatively less renal sinus fat (Fig. 7.5) (24, 25).

Small blood vessels and collecting structures may be seen coursing through the highly echogenic renal sinus fat. The renal vein may be prominent in normal patients and should not be mistaken for a dilated renal pelvis (Fig. 7.6). Previously, the ability to perceive the intrarenal collecting system was equated with dilatation of these structures. With current improved reso-

Table 7.1.
Renal medical diseases causing acute renal failure

I. Acute tubular necrosis
   A. Ischemic injury
   B. Nephrotoxic agents
II. Acute glomerulonephritis
   A. Poststreptococcal
   B. Subacute bacterial endocarditis
   C. Rapidly progressive glomerulonephritis
   D. Goodpasture's syndrome
   E. Systemic lupus erythematosus
   F. Polyarteritis nodosa
   G. Wegener's granulomatosis
III. Acute interstitial nephritis
   A. Drug reaction (i.e., methicillin)
   B. Idiopathic
IV. Small vessel disease
   A. Malignant hypertension
   B. Progressive systemic sclerosis
   C. Disseminated intravascular coagulation
   D. Thrombotic thrombocytopenic purpura
   E. Hemolytic-uremic syndrome
V. Major vessel disease
   A. Renal artery avulsion
   B. Renal artery thrombosis
   C. Renal artery embolism
   D. Renal vein thrombosis

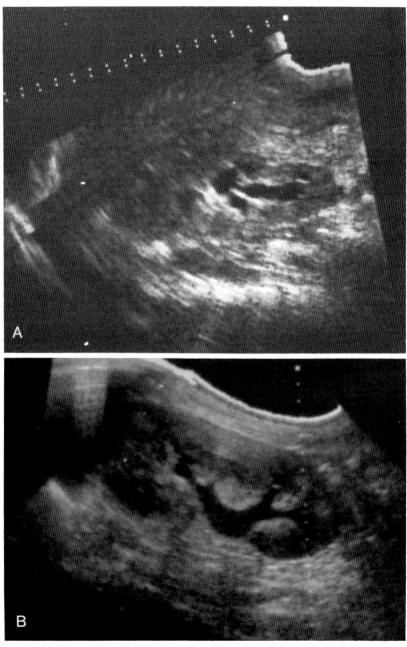

Figure 7.1. *A*, Supine longitudinal sonogram of the right kidney demonstrates anechoic fluid collections most probably representing dilated collecting system. *B*, Coronal image of the right kidney demonstrates unequivocal calyceal dilatation. In this projection the calyces, infundibula, and pelvis are seen in continuity.

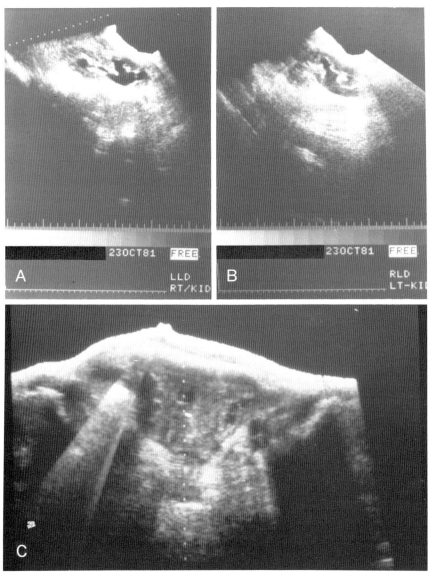

Figure 7.2. *A* and *B,* Coronal images of the right and left kidneys demonstrating bilateral pelvicaliectasis with dilatation of the left ureter. Under these circumstances ultrasound should be continued in search for the obstructing mass. *C,* Large solid neoplasm detected at the pelvic brim.

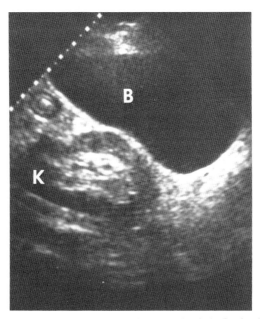

Figure 7.3. Patient without an identifiable kidney in the left flank. An ectopically positioned, nonhydronephrotic kidney (K) is found posterior to the distended urinary bladder (B).

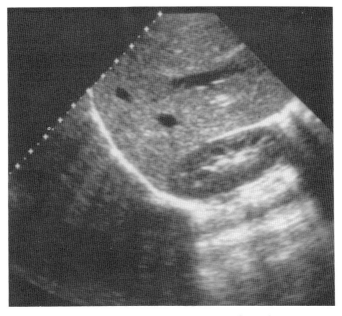

Figure 7.4. Longitudinal sonogram of the normal right kidney demonstrating good distinction between the cortical and medullary portions of the kidney.

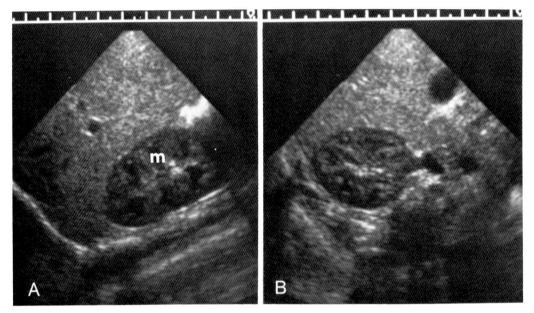

Figure 7.5.   Longitudinal (A) and transverse (B) sonograms of the kidney of a young child demonstrating the proportionately large medullary zones (m) of the kidney and comparatively less renal sinus fat than the adult.

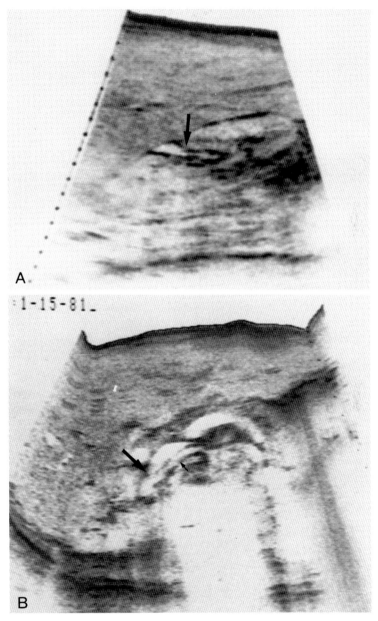

Figure 7.6.   *A*, Longitudinal scan of a kidney with a large renal vein (*arrow*) entering the renal hilus. This should not be mistaken for a dilated renal pelvis. *B*, Transverse sonogram demonstrating the renal artery (*small arrow*) and renal vein (*large arrow*) entering the renal hilus.

lution one must not make this broad sweeping statement (Fig. 7.7).

The presence or absence of urinary tract dilatation is the single most important issue that must be addressed in patients with ARF. Sonography has rightfully become the diagnostic modality of choice to screen patients in ARF for urinary tract dilatation. With minimal dilata-

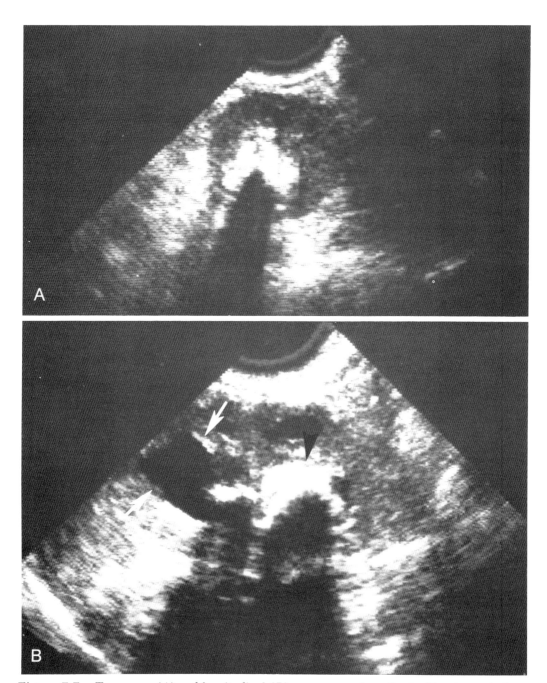

Figure 7.7.   Transverse (*A*) and longitudinal (*B*) sonograms of a patient with a large staghorn calculus. On the longitudinal scan, a dilated upper calyx (*white arrows*) and infundibulum are seen. The remainder of the collecting system is shadowed by the calculus (*arrowhead*).

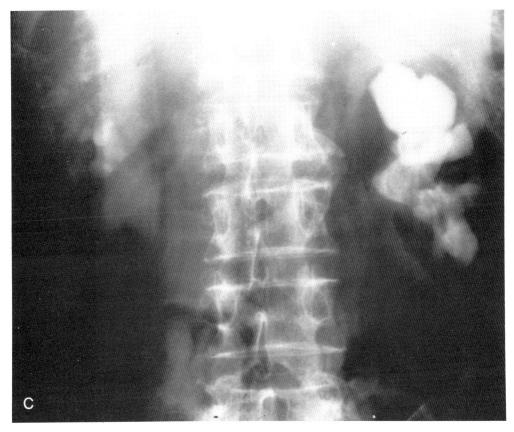

Figure 7.7. *C*, Excretory urogram documenting the large left staghorn calculus and the dilated upper pole calyces and infundibula.

tion, calyces and minor infundibula become readily visible and can be demonstrated in continuity (2) (Figs. 7.1 and 7.2). More marked dilatation produces bulbous enlargement of the calyces, infundibula, and renal pelvis (26). Judgments regarding the severity of dilatation are similar to those employed in excretory urography. While ultrasound accurately assesses dilatation of the intra- and extrarenal collecting system, the degree of dilatation does not necessarily reflect either the presence or the severity of an obstruction. Dilatation of the collecting system is a complex balance of the amount of urine produced, compliance of the collecting system, and degree of outflow obstruction. Therefore, when urinary obstruction is clinically suspected, even minimal dilatation of the pelvicalyceal system should be assessed by additional diagnostic procedures, such as an antegrade or retrograde pyelogram.

The sensitivity of sonography for the diagno-sis of urinary dilatation has ranged from 90 to 100% (4, 9, 11, 16, 17). One early study showed a relatively low specificity of 74% (9), but subsequent studies have all shown greater than 90% specificity (4, 11, 16, 17).

A normal ultrasound examination does not totally exclude urinary obstruction. Urinary dilatation has been missed in patients with large calculi in the renal pelvis (Fig. 7.7) (4). Such calculi are easily recognized by sonography, and their presence should forewarn the sonologist of the potential for the stone to mask associated dilatation. Early (4, 17) or partial obstruction (27) may only be identified when the patient is stressed with fluid or diuretics. This has been a particular pitfall in patients with retroperitoneal fibrosis (21). Rarely, there will be little or no dilatation even with established high grade urinary obstruction, presumably because of reduced glomerular filtration combined with some mechanism for urine resorption (28). For these reasons, nephrotomography or retrograde urography has been recommended for ARF patients with nondilated, normal to large kidneys by ultrasound (28). This concept provides the ultimate in safety, but it is impractical since one anticipates that the vast majority of patients with ARF will have normal-sized kidneys without upper tract dilatation.

Urinary dilatation may be mistakenly diagnosed using sonography. Patients with polyuric ARF are usually not suspected of having urinary tract obstruction. In these rare individuals, it is helpful to recall that dilatation does not equate with obstruction. However, if dilatation is marked in such a patient, this would constitute a clear indication for further, more invasive evaluation. Pregnant women with ARF are particularly difficult to evaluate since hydronephrosis is to be anticipated in gravid females. Because sonography is employed in a screening role, it is probably best to err on the false positive side (26).

Additional false positive diagnoses result from incorrect identification of renal and pararenal abnormalities. Peripelvic cysts in particular (Fig. 7.8) (29), as well as vascular aneurysms and arteriovenous malformations (21, 30), have been mistaken for urinary tract dilatation. Parapelvic cysts (i.e., single cyst in the renal hilus) can be distinguished from a dilated renal pelvis by careful scanning (Fig. 7.9) (2).

Adult polycystic kidney disease (APKD) and multicystic dysplastic kidney (MCDK) are other entities that have been reported to simulate urinary dilatation (31, 32). We believe that this problem is overstated. In both APKD and MCDK, the renal cysts are randomly distributed throughout the kidney and the renal contour is distorted in MCDK, whereas a hydronephrotic kidney usually maintains a reniform shape with a pattern of dilated calyces radiating from a larger central fluid collection, the renal pelvis (Fig. 7.10) (31). Furthermore, in APKD, identification of cysts in the liver or pancreas confirms the correct diagnosis (Fig. 7.11). The presence of renal cystic disease does not preclude simultaneous recognition of pelvicaliectasis (Fig. 7.11B).

There are a variety of nonobstructive causes of urinary dilatation which may occur in association with or precede ARF. These include diabetes insipidus, vesicoureteral reflux, postobstructive atrophy, atony associated with infection, postinflammatory calyceal clubbing, congenital megacalyces, and papillary necrosis (2,

17, 20, 30). Using ultrasound alone, it is impossible to differentiate between obstructive and nonobstructive urinary dilatation. Furthermore, in patients with obstructive urinary dilatation, it is frequently impossible to define the level of obstruction using sonography (2, 16), although attempts should be made to evaluate the ureters and bladder (Fig. 7.12) (2, 30). Therefore, when urinary dilatation is demonstrated by sonography, a further study (antegrade or retrograde pyelography) is recommended (2, 4, 29) to establish the existence of obstruction and to define its site and probable etiology.

Renal Medical Diseases

Once urinary dilatation as a cause of ARF has been excluded, sonography plays a relatively minor role. In our experience, in the vast majority of cases of acute renal failure caused by renal medical disease, the renal sonogram is unremarkable. Specifically, in a patient with uncomplicated acute tubular necrosis, the echo characteristics of the renal parenchyma are normal. The kidney may be globular in appearance, and the renal size can be normal or enlarged (10, 23). However, it has been reported in the literature that ATN may demonstrate increased cortical echogenicity with preservation of the cortical medullary boundary (22, 32). In our experience increased cortical echogenicity in acute renal failure was seen in cases of ARF caused by acute interstitial nephritis (Fig. 7.13) (10). Histologically, interstitial nephritis shows diffuse infiltration of the interstitium with lymphocytes, macrophages, plasma cells, and polymorphonuclear leukocytes (Fig. 7.13B). Increased cellular infiltration of the interstitium is probably responsible for the increased echogenicity seen sonographically. The ultrasonic appearance of acute poststreptococcal glomerulonephritis, as reported by Rochester et al. (33), may resemble multiple solid renal masses within an enlarged kidney. However, LeQuesne (34) reported a diffuse increase in the cortical echogenicity during acute poststreptococcal glomerulonephritis, similar to the appearance of interstitial nephritis. After the renal function had returned to normal, the cortical echogenicity reversed to normal as well (34). It is of interest that, when acute glomerulonephritis is found as a part of streptococcal septicemia, a large number of polymorphonuclear cells are present in the interstitium, in addition to typical changes in the glomeruli. Increased echogenicity during the acute

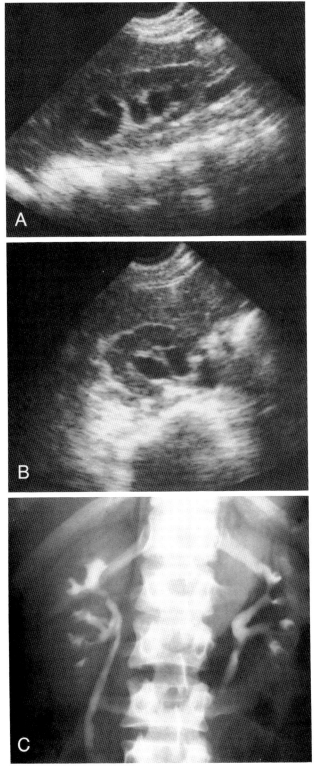

Figure 7.8. Longitudinal (*A*) and transverse (*B*) sonograms that strongly resemble calyceal dilatation. This patient has multiple peripelvic cysts which are illustrated by the excretory urogram (*C*).

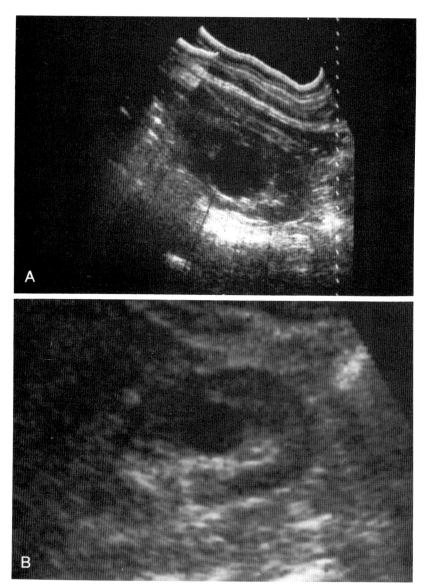

Figure 7.9.   Longitudinal (A) and oblique (B) scans of a patient with a large parapelvic cyst. The combination of these scans clearly discloses a centrally positioned fluid collection to be a discrete cyst rather than a dilated intrarenal collecting system.

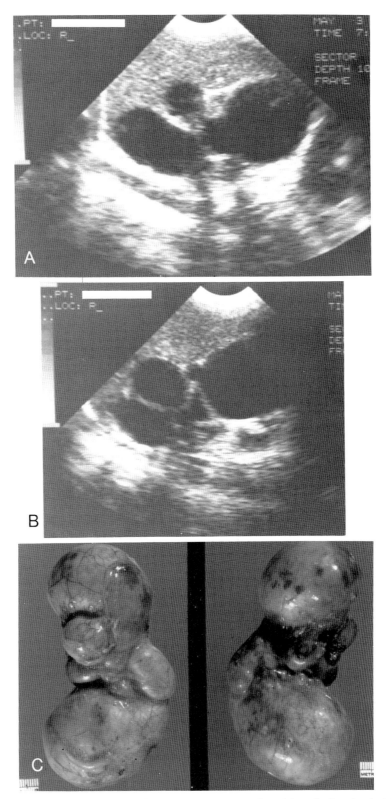

Figure 7.10. *A* and *B*, Two longitudinal scans of a typical multicystic dysplastic kidney. Note the disparity in the size of the cysts, the lack of communication between the cysts, and the absence of parenchymal tissue at the periphery of the cysts. *C*, Pathological specimen demonstrating the close correlation of the ultrasound appearance to the gross pathology of this malformation.

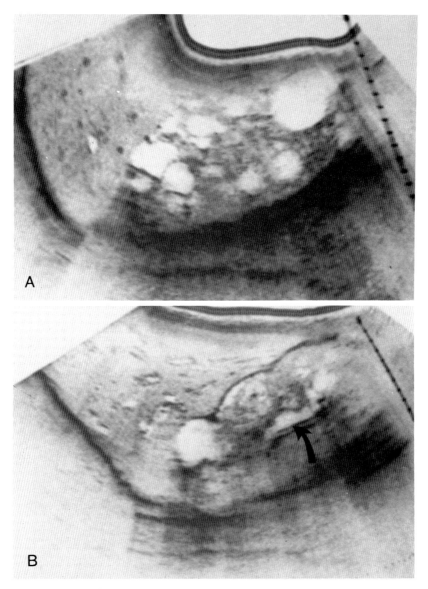

Figure 7.11. *A*, Longitudinal sonogram of a patient with typical polycystic kidney disease. Note that the kidney is markedly enlarged, the cysts are variable in size, and are randomly distributed through the renal parenchyma. *B*, Despite the presence of numerous cysts, a dilated intrarenal system is detected (*arrow*).

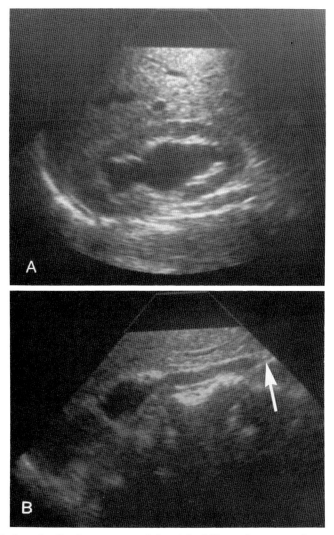

Figure 7.12. *A*, Longitudinal sonogram of the right kidney demonstrating severe pelvicalyceal dilatation. *B*, The ureter could be traced to its mid-portion where a tapered obstruction (*arrow*) was detected.

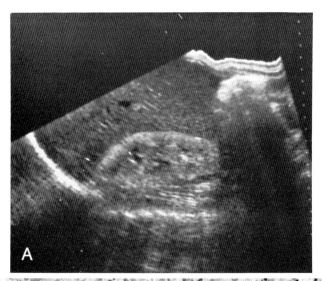

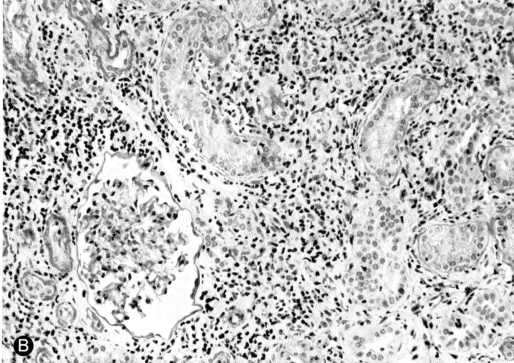

Figure 7.13.   *A*, Longitudinal sonogram of the right kidney in a patient with acute interstitial nephritis. Note the marked increase in cortical echogenicity. *B*, Histological specimen documents marked interstitial infiltration with lymphocytes, macrophages, and polymorphonuclear leukocytes.

stage of glomerulonephritis supports the premise that interstitial cellularity influences renal parenchymal echogenicity (22, 23).

Aside from those sporadic cases, the vast majority of patients with medically caused acute renal failure display a normal sonogram. Therefore, visualization of abnormal renal parenchyma should raise the possibility of chronicity of the renal failure. Importantly, if the renal parenchyma is abnormal, even unilateral obstruction may have resulted in a significant worsening of renal failure (Fig. 7.14). Not uncommonly, a patient with abnormal renal function cannot be clinically judged with regard to chronicity. Chronic renal failure is often insidious, the patient only recognizing symptoms in the recent past. Patient denial of disease is common. Sonographic assessment of renal vol-

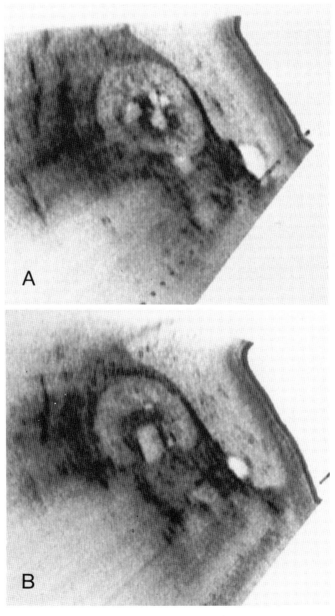

Figure 7.14. Two transverse images of the right kidney demonstrating an abnormal increase in renal cortical echogenicity. Note that this patient has moderate pelvicaliectasis. In such patients even unilateral hydronephrosis should be viewed with suspicion.

ume may help to differentiate acute (normal to large kidneys) and chronic (small kidneys) renal disease in patients with unrevealing histories (35). However, in some chronic conditions, such as membranoproliferative glomerulonephritis, the kidney remains of normal size.

When the ARF is caused by acute bilateral renal vein thrombosis (RVT), sonography may reveal bilateral renal enlargement and decreased echogenicity, probably reflecting edema. In the subacute phase (10 days to 3 weeks), there is usually increased cortical echogenicity with preserved corticomedullary definition (36, 37). A more specific sonographic finding of RVT is direct visualization of thrombus in the renal vein and inferior vena cava (38).

The Solitary Kidney

Although all of the aforementioned renal and postrenal causes of ARF can affect a solitary kidney, their relative frequencies change. Urinary tract obstruction becomes the most com-

mon cause of ARF (7, 16, 39), and etiologies of unilateral obstruction, such as calculi and sloughed papillae, assume a more prominent role. Unexpected entities can produce ARF in a solitary kidney, such as obstruction by a polyhydramniotic gravid uterus (40). A single kidney is also more susceptible to major renal vessel disease, either arterial or venous (7, 16, 26, 39).

In the setting of ARF of a solitary kidney, additional entities must be considered as well. Acute pyelonephritis is usually unilateral, and thus rarely causes ARF when two functioning kidneys are present (10). Renal sonography in a patient with acute pyelonephritis is often normal (21), but it may reveal renal enlargement with hypoechoic parenchyma and increased through transmission of sound (Fig. 7.15) (10, 41). ARF of a solitary kidney may also result from an extensive renal neoplasm, particularly when there is invasion of the renal vein. Perirenal abnormalities, such as abscess or hematoma, may also result in ARF in this setting (7, 16, 26, 39).

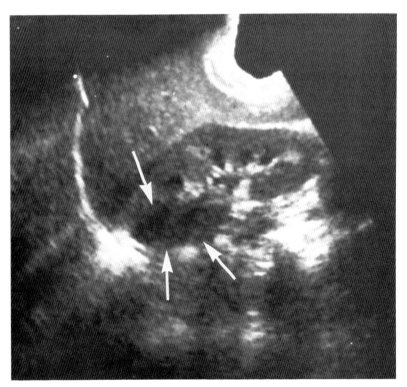

Figure 7.15.   Longitudinal sonogram of a solitary right kidney in a patient with symptoms of acute pyelonephritis. Note that the kidney is enlarged, and there is compression of the central sinus fat echoes, minimal dilatation of the renal pelvis, and a focal area of hypoechogenicity (*arrows*) at the posteromedial aspect of the kidney. The latter is presumably an area of focal bacterial nephritis.

Pediatric Acute Renal Failure

ARF in the pediatric population may be prerenal, renal, or postrenal in etiology, just as in the adult. As in the adult, the primary role of sonography in a child with ARF is to exclude urinary dilatation. Pelvic neoplasms, retroperitoneal fibrosis (42), and sloughed papillae all may cause urinary obstruction in children, but calculi and blood clots play a proportionately greater role than in adults (43). Congenital anomalies, such as posterior urethral valves, also deserve consideration, particularly in infants (44).

As for renal medical disease, many of the same entities that cause ARF in the adult, such as ATN, acute glomerulonephritis, and RVT, have similar sonographic manifestations in children. One important difference in pediatric RVT is the clinical setting. Unlike adults, infants with RVT have normal underlying kidneys, usually developing RVT secondary to dehydration (15, 43).

Other renal medical diseases must also be considered in the pediatric population. Hemolytic-uremic syndrome, a thrombotic disease of the small intrarenal vessels (1), is an important cause of pediatric ARF (45) that may present with sonographically normal kidneys (46). Infantile polycystic kidney disease (IPKD) is an autosomal recessive disorder characterized by multiple small renal cysts and hepatic periportal fibrosis. Depending on the extent of renal involvement, ARF may be a prominent clinical feature (43). Sonographically, the kidneys are enlarged with increased parenchymal echogenicity obliterating the corticomedullary junction (Fig. 7.16) (34, 47).

In infants with ARF, renal hypoplasia should be considered. Bilateral hypoplasia is a rare anomaly in which the total mass of renal tissue is insufficient to maintain normal growth and development (43). Obviously, hypoplasia indicates some element of chronicity, but the child is usually first evaluated in a setting which corresponds to ARF. Sonographically, hypoplasia manifests as decreased renal size usually associated with increased parenchymal echogenicity (Fig. 7.17). In one series (48), hypoplasia accounted for 3 of 10 infants with renal failure.

A rare cause of ARF that has a specific sonographic appearance is primary hyperoxaluria. In this hereditary disorder, there is increased excretion of calcium oxalate crystals which are deposited in the renal parenchyma (43). Sonography demonstrates remarkably increased parenchymal echogenicity, greater than that seen in IPKD. Unlike IPKD, in primary hyperoxaluria the corticomedullary distinction is preserved (49). The ultrasound appearance is probably distinctive enough, combined with the clinical setting, to render renal biopsy unnecessary.

Sonographically Guided Intervention

As previously mentioned, the sonographic diagnosis of urinary dilatation does not establish

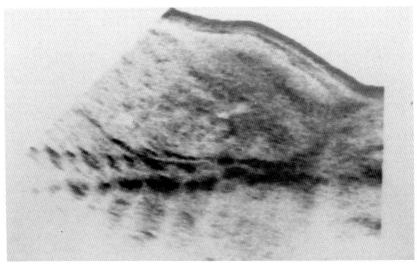

Figure 7.16. Typical appearance of infantile polycystic disease in a newborn with severe renal malfunction. The kidney is markedly enlarged and shows diffuse echogenicity of the central portion. This diffuse echogenicity obliterates all medullary detail.

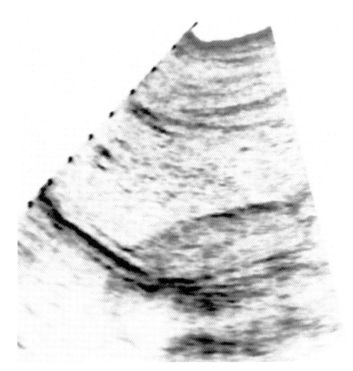

Figure 7.17. Longitudinal sonogram of a young child demonstrating a hypoplastic kidney. Note the marked increase in parenchymal echogenicity and the loss of intrarenal architectural detail.

the presence of urinary obstruction, nor does it define the nature of the abnormality if obstruction exists. In this setting, antegrade pyelography guided by ultrasound and fluoroscopy provides excellent detail of the collecting structures (2). Using local anesthesia and ultrasound guidance, a 22-gauge Chiba needle is passed into the dilated renal pelvis from a posterolateral approach. Once urine is aspirated, contrast is injected to opacify the collecting system. If urinary obstruction is demonstrated, an 18-gauge needle is passed under fluoroscopic guidance. Percutaneous urinary drainage then can be accomplished by passing a guidewire through the 18-gauge needle and then inserting a pigtail catheter over the guidewire. No significant complications have resulted from bilateral antegrade pyelography (2), and, with combined sonographic and fluoroscopic guidance, percutaneous nephrostomy insertion has been successful in well over 90% of patients (50). Ultrasound guidance also facilitates renal biopsy in patients without urinary dilatation (51).

CONCLUSION

In summary, sonography is easy, rapid, inexpensive, and noninvasive. Its ability to detect

surgically correctable acute renal failure without the administration of potentially harmful contrast agents makes it the examination of choice for patients with ARF. Sonography has the added advantage of being able to direct interim percutaneous urinary drainage, allowing for stabilization of the ARF patient prior to definitive therapy.

References

1. Kerr DNS: Acute renal failure. In Black D, Jones NF: *Renal Disease.* Oxford, Blackwell Scientific Publications, 1979, pp 437–493.
2. Hricak H: Ultrasound and the azotemic patient. In Margulis AR, Gooding CA: *Diagnostic Radiology.* San Francisco, University of California School of Medicine, 1982, pp 385–392.
3. Griffiths HJ: *Radiology of Renal Failure.* Philadelphia, WB Saunders, 1976, p 23.
4. Talner LB, Scheible W, Ellenbogen PH, Beck CH Jr, Gosink BB: How accurate is ultrasonography in detecting hydronephrosis in azotemic patients? *Urol Radiol* 3:1–6, 1981.
5. Damascelli B, Lattuada A, Musemci R, Severini A: Two-dimensional ultrasonic investigations of the urinary tract. *Br J Radiol* 41:837–843, 1968.
6. Sanders RC, Bearman S: B-scan ultrasound in the diagnosis of hydronephrosis. *Radiology* 108:375–382, 1973.
7. Sanders RC: The place of diagnostic ultrasound

in the examination of kidneys not seen on excretory urography. *J Urol* 114:813–821, 1975.

8. Sanders RC, Jeck DL: B-scan ultrasound in the evaluation of renal failure. *Radiology* 119:199–202, 1976.

9. Ellenbogen PH, Scheible RW, Talner LB, Leopold GR: Sensitivity of gray scale ultrasound in detecting urinary tract obstruction. *AJR* 130:731–733, 1978.

10. Hricak H: Renal medical disorders—role of sonography. In Sanders RC: *Ultrasound Annual.* New York, Raven Press, 1982, pp 43–80.

11. Malave SR, Neiman HL, Spies SM, Cisternino SJ, Adamo G: Diagnosis of hydronephrosis: comparison of radionuclide scanning and sonography. *AJR* 135:1179–1185, 1980.

12. Schrier RW: Acute renal failure: pathogenesis, diagnosis, and management. *Hosp Practice* 16:93–112, 1981.

13. Robbins SL, Cotran RS: *Pathologic Basis of Disease.* Philadelphia, WB Saunders, 1979, pp 1149–1152.

14. Epstein FH: Acute renal failure. In Wintrobe MM, Thorn GW, Adams RD, Braunwald E, Isselbacher KJ, Petersdorf RG: *Harrison's Principles of Internal Medicine.* New York, McGraw-Hill, 1974, pp 1383–1388.

15. Clark RA, Wyatt GM, Colley DP: Renal vein thrombosis: an underdiagnosed complication of multiple renal abnormalities. *Radiology* 132:43–50, 1979.

16. Behan M, Wixson D, Kazam E: Sonographic evaluation of the nonfunctioning kidney. *J Clin Ultrasound* 7:449–458, 1979.

17. Lee JKT, Baron RL, Melson GL, McClennan BL, Weyman PJ: Can real-time ultrasonography replace static B-scanning in the diagnosis of renal obstruction? *Radiology* 139:161–165, 1981.

18. Thompson IM, Kovac A, Geshner J: Coronal renal ultrasound. II. *Urology* 17:210–213, 1981.

19. Bazzocchi M, Rizzatto G: The value of the posterior oblique longitudinal scan in renal ultrasonography. *Urol Radiol* 1:221–225, 1980.

20. Maklad NF: Ultrasound in acute renal failure. *Clin Diag Ultrasound* 7:166–181, 1981.

21. Rosenfield AT: Ultrasound evaluation of renal parenchymal disease and hydronephrosis. *Urol Radiol* 4:125–133, 1982.

22. Rosenfield AT, Siegel NJ: Renal parenchymal disease: histopathologic-sonographic correlation. *AJR* 137:793–798, 1981.

23. Hricak H, Cruz C, Romanski R, Uniewski MG, Levin NW, Madrazo BL, Sandler MA, Eyler WR: Renal parenchymal disease: sonographic-histologic correlation. *Radiology* 144:141–147, 1982.

24. Haller JO, Berdon WE, Friedman AP: Increased renal cortical echogenicity: a normal finding in neonates and infants. *Radiology* 142:173–174, 1982.

25. Hricak H, Slovis T, Alpers CE, Callen PE, Romanski RN: Neonatal kidneys—sonographic anatomic correlation. *Radiology* 147:699–702, 1983.

26. Sanders RC: Examination of kidneys not seen at excretion urography. In Resnick MI, Sanders RC: *Ultrasound in Urology.* Baltimore, Williams & Wilkins, 1979, pp 146–169.

27. Rosenfield AT: Renal and adrenal ultrasonography. In Syllabus for the categorical course in ultrasonography, presented at the annual meeting of the American Roentgen Ray Society, San Francisco, March 22–27, 1981, pp 27–58.

28. Curry NS, Gobien RP, Schabel SI: Minimal-dilatation obstructive nephropathy. *Radiology* 143:531–534, 1982.

29. Cronan JJ, Amis ES Jr, Yoder IC, Kopans DB, Simeone JF, Pfister RC: Peripelvic cysts: an imposter of sonographic hydronephrosis. *J Ultrasound Med* 1:229–236, 1982.

30. Rosenfield AT, Taylor KJW, Crade M, DeGraaf CS: Anatomy and pathology of the kidney by gray scale ultrasound. *Radiology* 128:737–744, 1978.

31. Ralls PW, Esensten ML, Boger D, Halls JM: Severe hydronephrosis and severe renal cystic disease: ultrasonic differentiation. *AJR* 134:473–475, 1980.

32. Babcock DS: Medical diseases of the urinary tract and adrenal glands. *Clin Diag Ultrasound* 8:113–134, 1981.

33. Rochester D, Aronson AJ, Bowie JD, Kunzmann A: Ultrasonic appearance of acute poststreptococcal glomerulonephritis. *J Clin Ultrasound* 6:49–50, 1978.

34. LeQuesne GW: Assessment of glomerulonephritis in children by ultrasound. In White D, Lyons EA: *Ultrasound in Medicine.* New York, Plenum Press, 1978.

35. Winston M, Pritchard J, Paulin P: Ultrasonography in the management of unexplained renal failure. *J Clin Ultrasound* 6:23–27, 1978.

36. Rosenfield AT, Zeman RK, Cronan JJ, Taylor KJW: Ultrasound in experimental and clinical renal vein thrombosis. *Radiology* 137:735–741, 1980.

37. Hricak H, Sandler MA, Madrazo BL, Eyler WR: Sonographic findings following acute renal vein thrombosis—experimental study. *Invest Radiol* 16:30–35, 1981.

38. Braun B, Weilemann LS, Weigland W: Ultrasonographic demonstration of renal vein thrombosis. *Radiology* 138:157–158, 1981.

39. Marangola JP, Bryan PJ, Azimi F: Ultrasonic evaluation of the unilateral nonvisualized kidney. *AJR* 126:853–862, 1976.

40. Homans DC, Blake GD, Harrington JT, Cetrulo CL: Acute renal failure caused by ureteral obstruction by a gravid uterus. *JAMA* 246:1230–1231, 1981.

41. Edell SL, Bonavita JA: The sonographic appearance of acute pyelonephritis. *Radiology* 132:683–685, 1979.

42. Birnberg FA, Vinstein AL, Gorlick G, Lee FA, Hales MS: Retroperitoneal fibrosis in children. *Radiology* 145:59–61, 1982.

43. Drummond KN: The urinary system. In Vaughan VC III, McKay RJ, Nelson WE: *Nelson Textbook of Pediatrics.* Philadelphia, WB Saunders, 1975, pp 1166–1258.

44. Glazer GM, Filly RA, Callen PW: The varied sonographic appearance of the urinary tract in the fetus and newborn with urethral obstruction. *Radiology* 144:563–568, 1982.

45. Teele RL: Ultrasonography of the genitourinary tract in children. *Radiol Clin North Am* 15:109–128, 1982.

46. Sumner TE: Pediatric ultrasonography. In Resnick MI, Sanders RC: *Ultrasound in Urology*. Baltimore, Williams & Wilkins, 1979, pp 275–302.

47. Metreweli C, Garel L: The echographic diagnosis of infantile renal polycystic disease. *Ann Radiol* 23:103–107, 1980.

48. Boineau FG, Rothman J, Lewy JE: Nephrosonography in the evaluation of renal failure and masses in infants. *J Pediatr* 87:195–201, 1975.

49. Brennan JN, Diwan RV, Makker SP, Cromer BA, Bellon EM: Ultrasonic diagnosis of primary hyperoxaluria in infancy. *Radiology* 145:147–148, 1982.

50. Stables DP, Johnson ML: Percutaneous nephrostomy: the role of ultrasound. *Clin Diag Ultrasound* 2:73–87, 1979.

51. Shkolnik A: B-mode ultrasound and the nonvisualizing kidney in pediatrics. *AJR* 128:121–125, 1977.

CHAPTER 8

Nonvisualized Kidney on Intravenous Pyelogram as Assessed by Sonography

ROGER C. SANDERS, M.D.

This relatively uncommon situation following high dose urography with tomography can be well assessed by sonography. Most cases are due to hydronephrosis, multicystic kidney, or small end-stage kidneys. Multicystic kidney and hydronephrosis are examined in detail in other chapters. A variety of other rarer lesions, mainly of vascular or tumorous origin, will be considered in the latter part of this chapter

Hydronephrosis is unquestionably the most common cause of a nonvisualized kidney on urography. The appearances are the same on a unilateral basis as those described in Chapter 7. If the kidney is not visible on urography because of hydronephrosis, it is almost always severely and permanently damaged. The amount of remaining renal parenchyma will be minimal. Either a large, single, cystic structure with minimal border lobulations will be seen or, more commonly, the calyces will be visible separated by apparent septa and connected to a large renal pelvis. The dilated ureter may be traceable toward the true pelvis from the renal pelvis.

If a nonfunctioning hydronephrotic kidney is found, several possible associations should be considered. The contents of the collecting system should be examined in some detail because if the patient is febrile with local pain, pyonephrosis is a possibility. Pus can either form low level echoes within the urine, develop a fluid-fluid level, or, rarely, look completely sonolucent (1). Another possibility is xanthogranulomatous pyelonephritis, which in its most common form is seen as a centrally located calculus with secondary hydronephrosis. Typically, the pelvis becomes contracted while the calyces remain quite large (Fig. 8.1).

Another entity associated with hydronephrosis is ureterocele. A dilated ureter will be traceable from the kidney toward the pelvis, and

examination of the bladder will show the typical cobra-headed deformity of an ectopic ureterocele (2, 3).

A second cause of unilateral nonvisualizing kidney on urography is the small kidney. A variety of different lesions cause a small kidney, but they are difficult to separate pathologically, radiologically, and sonographically. A small kidney may, for example, be a consequence of postobstructive atrophy, "hypoplasia," long-standing renal venous occlusion, chronic pyelonephritis, renal artery stenosis, or gouty nephritis. The sonographic appearances of the first three lesions are similar (Fig. 8.2), but it may be possible to see areas of focal parenchymal deficiency due to scarring with infarct or infection (Fig. 8.3). Whereas bilateral small end-stage kidneys cause uremia and compel the patient to present with symptoms when the kidneys shrink to approximately 6 to 8 cm in length, a unilateral small kidney may decrease to a tiny size (less than 2 cm) before symptoms occur or may always be symptom free. Such kidneys, however, may cause hypertension or chronic infection. It is usually possible to distinguish the sinus echoes from the renal parenchyma even when the kidney is small; the parenchyma in unilateral small kidneys can become echogenic but rarely to the point of a loss of visualization of renal anatomy.

Even with modern real-time scanners it may be difficult to distinguish a very small end-stage kidney from renal agenesis with a loop of bowel where the kidney should be (Fig. 8.4). The sonolucent bowel wall can resemble the renal parenchyma, and the echoes at the center of an empty bowel loop resemble the renal pelvis. In left renal agenesis, the splenic flexure falls into the site where the kidney normally lies (4). Renal agenesis is associated with such genital anoma-

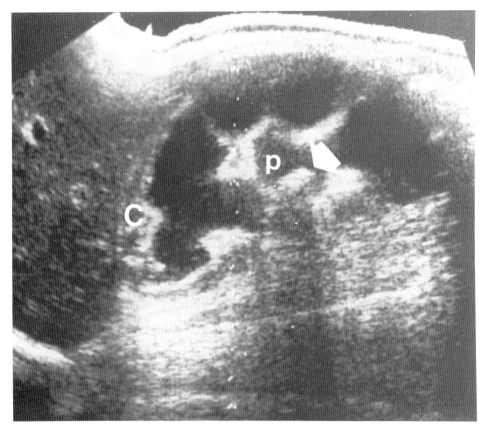

Figure 8.1.   Longitudinal section. Xanthrogranulomatous pyelonephritis. Although the kidney shows evidence of hydronephrosis, the pelvis (*p*) is relatively small. Note the calculus (*arrow*) at the center of the kidney. There is virtually no renal cortex (*C*).

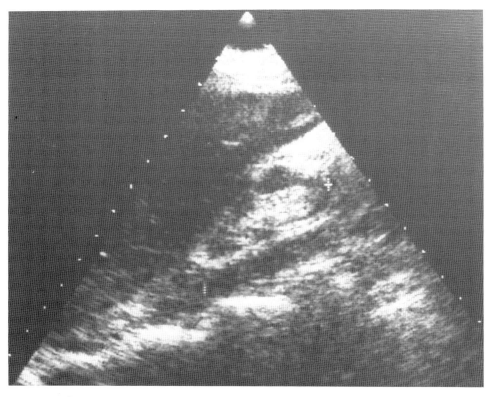

Figure 8.2.   Small end-stage kidney due to vascular disease. Note the relative symmetry of the renal parenchyma.

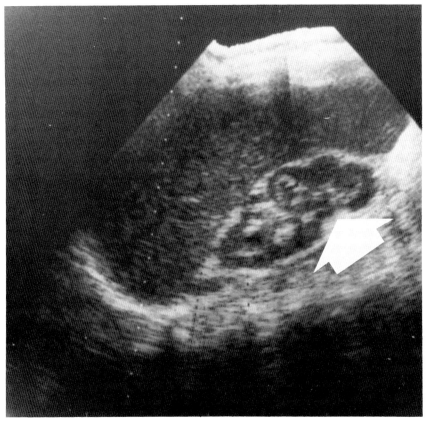

Figure 8.3. Small kidney damaged by chronic pyelonephritis. Note the scarring (*arrow*) and varying parenchymal depth.

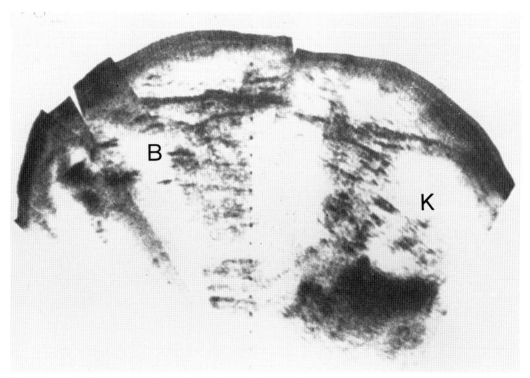

Figure 8.4. Transverse view of a patient with renal agenesis; a left kidney was thought to be present at the time of the study (*B*). At laparotomy, the supposed kidney was shown to be due to the colon. *K*, right kidney.

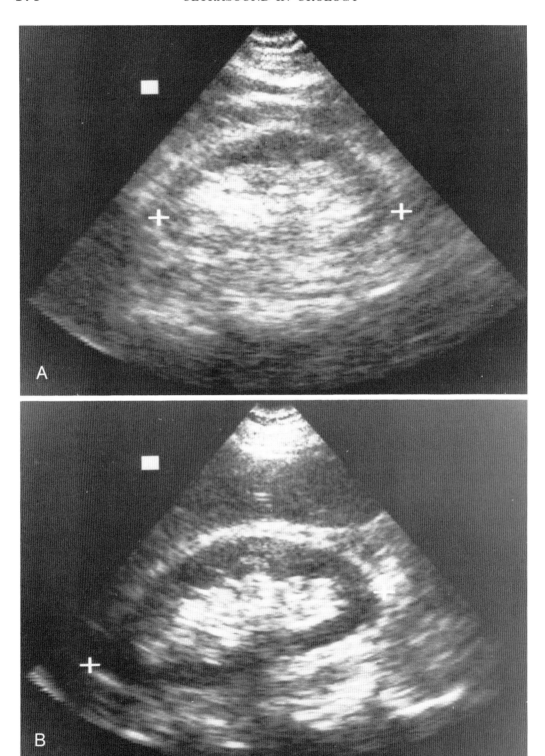

Figure 8.5. Renal artery occlusion due to a bicycle accident. Longitudinal section of left kidney. Note the slight shrinkage in the renal parenchyma but the normal-appearing sinus echoes. This sonogram was performed about 2 weeks after injury. *B*, Sonogram of the normal right kidney. Note normal thickness of the renal parenchyma. *C*, Renal arteriogram showing complete left renal artery occlusion.

lies as uterovaginal atresia or double uterus and vagina and seminal vesicle cyst (5).

Renal vascular problems may be responsible for nonvisualization of the kidney. In renal artery occlusion, the initial response of the kidney is renal enlargement due to edema. There is a slow decrease in renal size; it takes weeks or months for the kidney to decrease to the small size that is characteristic of renal artery occlusion. The diagnostic findings in acute renal artery occlusion will be an inconsistency between the intravenous pyelogram and the sonographic appearances (Fig. 8.5, *A* to *C*). An enlarged, normal-sized, or small kidney will be seen on the sonogram. There will be an overall normal configuration but no renal visualization on the intravenous urogram or on the nuclear medicine scan (6). Such absence of renal function does not necessarily mean a complete renal infarct. Occlusion of the dorsal or ventral renal artery can lead to complete nonfunction of the kidney, although only half of the kidney is infarcted. Focal renal infarcts usually initially give rise to a zone of hypoechoic renal parenchyma (7), but a few echogenic lesions have been described (8)

(Fig. 8.6). This appears to be a later finding (9). Such an echogenic area may represent a hemorrhagic infarct. Theoretically the demonstration of thrombus in the renal artery is possible, but this has not been achieved in practice.

Renal vein thrombosis is a confusing entity from a sonographic viewpoint. This condition usually occurs in infants and small children and is associated with vomiting, diarrhea, sepsis, and dehydration. It may lead to or be a consequence of membranous glomerulonephritis (10) with the nephrotic syndrome. In older individuals it may be secondary to trauma, tumor, or pregnancy related. It is three times as common on the left due to the long course of the left renal vein and the "nutcracker" effect as the left renal vein is compressed between the superior mesenteric artery and the aorta. Varicoceles are a common consequence of left renal vein partial obstruction (11).

The kidney enlarges in acute renal vein thrombosis and slowly contracts with long term thrombosis. The central sinus and parenchymal echoes are not predictably distorted by venous thrombosis (12). In some instances the sinus

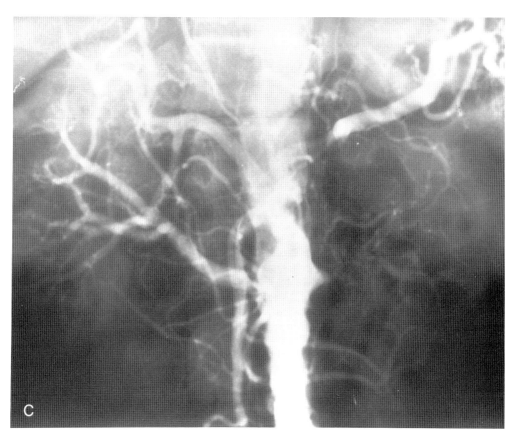

Figure 8.5C.

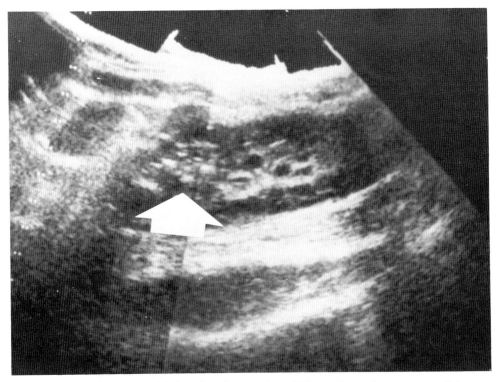

Figure 8.6. Renal infarct of left pole of transplant kidney shown by an area of increased echogenicity (*arrow*).

echoes increase in size (Fig. 8.7, *A to C*); in others there is a diminution and a disorganization of the sinus echoes (13). Presumably, the pattern variability relates to the amount of hemorrhage that occurs. The cortex is consistently less echogenic. Although the kidney is swollen in the first 2 weeks, it becomes more echogenic as it shrinks with time as fibrosis occurs (12). Recognition is easier with unilateral as opposed to bilateral renal vein thrombosis since size increase is the principal indication of abnormality. Focal sonolucent areas due to hematoma may occur. The sinus echoes may be distorted or displaced (9). Focal echogenic areas with renal vein thrombosis possibly represent small infarcts (10). Thrombus within the renal vein may be demonstrable with high quality real-time systems, particularly on the left (13, 14). Many examples of renal vein thrombosis have been described in association with renal tumors, particularly hypernephroma (15–17).

The usual cause of nonvisualization of the kidney with intravenous pyelography when tumor is present in renal vein thrombus; however, the tumor may involve the whole kidney (18).

Hypernephroma is by far the most common tumor that causes complete nonvisualization of the kidney.

Nonvisualization can also occur in transitional cell tumors since they are strategically centrally located and often cause hydronephrosis; other tumors, such as lymphoma or multiple angiomyolipomas, can rarely involve the whole kidney.

Severe acute pyelonephritis or multiple renal abscesses can cause nonvisualization on the intravenous pyelogram. The kidney swells and with focal infection, selective enlargement of one or other pole may be seen; the kidney in the involved area is also less echogenic. Multiple abscesses are seen as hypoechoic, well-defined areas within the renal parenchyma sometimes containing low level echoes. Ultrasound is of value in showing that the lesion contains fluid-filled areas compatible with pus (Fig. 8.8), as opposed to the more subtle changes seen with acute pyelonephritis (Fig. 8.9). The latter is usually treated with antibiotics, whereas abscesses are drained.

An important, although rare, cause of nonvi-

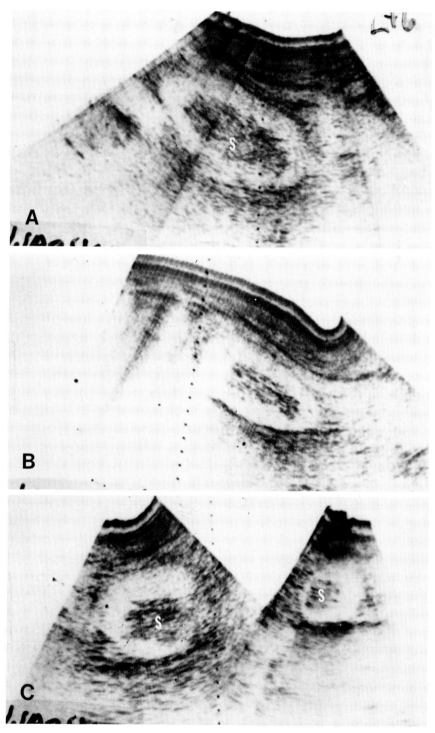

Figure 8.7. *A,* Longitudinal view. Acute renal vein thrombosis. Kidney is enlarged and has a prominent sinus echo pattern (*S*). *B,* Normal kidney in the same patient which is much smaller and with a smaller pelvic echo pattern. *C,* Transverse section shows the two kidneys side by side. Note the difference in size of the kidneys as a whole and of the pelvic echoes (*S*).

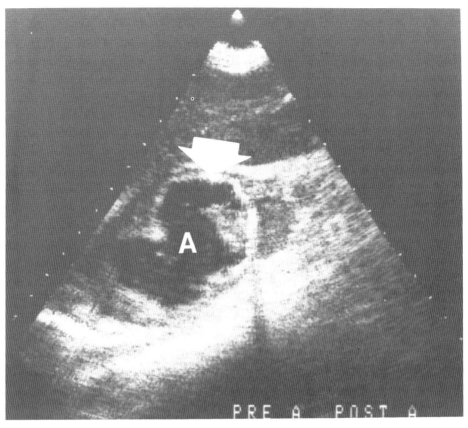

Figure 8.8.   Duplicated system with pyonephrotic upper segment (*A*). The pyonephrosis has a relatively dense echogenic rim (*arrow*). There are some echoes within the infected urine.

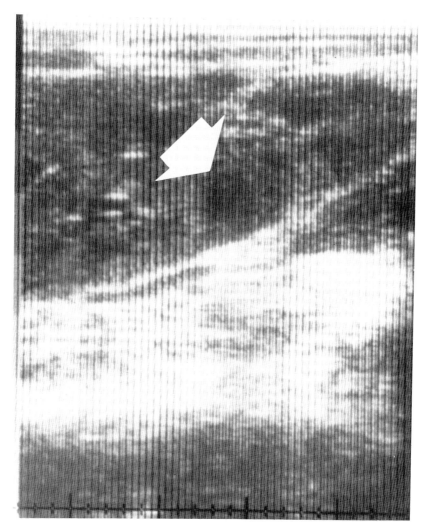

Figure 8.9. Acute pyelonephritis. Real-time longitudinal study. Hypoechoic area (*arrow*) is due to an area of acute pyelonephritis.

sualization of a kidney on a unilateral basis is Page kidney (Fig. 8.10). In this condition following trauma, hematoma deposition with subsequent fibrosis occurs around the kidney forming a shell so that the kidney is unable to expand. (There is normally considerable variability in kidney size with respiration and pulsation.) Some Page kidneys fail to function normally, and the patient becomes hypertensive. The perinephric collection of blood can have a variety of different appearances, but at the stage at which it causes hypertension it is usually mildly echogenic (19, 20).

Sonography is valuable in renal trauma, although it may be technically difficult due to overlying bandaging or wounds. Traumatic dam-

age to the kidney by gun or knife wound may involve the renal artery and can result in nonvisualization on the intravenous pyelogram if the artery is transected. Sonography will show a normal-appearing kidney if the renal artery has been interrupted between the aorta and kidney or evidence of renal damage if occlusion occurred in the kidney itself.

If there is a laceration of the kidney, it may be possible to see a line through the kidney at the fracture site and an irregular renal border (21, 22); a perirenal collection of blood and urine is usual. A fresh hematoma is usually echo free, but echoes rapidly develop within the collection. A combination of echo-free and echogenic areas in or around the kidney can indicate the pres-

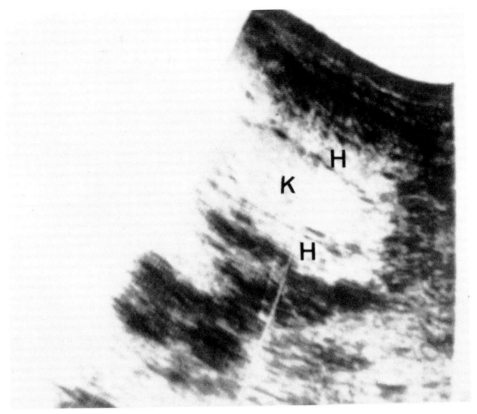

Figure 8.10. Decubitus view of a kidney (*K*) surrounded by a large well-organized hematoma (*H*) resulting in the Page kidney phenomenon. (Reprinted with permission from Conrad et al. (19).)

ence of urine and blood. Hematoma may be completely intrarenal or, as is usually the case, involve only the perinephric space. Management of renal lesions associated with trauma is not clear cut, but undoubtedly ultrasound is helpful in demonstrating whether a perirenal collection is expanding or decreasing in size on serial studies.

It is not uncommon for unexpected renal pathology to be revealed when trauma occurs. Wilms' tumor or severe hydronephrosis may not cause symptoms prior to trauma and be obvious on a sonogram after the injury.

References

1. Subramanyam BR, Raghavendra BN, Bosniak MA, et al: Sonography of pyonephrosis: a prospective study. *AJR* 140:991–993, 1983.
2. Sumner TE, Crowe JE, Resnick MI: Diagnosis of ectopic ureterocele using ultrasound. *Urology* 15:82, 1980.
3. Mascatello VJ, Smith EH, Carrera GF, et al: Ultrasonic evaluation of the obstructed duplex kidney. *AJR* 129:113–120, 1977.
4. Teele RL, Rosenfield AT, Friedman GF: Anatomic splenic flexure and ultrasonic renal impostor. *AJR* 128:115–120, 1977.
5. Cohen RC, Davey RB, LeQuesne GW: Ultrasonography in the diagnosis and management of unilateral hematometracolpos and associated renal agenesis. *Aust Paediatr J* 18:287–290, 1982.
6. Sanders RC, Menon S, Sanders AD: The complementary uses of nuclear medicine and ultrasound in the kidney. *J Urol* 120:521, 1978.
7. Allibone GW: Renal infarction presenting as a mass: diagnostic role of computerized tomography and ultrasound. *Urology* 19:98, 1982.
8. Erwin BC, Carroll BA, Walter JF, et al: Renal infarction appearing as an echogenic mass. *AJR* 138:759–761, 1982.
9. Hricak H, Sandler MA, Madrazo RL, et al: Sonographic manifestations of acute renal vein thrombosis: an experimental study. *Invest Radiol* 16:30, 1980.
10. Bradley WG, Jacobs RP, Trew PA, et al: Renal vein thrombosis: occurrence in membranous glomerulonephropathy and lupus nephritis. *Radiology* 139:571–576, 1981.
11. Zerhouni EA, Siegelman SS, Walsh PC, White RI: Elevated pressure in the left renal vein in patients with varicocele: preliminary observa-

tions. *J Urol* 123:512, 1980.

12. Lam AH, Warren PS: Ultrasonographic diagnosis of neonatal renal venous thrombosis. *Ann Radiol* 24:7–12, 1981.

13. Fowler JE, Paciulli J: Renal vein thrombosis: diagnosis by B-scan ultrasonography. *J Urol* 118:849, 850, 1977.

14. Braun B, Wilemann LS, Weigand W: Ultrasonographic demonstration of renal vein thrombosis. *Radiology* 138:157–158, 1981.

15. Thomas JL, Bernardino ME: Neoplastic-induced renal vein enlargement: sonographic detection. *AJR* 136:75–79, 1981.

16. Goldstein HM, Green B, Weaver RM: Ultrasonic detection of renal tumor extension into the inferior vena cava. *AJR* 130:1083–1085, 1978.

17. Walzer A, Weiner SN, Koenigsberg M: The ultrasound appearance of tumor extension into the left renal vein and inferior vena cava. *J Urol* 123:945–946, 1980.

18. Behan M, Wixson D, Kazam E: Sonographic evaluation of the nonfunctioning kidney. *J Clin Ultrasound* 7:449–458, 1979.

19. Conrad MR, Freedman M, Weiner C, et al: Sonography of the Page kidney. *J Urol* 116:293, 1976.

20. Chamorro HA, Forbes TW, Padkowsky GO, et al: Multiimaging approach in the diagnosis of Page kidney. *AJR* 136:620–621, 1981.

21. Afschrift M, de Sy W, Voet D, et al: Fractured kidney and retroperitoneal hematoma diagnosed by ultrasound. *J Clin Ultrasound* 10:335–336, 1982.

22. Kay CH, Rosenfield AT, Armm M: Gray-scale ultrasonography in the evaluation of renal trauma. *Radiology* 134:461–466, 1980.

CHAPTER 9

Retroperitoneal Pathology

ROGER C. SANDERS, M.D.

Examination of the retroperitoneum by ultrasound is not easy. Supine or supine oblique views on the right usually show the adrenal and immediate perinephric tissue well. The coronal view used for the left kidney shows the perirenal area adequately on the left, but the psoas muscles and quadratus lumborum muscles may need to be examined in the prone position. The prone position is also required for the area inferior to the kidney which may otherwise be invisible due to overlying gas. The area in front of the sacrum where retroperitoneal fibrosis occurs can sometimes be seen on supine views but may be inaccessible due to gas.

The retroperitoneal area around the kidney is divided by fascial planes into a number of spaces (Fig. 9.1); two muscles also lie in the area—the psoas muscle and quadratus lumborum (Fig. 9.2). The capsule around the kidney is defined by an echogenic line which principally represents fat. This interface also indicates the margin between the peritoneum and the retroperitoneum and extends inferior and superior to the kidney; it is particularly obvious on the right and becomes quite sizable when there is significant perinephric fat around the kidney. Within the retroperitoneum; the fascial planes defining anterior pararenal and posterior pararenal spaces and Gerota's fascia are not easily distinguished by ultrasound but can be seen in some obese people when outlined by fat (1) (Fig. 9.3). Such fat has a variable acoustic pattern. Sometimes it is relatively echogenic (Fig. 9.4A); in other individuals, it is less echogenic so the fascial planes can be seen better (Fig. 9.3). Perirenal fat can reach such a size that it can be thought to represent a retroperitoneal mass (Fig. 9.4, A and B).

Collections and masses in the retroperitoneum in the vicinity of the kidney can develop in one of seven potential spaces around the kidney.

It is worthwhile recognizing which of the potential spaces a collection occupies because it

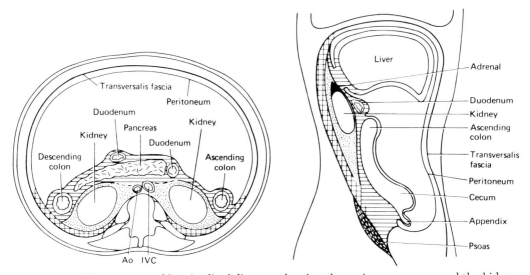

Figure 9.1. Transverse and longitudinal diagram showing the various spaces around the kidney. The *dotted area* is the perinephric space within Gerota's capsule. *Transverse strips* represent the anterior pararenal space, and the *cross-hatched* area is the posterior pararenal space. (Reproduced with permission of M. Meyers.)

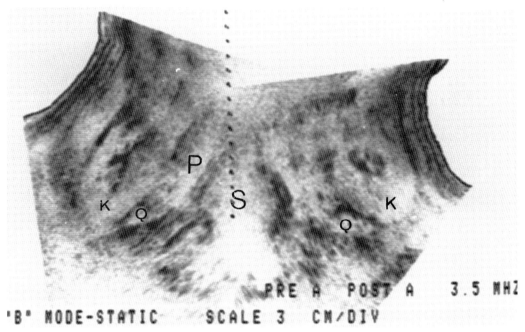

Figure 9.2. Transverse view showing the kidneys (*K*), the psoas muscles (*P*), and the quadratus lumborum muscles (*Q*) on either side of the spine (*S*). Note echogenic line around the kidneys (the capsule).

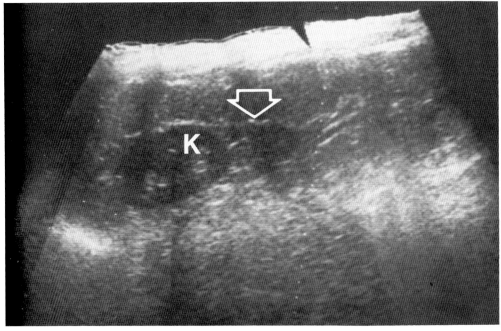

Figure 9.3.   Longitudinal prone section through kidney (*K*) which is surrounded by fat. Gerota's fascia (*arrow*) can be seen.

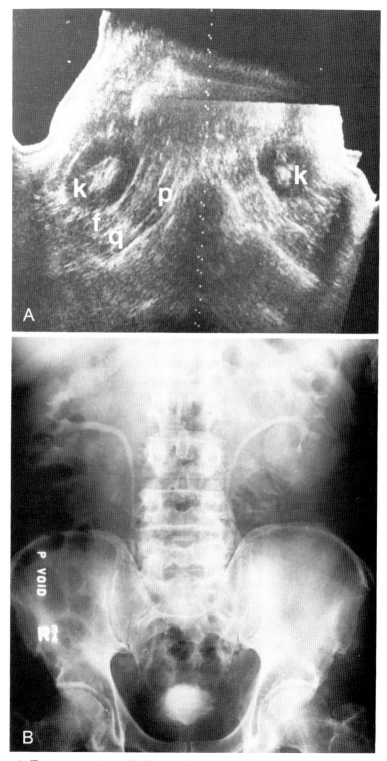

Figure 9.4.   *A,* Transverse view of kidneys (*k*) surrounded by much fat (*f*). In this case the fat is relatively echogenic. *p,* psoas; *q,* quadratus lumborum. *B,* Same case. The intravenous pyelogram had been interpreted as showing a perinephric mass with ureteric deviation. The supposed mass was actually due to fat.

can give a clue to the organ of origin (e.g., an anterior pararenal abscess may originate from pathology in the pancreas or stomach) or to potential complications (e.g., Page kidney).

1. Subcapsular. Subcapsular collections lie between the kidney and the capsule (Fig. 9.5, *A* and *B*). Such collections have a typical ultrasonic appearance, being rounded at both ends; they can be seen to distort and squash the kidney while encircling it. They may lie both anterior and posterior to the kidney simultaneously on ultrasonic examination and are surrounded by a well-defined line representing the renal capsule. Most commonly such collections are hematomas.

2. Posterior pararenal space. The posterior pararenal space lies posterior and extends lateral to the kidney (Fig. 9.6). It is posterior to Gerota's fascia and bordered by the lateroconal fascia. It extends far into the flanks and is long and lean in shape. A large lateral extension suggests the presence of a collection in this space.

3. Anterior pararenal space. The anterior pararenal space is continuous with the pancreas and passes across the midline (Fig. 9.7). It contains the pancreas, splenic and hepatic arteries, and the ascending and descending colon. An abscess originating in the epigastric area due to pancreatitis or a perforated ulcer can migrate a good distance in this space eventually to lie inferior to the kidney. Abscesses following trauma may occur in this area. The kidney shape is not altered.

4. Perirenal space. Gerota's fascia encloses a cone-shaped space—the perirenal space—which is open ended inferiorly and contains the kidney and adrenal glands. A large collection in this area may spread into the other spaces (Fig. 9.8). Most collections in this area are renal in origin, but pancreatic pseudocysts and aortic aneurysm leaks have been reported penetrating into the space. Really large perinephric collections can squash the kidney in a fashion similar to a subcapsular lesion, but this is most unusual.

5. Subhepatic space. Morrison's pouch is a portion of the peritoneal cavity which forms a recess anterior to the kidney and posterior to the liver. It is quite a common site of collections bulging and expanding what is normally only a potential space (Fig. 9.9).

6. Psoas muscles. The psoas muscles lie medial to the kidney and may be the site of an abscess or hematoma. Both processes can track along the muscle into the upper part of the thigh (Fig. 9.10, *A* and *B*).

7. Quadratus lumborum muscles. A less common site for a collection is within the quadratus lumborum and transversalis abdominus muscles posterior to the kidney. The quadratus lumborum muscle itself can be mistaken for an abscess (2) (Fig. 9.11); comparison to the contralateral muscle will show a similar acoustic texture. It can be distinctly less echogenic than the psoas muscle.

A number of organs lie in the vicinity of the kidneys.

Stomach and duodenum. One can often see evidence of the stomach anterior to the left kidney; it may appear as a sonolucent cystic area with high level echoes due to food posteriorly. If one suspects that a mass anterior to the left kidney is the stomach, a simple test is available. The patient drinks freshly run water through a straw. There will be the transitory creation of numerous microbubbles within the stomach contents; the gas within the bubbles prevents the transmission of sound, so one no longer sees the cystic organ. Within a few minutes the microbubbles disappear and the mass becomes visible again (3). Neoplasms of the stomach wall can be detected sonographically. If the stomach contains mucus but no fluid, one sees central echoes which, together with the sonolucent wall, create a typical "doughnut"-like pattern (4).

The duodenum has a medial anterior relationship to the right kidney and can resemble a cystic mass, although more commonly it is echo filled.

Colon. A difficult sonographic problem is the colon filled with fluid or fecal material. This can closely mimic a true mass. As yet no satisfactory method exists of proving that a mass is a colon full of intestinal contents—if real-time does not reveal peristalsis or if a high water enema is unhelpful—short of the performance of a repeat sonographic examination.

Liver. Anterior to and usually completely covering the kidney is the liver. The latter is separated from the kidney by the retroperitoneal fat line, so, as a rule, it is relatively easy to distinguish renal or retroperitoneal from hepatic masses (Fig. 9.12, *A* and *B*). However, hepatic pathology can secondarily invade the kidney if it is neoplastic. Hepatomegaly or intrahepatic masses can squash the kidney in such a fashion that the intravenous pyelogram gives the

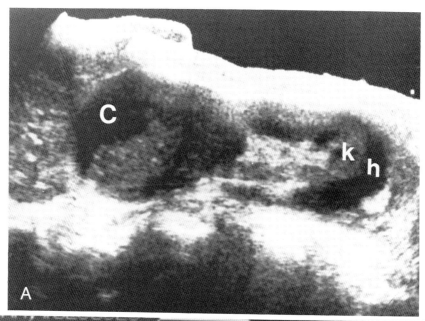

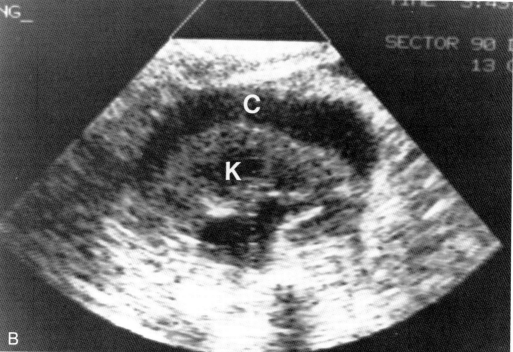

Figure 9.5. *A,* Subcapsular hematoma. Left semi prone view. The kidney (*k*) is deformed by a large infected hematoma (*h*) which is within the capsule. There is also a hemorrhage into an upper pole renal cyst (*C*). *B,* Left coronal view. Real-time. The subcapsular hematoma (*C*) can be seen around the kidney (*K*).

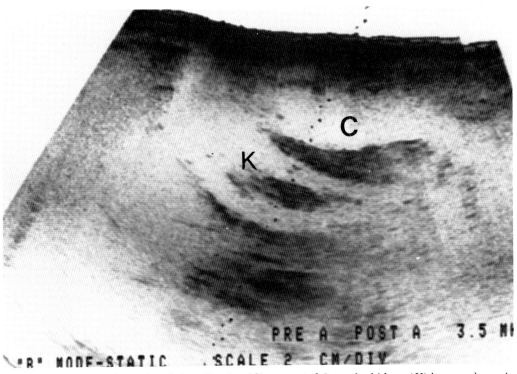

Figure 9.6. Posterior perinephric collection (*C*) separated from the kidney (*K*) by an echogenic structure presumed to represent Gerota's fascia and the renal capsule.

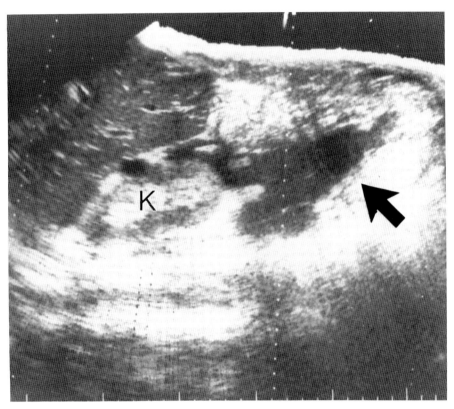

Figure 9.7. Anterior perinephric collection (*arrow*) which arose in the pancreas. It lies anterior and inferior to the kidney (*K*).

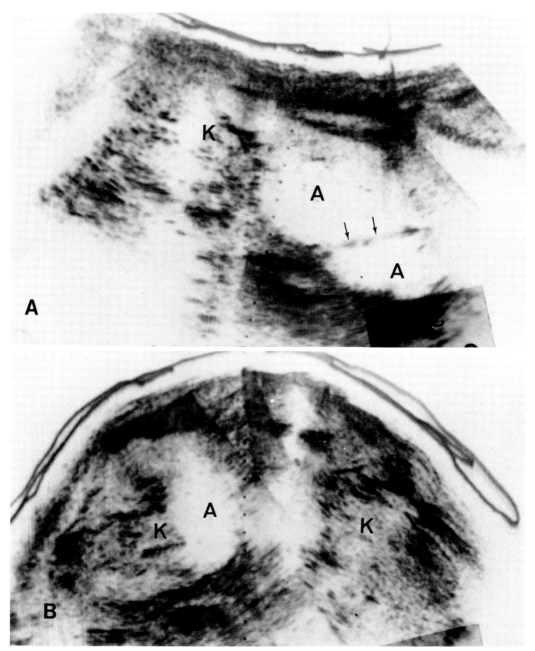

Figure 9.8. Prone (A) longitudinal and (B) transverse sections through an abscess which lies posteromedial to the kidney and extends in a cone-shaped fashion into the pelvis. Since the collection extended inferiorly, some of the abscess (A) had tracked outside Gerota's fascia and now lies in the anterior pararenal space (A) as well as within Gerota's fascia. The abscess followed a renal biopsy. K, kidney. Gerota's fascia is shown by *arrows*.

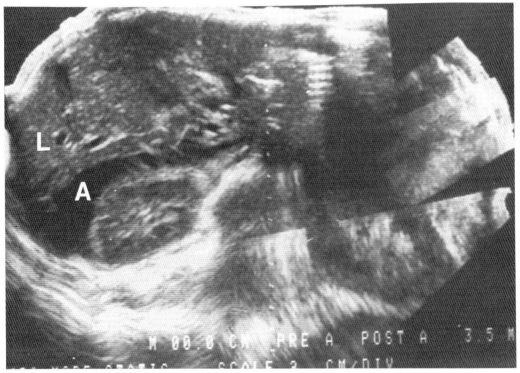

Figure 9.9.   Collection in Rutherford Morison's pouch (*A*) in the peritoneum (loculated ascites). *L*, liver.

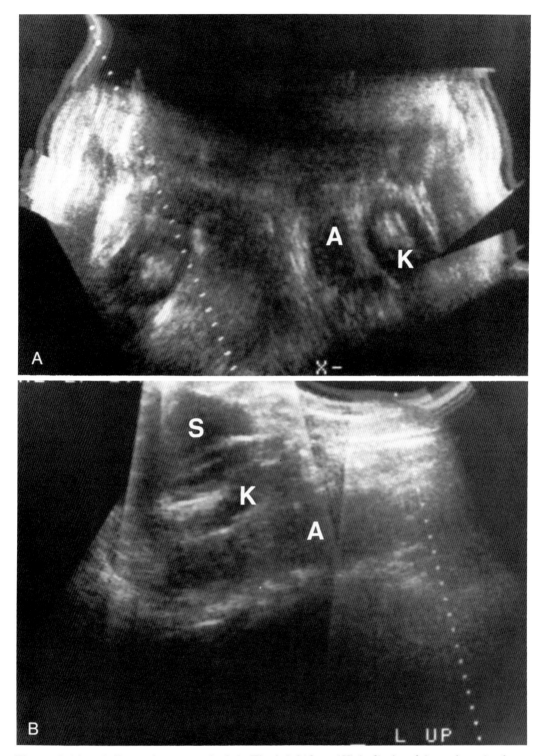

Figure 9.10.   *A*, Psoas abscess on the left. The left kidney (*K*) is displaced from the spine by a collection (*A*) within the muscle. *B*, Same case. Longitudinal section angling medially showing the kidney (*K*) and an enlarged psoas muscle containing the abscess (*A*). *S*, spleen.

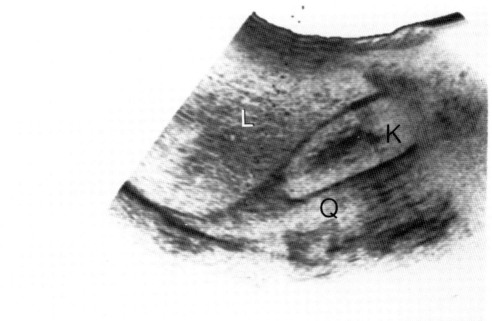

PRE A   POST A   3.5 MHZ

"B" MODE-STATIC   SCALE 3   CM/DIV

Figure 9.11.   Quadratus lumborum muscle (*Q*) appearing as relatively sonolucent area mimicking a collection. A normal variant. *L*, liver; *K*, kidney.

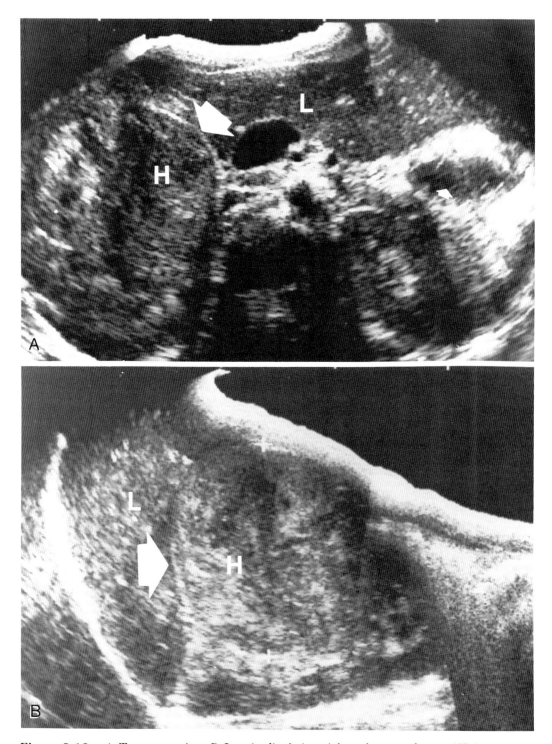

Figure 9.12. *A*, Transverse view. *B*, Longitudinal view. A large hypernephroma (*H*) in 15-year-old displacing the retroperitoneal fat line (*arrow*) anteriorly indicating a renal origin. *L*, liver.

impression that there is an intrarenal mass (Fig. 9.13). Sonography clearly outlines the expanding liver as being extrarenal in location.

Spleen. The spleen normally lies lateral and superior to the left kidney. However, when it enlarges, it extends inferomedially and covers the anterior portion of the left kidney. If there is considerable enlargement, an apparent intrarenal mass may be thought to be present on the intravenous pyelogram, but it is readily revealed to be due to extrinsic pressure of splenic origin by the sonogram.

Pancreas.. The tail of the pancreas has a variable relationship to the left kidney. It usually lies in contact with the upper pole and may pass anterior to it. Therefore, it is not surprising that processes that originate in the pancreas, such as carcinoma of the pancreas or pancreatic pseudocyst, can invade and involve renal parenchyma and even be thought to be intrarenal in origin (Fig. 9.14).

Gallbladder. Although the gallbladder can lie in very close relationship to the right kidney, I have not yet seen an example of gallbladder disease involving the kidney, presumably because the two structures are separated by two layers of peritoneum. A distinct wall to this typically cystic structure can be discerned. It has the shape of a lopsided pear and contracts if fat is administered.

PATHOLOGY
Fluid Collections

Fluid collections in the retroperitoneum are notoriously treacherous and difficult to detect

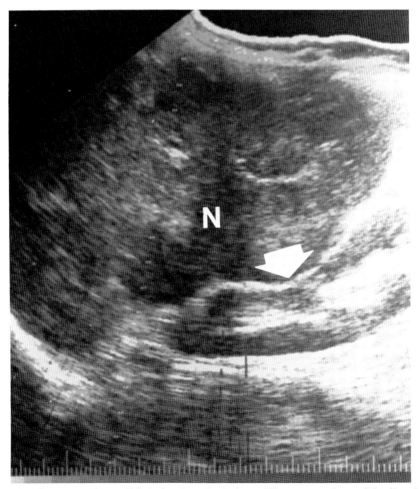

Figure 9.13.   Liver neoplasm (*N*) indenting the kidney. The retroperitoneal fat line (*arrow*) is displaced posteriorly.

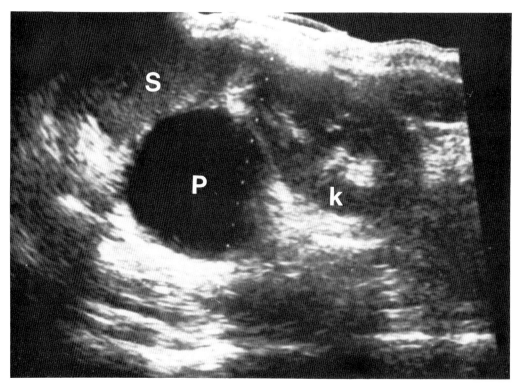

Figure 9.14. Pancreatic pseudocyst (P) indenting the superior pole of the kidney (k) and spleen (S). On the intravenous pyelogram one had the impression of a mass of renal origin.

by conventional radiological procedures, but they stand out on sonography, whatever their nature (5, 6). Perinephric fluid collections not associated with any organ or mass are of seven different types: abscesses, urinoma, hematomas, lymphoceles, seromas, pancreatic pseudocysts, and uriniferous pseudocysts. The latter are cysts apparently the result of a previous unrecognized urinoma or perhaps congenital cysts of the kidney which have become divorced from their primary source. Such fluid collections may develop in any of the potential spaces around the kidney (Fig. 9.1). Although every type of potential fluid collection can give a totally cystic appearance, some fluid collections, notably abscesses and hematomas, sometimes have a more typical acoustic appearance.

Acoustic features of the various fluid collections will be described.

ABSCESSES

Perinephric abscesses usually develop as a consequence of an intrarenal infection. As recently as 1969, less than 45% of retroperitoneal abscesses were discovered prior to autopsy or operation (7, 8). Perinephric abscesses vary in sonographic appearance depending on age and "ripeness"—the amount of pus within the abscess (9). When inflammation first occurs, there are decreased echoes without cystic areas. At a later stage when pus formation has occurred, a "cyst" may develop surrounded by zones of decreased echoes. There may well be more than one pus collection, and each individual loculation will be seen as a distinct cystic area separated by a zone of decreased echoes. The echogenicity of the abscess varies depending on the amount of the protein aggregates within the abscess (10) (Figs. 9.8 and 9.10). Pus is sometimes quite echogenic if it is relatively thick. If the abscess contains gas, acoustic shadowing will occur within the abscess (11). Abscesses may track along with psoas and cause lateral displacement of the kidneys. Supine views in the pelvis may help to show psoas abscesses (6).

Attempted surgical release of the pus, particularly if the abscess is not acoustically ripe, may well be incomplete, and postoperative ultrasound can show residual pus collections (5).

Percutaneous drainage under ultrasound control has become a popular therapeutic approach (see Chapter 16).

URINOMA

Urinomas around the kidney occur as a result of trauma or surgery or in relation to a renal transplant. A urinoma is a well-delineated, fluid-filled structure with essentially no internal echoes within it, although there may be one or two septa. In general, they have smooth walls, although the smoothness depends upon the tissue that borders on the urinoma.

HEMATOMAS

Hematomas are of considerable interest because they vary greatly sonographically. The acoustic pattern depends upon the phase at which they are seen (12). Within the first few hours after they develop, hematomas are liquid and, therefore, cystic (Fig. 9.15). Later they clot and develop internal echoes to a variable extent (Fig. 9.16). Eventually they may liquify once

again and become cystic; in other instances they become organized and develop low level echoes within. Sonographic recognition of the presence of a hematoma surrounding the kidney is important because if it is subcapsular or within Gerota's fascia it can cause hypertension and be responsible for the Page kidney phenomenon (13, 14) (Fig. 9.17). When clot formation occurs there can be relatively dense, large echoes dispersed within the hematoma. Large echo-free hematomas in the perinephric area within the psoas muscle grow in hemophiliacs (15). Hematomas have occurred around the kidney following performance of renal biopsy.

Hematomas can develop in any one of the various spaces that develop around the kidney; they differ from abscesses in that they remain in that space and do not tend to disrupt the fascial boundary if no surgery has been performed. Perinephric hematomas tend to be relatively thin and elongated in shape since they more or less conform to the outline of the space that they occupy. Such hematomas form different shapes around the transplant kidney or after

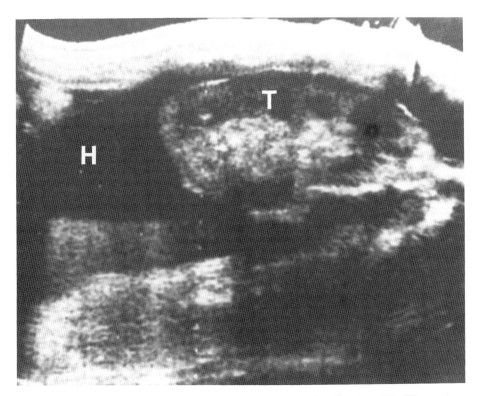

Figure 9.15. Transplant (*T*) surrounded by a superior fluid collection (*H*). These views were obtained 12 hours after operation.

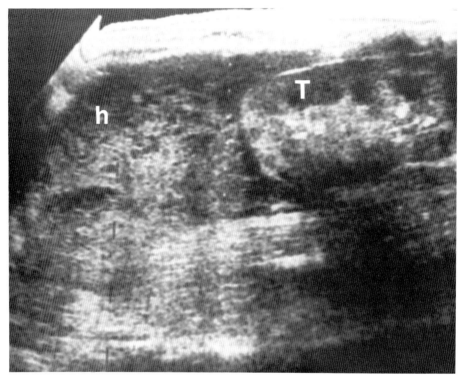

Figure 9.16.   The same case was re-examined 12 hours later. The hematoma (*h*) has now become echogenic presumably because it has developed clot within. *T*, transplant.

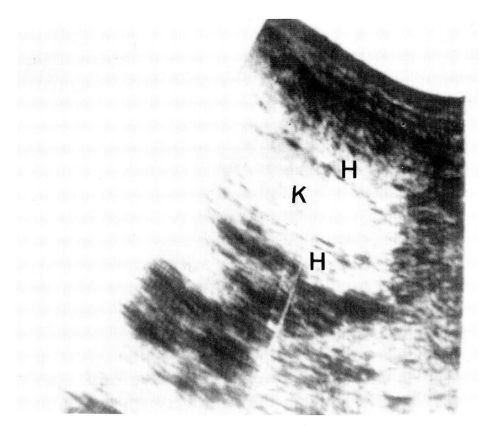

Figure 9.17. Decubitus view of a kidney (*K*) surrounded by a large, well-organized hematoma (*H*) resulting in the Page kidney phenomenon. (Reprinted with permission from Conrad et al. (13).)

trauma because the natural tissue boundaries have been disturbed (Figs. 9.15, 9.16, and 9.18). Abscesses and hematomas represent the only two of the various liquid collections that may develop around the kidney which often contain internal echoes.

Adrenal Hematoma (See Chapter 13)

Although rare in adults, hematomas are a common development in the adrenal gland immediately after birth when they can present as a fairly large palpable mass (Fig. 9.19, A and B). Later they become calcified, and the only evidence that they ever occurred is the presence of a small patch of calcification in the adrenal gland in a somewhat older child. At birth a large generally echo-free mass with an irregular shape is found sonographically located superior to the kidney (16).

LYMPHOCELES

Lymphoceles are rare around the kidney unless they are related to a renal transplant. In this situation they are quite common because of the disturbance to the lymphatic drainage that takes place when the transplant is performed. Similar to urinomas, they generally lack internal echoes. However, their border is relatively irregular, and one or two examples have been seen in which a lymphocele dissected through the tissues and caused the creation of a space with low level echoes resembling gut. Septa are quite common (Fig. 9.20). When secondarily infected, their acoustic pattern changes and they develop internal echoes. An example is shown of an infected lymphocele that developed a fluid-fluid level (Fig. 9.21).

SEROMAS

Seromas are a rare cause of a perinephric collection and are mainly seen in relationship to a transplant in the acute period following operation. They do not have any specific features, being echo-free with relatively smooth borders. Indeed one seroma was mistaken for the bladder when the bladder was empty.

PANCREATIC PSEUDOCYSTS

Particularly on the left, pancreatic pseudocysts can burrow around the kidney in virtually every direction, both medial, lateral, superior, and inferior (Fig. 9.22). They are not limited by

the fascial spaces previously described and may be difficult to visualize at ultrasonography; as an uncommon feature they can contain low level echoes. Part of the pancreatic pseudocyst may lie out of the area that is easily visualized by sonography, i.e., between the costal margins and the iliac crest. Therefore, one may underestimate the size of a pancreatic pseudocyst by sonography. They can expand and squash the kidney and be so intimately associated with the kidney that they can be confused with a renal cyst on conventional x-ray examination (Fig. 9.14). However, sonographic visualization of the cyst in cross-sectional fashion generally reveals that the suspect lesion is of pancreatic origin. The right kidney is very rarely affected by pancreatic pseudocysts.

Pancreatic pseudocysts vary markedly in acoustic texture, most being sonolucent, but some having internal echoes or a fluid-fluid level. Their walls may be spherical and smooth or quite jagged.

SIMPLE CYSTS (URINEPHEROUS PSEUDOCYSTS)

Occasionally, a simple cystic lesion is found in the perinephric space within Gerota's fascia. It is never quite certain whether this is a congenital lesion or the result of previous trauma with loculation of a small urinoma. The ultrasonic features are similar to those described for simple cysts in Chapter 5.

Spleen

As already mentioned, perhaps the commonest pathological way in which the spleen impinges on the perirenal area is when it is large and squashing the kidney, causing an apparent intrarenal mass on the intravenous pyelogram. Splenic cysts are uncommon congenital cystic lesions that occur in the left upper quadrant and which may be the result of trauma (17); indeed they may originate as pancreatic pseudocysts dissecting into the spleen (18). The only sure way of identifying a lesion preoperatively as a splenic cyst is by identifying its border with the spleen and noting that it is entirely surrounded by splenic parenchyma. Splenic cysts, although generally echo free, may contain internal echoes.

Aortic Aneurysms

Aortic aneurysms can enlarge asymmetrically and displace the kidneys laterally. On other

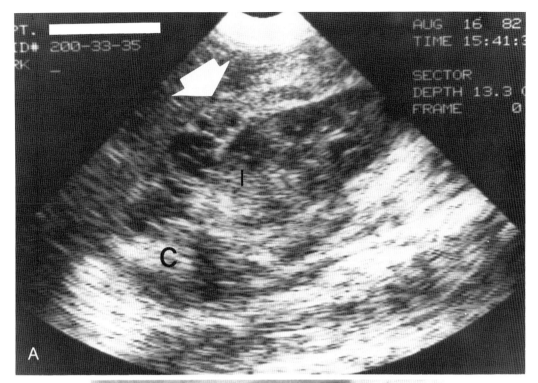

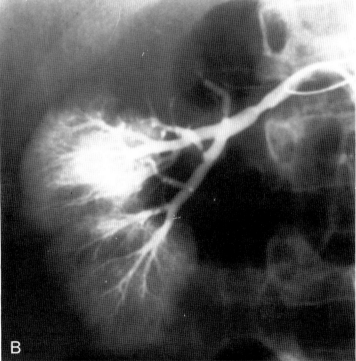

Figure 9.18. *A*, Child involved in a bicycle accident. A collection (*C*) consisting of a mixture of blood and urine surrounds the upper pole of the kidney. The upper pole of the kidney is infarcted, causing an echogenic area (*I*). The collection lies within Gerota's fascia (*arrow*). *B*, Same case. An arteriogram showed no vascular supply to the upper pole of the kidney.

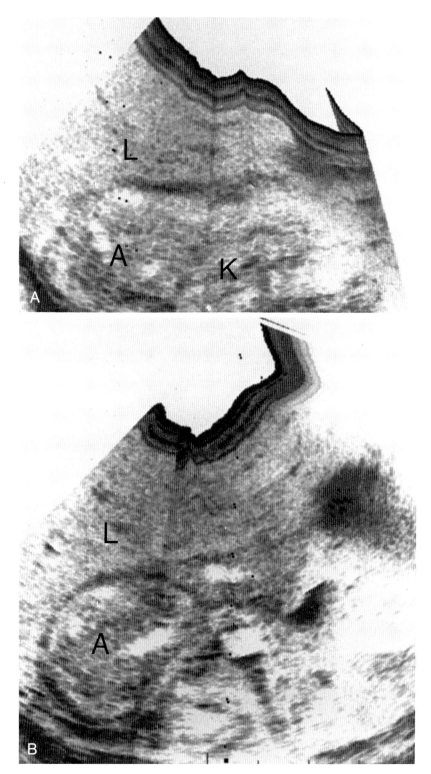

Figure 9.19. *A*, Adrenal hematoma. The large mass (*A*) superior to the kidney (*K*) represents an adrenal hematoma in this 3-day-old neonate. *L*, liver. *B*, A transverse view showing some sonolucent areas within the hematoma (*A*). *L*, liver.

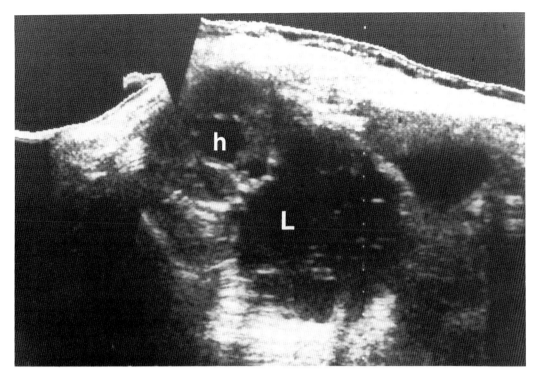

Figure 9.20. A large lymphocele (*L*) lies adjacent to a transplant kidney and is causing some hydronephrosis (*h*). Note that the lymphocele contains some septum.

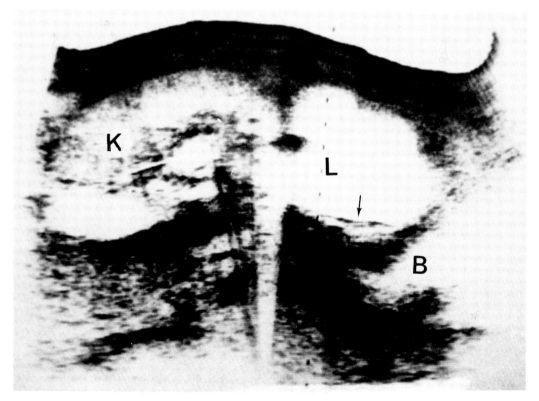

Figure 9.21. Lymphocele (*L*) which has become infected and developed low level echoes forming a fluid-fluid (*arrow*) level within it. Fluid-fluid levels are associated with abscess and hematoma. *K*, kidney; *B*, bladder.

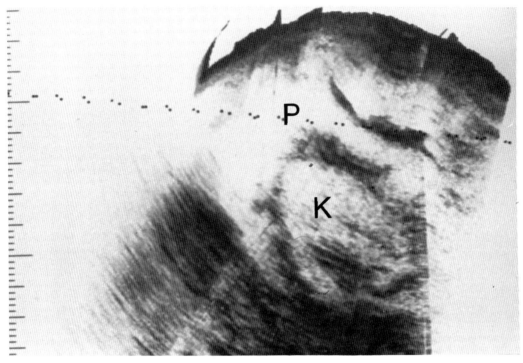

Figure 9.22.   A left side up transverse view shows a pancreatic pseudocyst (P) surrounding the left kidney (K).

occasions, there can be an asymmetrical enlargement and an aneurysm apparently connected to the aorta by a branch only; this type of aortic aneurysm can squash the kidney. The aneurysm is then difficult to recognize as an aneurysm— it appears to be a separate mass. Usually the sonographic appearance of an aneurysm is that of a large sonolucent cystic mass in contact with a normal-sized aorta at either end and often containing some organized low level echoes due to clot. If the aneurysm is more or less separate from the aorta with a small connecting orifice, a real-time scanner is helpful in showing the mass to be pulsatile; a local connection between the aneurysm and the rest of the aorta can usually be demonstrated.

Dissection can best be shown satisfactorily with a real-time system. A pulsatile line within the aorta is seen. On some occasions aortic aneurysms rupture, and the consequent hematoma accumulates adjacent to the kidney (Fig. 9.23).

Retroperitoneal Fibrosis

Retroperitonal fibrosis is a somewhat mysterious entity which has been associated with a number of different causes. It is known to be a response to ergot treatment for migraine and has been associated with infection and neoplasm, but in other instances no etiology is ever discovered. Fibrous tissue is deposited in a paraspinous location, usually starting at the sacral promontory in a fashion that eventually leads to obstruction of the ureters (19–21) (Fig. 9.24). The major sites of fibrous tissue deposition are along the psoas and iliacus muscles and around the aorta and inferior vena cava. The process can extend into the pelvis or toward the renal hilum. The sonographic appearances are of a smooth-bordered subtle preaortic mass sometimes associated with hydronephrosis.

Retroperitoneal Nodes

Node deposition alongside the aorta, between the aorta and the spine, and in front of the aorta in a retroperitoneal location is commonplace. Such nodes, if due to lymphoma, are almost always echopenic. If due to other processes, such as metastases, they can be more echogenic. Nodes are also deposited along the iliacus muscle directly adjacent to the psoas muscle toward the pelvis. Node deposition in a perirenal area

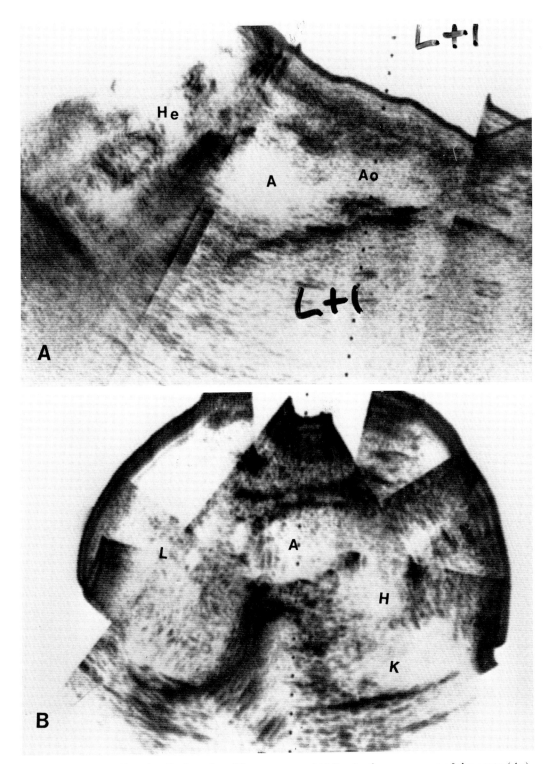

Figure 9.23. *A*, Longitudinal supine. The aneurysm (*A*) lies in the upper part of the aorta (*Ao*). *He*, heart. *B*, Transverse supine (same patient). Leaking aortic aneurysm (*A*) with large clot (*H*) adjacent to the left kidney (*K*). *L*, liver.

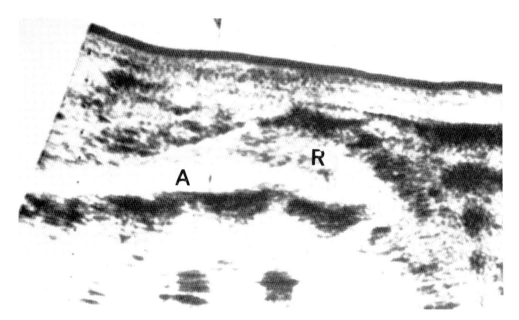

Figure 9.24.   Longitudinal section. Patient with retroperitoneal fibrosis with a deposit of fibrous tissue (*R*) anterior to the aorta (*A*).

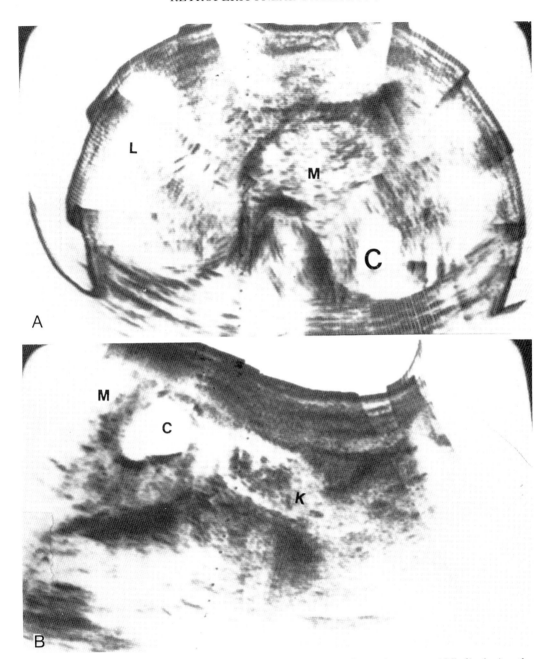

Figure 9.25.   *A* and *B,* Left side up superior view of retroperitoneal sarcoma (*M*) displacing the kidney (*K*) inferiorly and the spleen laterally. It has an area of necrosis (*C*) within it. *L,* liver.

within the kidney is unusual but does occur. Secondary hydronephrosis due to ureteric compression by nodes is commonplace.

Retroperitoneal Neoplasms

Neoplasms may arise from the fibrous tissues, nodes, blood, and lymph tissue around the kid-

neys, giving rise to neurogenic tumors, pheochromocytoma, leiomyosarcoma, and teratoma (22). These masses often reach a very large size before they are discovered (Fig. 9.25) and invade the neighboring tissues, including the kidneys, spleen, adrenals, etc. They usually have relatively low level echoes within them. A typical pattern is seen with leiomyoblastoma when large sonolucent holes occur within the mass.

Sonography is especially valuable in the perinephric area because this is a site in which conventional radiographic techniques are of little or no value. On the whole, examination of this area is easy by sonography, although computed tomography often produces a more complete view of the area because ribs and lungs do not interfere.

References

1. Weill FS, Perriguey G, Rohmer P: Sonographic study of the juxtarenal retoperitoneal compartments. *J Ultrasound Med* 1:307–310, 1982.
2. Callen P, Filly R, Marks W: The quadratus lumborum muscle: a possible source of confusion in sonographic evaluation of the retroperitoneum. *J Clin Ultrasound* 7:349–352, 1979.
3. Yeh HC, Wolf BS: Ultrasonic contrast study to identify stomach with tap water microbubbles. *J Clin Ultrasound* 5:170, 1976.
4. Mascatello VJ, Carrera GF, Teele RL, Berger M, Holm HH, Smith EH: The ultrasonic demonstration of gastric lesions. *J Clin Ultrasound* 5:383, 1977.
5. McCullough DL, Leopold GR: Diagnosis of retroperitoneal fluid collections by ultrasonography: a series of surgically proved cases. *J Urol* 115:656, 1976.
6. Laing FC, Jacobs RP: Value of ultrasonography in the detection of retroperitoneal inflammatory masses. *Radiology* 123:169–172, 1977.
7. Stevenson EOS, Ozeran RS: Retroperitoneal space abscesses. *Surg Gynecol Obstet* 128:1202, 1969.
8. Malgieri JJ, Kursh ED, Persky L: The changing clinicopathological pattern of abscesses in or adjacent to the kidney. *J Urol* 118:230, 1977.
9. Hill M, Sanders RC: Gray scale B-scan characteristics of intraabdominal cystic masses. *J Clin Ultrasound* 6:217–222, 1978.
10. Cunningham JJ, Wooten W, Cunningham MA: Gray scale echography of soluble protein and protein aggregate fluid collections (in vitro study). *J Clin Ultrasound* 4:417, 1976.
11. Kressel HY, Filly RA: Ultrasonographic appearance of gas-containing abscesses in the abdomen. *AJR* 130:71, 1978.
12. Kaplan GN, Sanders RC: B-scan ultrasound in the management of patients with occult abdominal hematomas. *J Clin Ultrasound* 1:5, 1973.
13. Conrad MR, Freedman M, Weiner C, et al: Sonography of the Page kidney. *J Urol* 116:293, 1976.
14. Chamorro HA, Forbes TW, Padkowsky GO, et al: Multiimaging approach in the diagnosis of Page kidney. *AJR* 136:620–621, 1981.
15. McVerry BA, Vicary FR, Voke J, et al: Ultrasonography in the management of haemophilia. *Lancet* 2:872–874, 1977.
16. Pond GD, Haber K: Echography: a new approach to the diagnosis of adrenal hemorrhage of the newborn. *J Assoc Can Radiol* 27:49, 1976.
17. Wright FW, Williams EW: Large post-traumatic splenic cyst diagnosed by radiology, isotope scintigraphy and ultrasound. *Br J Radiol* 47:454, 1974.
18. Dembner AG, Taylor KJW: Gray scale sonographic diagnosis: multiple congenital splenic cysts. *J Clin Ultrasound* 6:173, 1978.
19. Fagan CJ, Amparo EG, Davis M: Retroperitoneal fibrosis. *Semin Ultrasound* 3:123, 1982.
20. Center S, Schwab R, Goldberg BB: The value of ultrasonography as an aid in the treatment of idiopathic retroperitoneal fibrosis. *J Ultrasound Med* 1:87–89, 1982.
21. Sanders RC, Duffy T, McLoughlin MG, et al: Sonography in the diagnosis of retroperitoneal fibrosis. *J Urol* 118:944–946, 1977.
22. Karp W, Hafstrom LO, Johsson PE: Retroperitoneal sarcoma: ultrasonographic and angiographic evaluation. *Br J Radiol* 53:525–531, 1980.

CHAPTER 10

Ultrasonography of the Urinary Bladder

DONALD BODNER, M.D.
PATRICK J. BRYAN, M.D.
JOSEPH P. LiPUMA, M.D.
MARTIN I. RESNICK, M.D.

Although not as widely used in the evaluation of diseases of the lower urinary tract as for those of the kidney and retroperitoneum, ultrasonography has been shown to be of value in the diagnosis and management of specific disorders of the bladder. Disorders of the bladder are not uncommon, and, due to its position deep within the pelvis, it is often difficult to evaluate by usual diagnostic techniques. Endoscopy, particularly with the recent development of new lens systems, is useful in detecting abnormalities of the bladder wall. Radiographic procedures (intravenous urography, cystography, lymphangiography, and arteriography) are helpful in assessing abnormalities of the bladder, but tumor staging by these techniques alone is inaccurate and similarly often gives a poor assessment of disease processes. In addition, triple contrast studies, although often helpful, are difficult to perform and are often impractical. Rectal examination and bimanual examination are used in the staging of bladder malignancies but, like the other studies mentioned, are recognized to be inaccurate, and understaging is not uncommon (1). Computed tomography is valuable in showing extension of tumor beyond the bladder or prostate but cannot show the depth of invasion in the bladder wall by bladder carcinoma or prostatic tumors which are confined within the gland.

Ultrasonography of the pelvis is of value in assessing diseases of the bladder. Soft tissue structures can be studied, and often the information gained cannot be obtained by the other diagnostic modalities available. In addition, distortion or invasion of the bladder from tumors arising in contiguous organs can often be detected.

TECHNIQUES OF EXAMINATION

Several ultrasonic techniques can be used for the evaluation of disorders of the bladder. Basically three types of examinations can be employed: transabdominal, transrectal, and, most recently, transurethral. As emphasized previously, ultrasonic studies of the pelvic structures should be considered as one diagnostic procedure among many, and the data obtained require correlation with the information derived from other diagnostic studies, i.e., physical examination, intravenous urography, urinary cytology, cystoscopy, and panendoscopy. The examiner should have some concept of the patient's difficulties so that attention can be directed at specific structures.

When the lower urinary tract is evaluated, it is advisable to study all pelvic structures. Contiguous structures, such as the bladder, seminal vesicles, prostate, rectum, and uterus, should be routinely imagined. At times disease processes of one structure can involve other closely related organs.

Transabdominal Scanning

Bladder distention, either by having the patient not void prior to the examination or by catheterization and instillation of a fixed amount of fluid, is the only preparation required for adequate pelvic ultrasonography. When transabdominal studies are performed, it is not necessary to restrict diet or use catheters or enemas to reduce intestinal contents and air. Studies should precede radiographic examinations of the upper and lower intestinal tract because the presence of barium will interfere with satisfactory imaging. It is generally useful to image the bladder initially both in the transverse and longitudinal directions (Fig. 10.1, *A* and *B*). Routinely, transverse scans are made from the symphysis toward the umbilicus at 1- to 2-cm intervals. Longitudinal scans are obtained from the umbilicus to the symphysis at 1- to 2-cm intervals from the midline. Generally a 3.5-MHz transducer is used, and in most instances it is adequate to visualize all pelvic structures clearly. As with renal scanning, either mineral oil or another suitable coupling agent is used on the skin surface. The patient is placed supine during all studies, and only occasionally is it necessary to change to the oblique position. The development of high quality real-time sector scanners has made bladder scanning very simple, and a thorough examination of the bladder can be done in a few minutes using a real-time scanner.

The bladder should normally appear as a sonolucent structure with sharply demarcated walls. With abdominal scanning it is not unusual to have reverberation echoes present anteriorly. If the Foley catheter is in place it can often be well visualized, and it is a useful landmark to localize the bladder neck.

Transrectal Scanning

The basic technique for transrectal ultrasonography was developed by Watanabe and associates and consists of a transrectal transducer, radial scanner, and imaging screen (2, 3). Originally performed with the patient in the sitting position in a special chair allowing for placement of the probe, examinations have also been carried out with placement of the probe while the patient is in the lithotomy position (4, 5). A major advance in transrectal scanning was the development of gray-scale imaging.

Present instrumentation consists of a two-part probe: an outer stationary unit and a freely movable inner assembly. The outer stationary unit provides inflow and outflow parts for the fluid interface and a polyethylene cover to protect the rectal mucosa. The inner assembly is free to move in longitudinal and rotational directions. Longitudinal movement provides an infinite number of serial sections of the bladder, and the rotational movement provides sonotomograms of it (Fig. 10.2, *A* and *B*). An ultrasonic beam is emitted at right angles to the probe, and the transducer receives the echoes and transmits them to the gray-scale unit.

In preparation for the scan the patient is given an enema to cleanse the rectum just prior to the study. If the patient has recently voided, a Foley catheter is inserted and 200 ml of sterile saline are instilled into the bladder. Often the Foley catheter is left in place during the study because the balloon serves as a useful landmark in localizing the bladder neck. Prior to rectal insertion, the transducer is covered with a rubber condom; after insertion, it is filled with approximately 100 ml of water until it is airtight against the rectal mucosa. This procedure interposes an aqueous interface between the sonic disc and the rectum to ensure uniformity of the conducting media in the area. The probe is lubricated with a suitable coupling agent, such as water-soluble jelly, and is inserted 8 to 9 cm above the anal verge with the patient in the lithotomy position. The probe must be inserted with care to avoid rectal injury. Only occasionally can a study not be performed because of the presence of an excessively enlarged prostate or perianal disease (fissures or hemorrhoids). Several transverse tomograms are then obtained beginning at the level of the bladder and progressing distally at 0.5- to 1.0-cm increments. The entire examination usually takes approximately 15 to 20 minutes and results in only minimal patient discomfort.

Major areas of improvement will be in the development of higher frequency transducers to provide enhanced resolution. Currently available instruments have a concave oscillating barium titanate disc fitted at the end of the rotating assembly, and only recently have other transducers become available. Transrectal scanning equipment currently in the developmental stage employs two piezoelectric transducer elements on a single shaft (R. Hileman, personal communication). One transducer element, resonant at 7 MHz, is optimized for depth ranges up to 5 cm for examining the prostate and seminal vesicles; the other is resonant at 3.5 MHz and is optimized for ranges to 10 cm for examining the fluid-filled balloon.

Transurethral Scanning

Transurethral scanning of the bladder offers great potential for improved staging of bladder tumors. Transabdominal and transrectal routes of scanning have been helpful for differentiating stage A from stage C disease but have proven less helpful in defining stage B disease. Recent

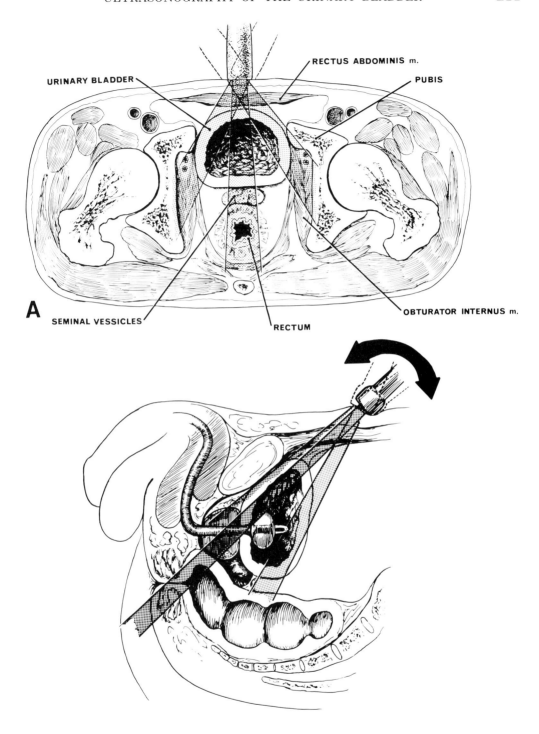

Figure 10.1. Transabdominal pelvic ultrasonography. *A*, Transverse scan. *B*, Longitudinal scan.

experience suggests that the bladder can best be visualized by transurethral scanning (6, 7).

Transurethral scanning was first employed when von Micksy (8) utilized a transurethral probe to image the female structures. He used a linear scanner consisting of a small ultrasonic transducer combined with a cystoscope and a precision scanning bridge. The device allowed

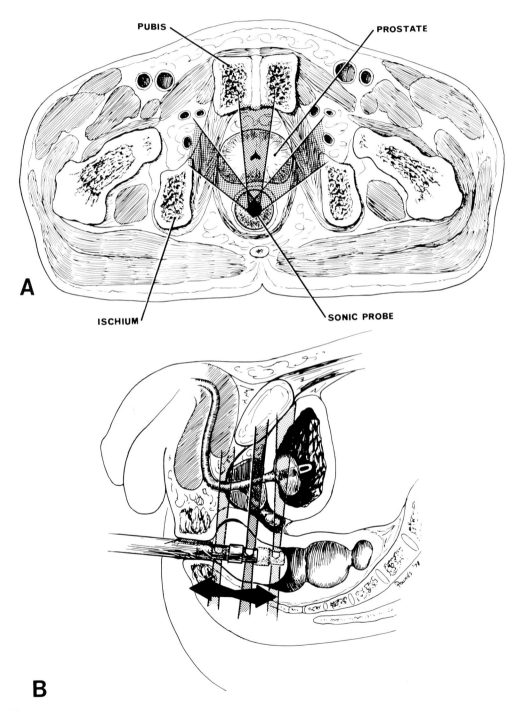

Figure 10.2.   Transrectal pelvic ultrasonography. *A*, Transverse scan. *B*, Longitudinal scan.

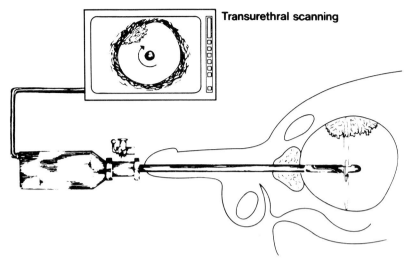

Transurethral scanning

Figure 10.3.   Transurethral ultrasonography. (Reprinted with permission from Gammelgaard and Holm (6).)

for direct visualization of the bladder and subsequent scanning of points of interest; it had application in the staging of cervical malignancies and in the evaluation of recurrence and spread of other pelvic tumors. Holm and Northeved (6, 9) described a transurethral ultrasonic scanner that was interchangeable with the optic system of a resectoscope. Subsequent improvements have made transurethral ultrasound scanning an integral part of routine cystoscopy (Fig. 10.3).

The scanner for transurethral ultrasonography consists of a motor that rotates a long rod which is connected at the opposite end to an interchangeable transducer. The scanner fits within a standard resectoscope sheath.

The scanner can be sterilized before use. When further information is desired during cystoscopy, the optics can be removed from the sheath and replaced with the transurethral scanner. The bladder is inflated with sterile water and the motor activated. Dynamic scans of the bladder are obtained at different angles, positions, and different degrees of inflation to view all surfaces of the bladder. The seminal vesicles in males, the bladder neck, and the ureteral orifices serve as landmarks in localizing abnormalities in the bladder. The procedure need not be performed under general anesthesia if the cystoscopy can be obtained under local anesthesia. The procedure is sterile, rapid, and can greatly enhance the information gained at cystoscopy.

NORMAL BLADDER

Typically the bladder is seen as a global structure, and the interface between the fluid medium (urine) and bladder wall is distinct. The bladder wall normally appears as a symmetrical, smooth, gently curved surface. Scans obtained during different phases of filling clearly reveal the distensibility of the walls, and areas of fixation are readily identifiable.

When viewed abdominally the bladder shows some variability in shape depending upon the amount of fluid present, changes in intrapelvic pressure, patient position, and the position of the probe (Fig. 10.4, *A* and *B*). Longitudinal scans reveal there to be a tapering of the bladder anteriorly with an orientation toward the umbilicus. Frequently, parallel reverberation echoes arise from the interface of the bladder wall and urine and are readily distinguishable from echo patterns arising from tumors. Transverse scans reveal variations in the shape of the bladder ranging from almost circular to almost square; but, as with the longitudinal scans, they are also affected by degree of filling and intrapelvic pressures. Real-time has allowed visualization of urine as it enters the bladder from the ureters. Urine normally squirts into the bladder intermittently, forming the "jet" effect (10, 11).

Transrectal scans provide similar information about the bladder contour to the transabdominal study (Fig. 10.5). Reverberation echoes are also frequently seen but are located posteriorly. Ex-

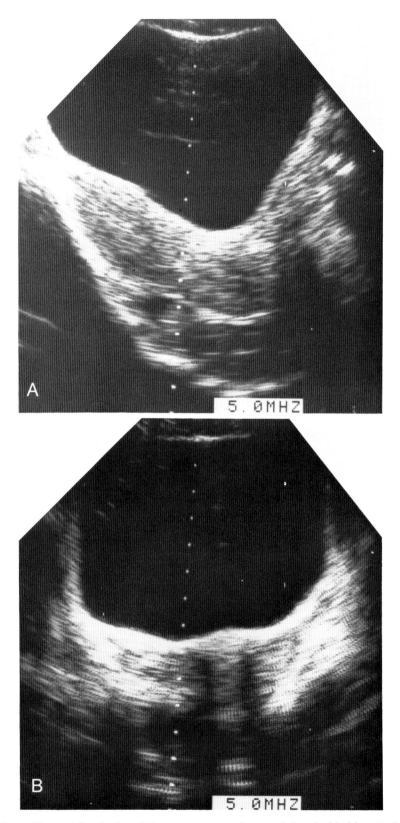

Figure 10.4. Transabdominal real-time sonogram of normal female bladder. *A*, Longitudinal scan. *B*, Transverse scan.

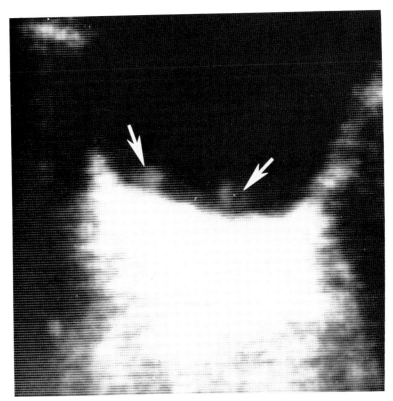

Figure 10.5.   Urine jets (*arrows*) are seen emerging from the urethral orifices on this real-time scan. Echoes from such urine jets are frequently seen on real-time studies. The echoes are thought to be due to an acoustic mismatch caused by a lower specific gravity of the urine emerging from the ureters compared to the urine already in the bladder in patients who have been given a water load.

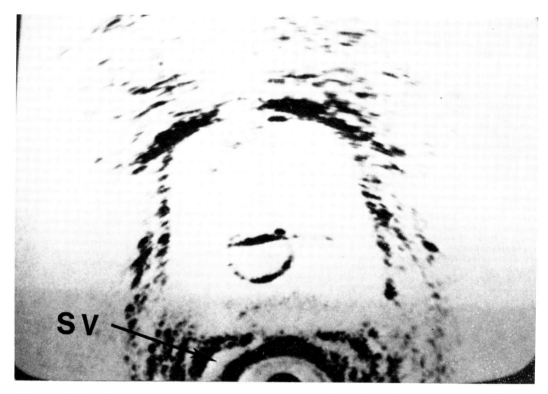

Figure 10.6. Transrectal gray-scale sonogram of normal bladder. Seminal vesicles (*SV*) are visualized posteriorly.

perience reveals that the methods of scanning are comparable; however, abdominal scanning offers the advantage of assessing pelvic lymph nodes (12, 13), psoas muscle, and other intra-abdominal and pelvic structures that are not accessible by the transrectal technique.

Transurethral scans provide similar information to transabdominal and transrectal studies (Fig. 10.6). Recent experience suggests that the transurethral scan best visualizes the bladder as the ultrasonic beam examines the bladder circumferentially at right angles (6).

BLADDER TUMORS

Understaging of bladder malignancies is a problem associated with the evaluation of patients with carcinomas of the bladder. Staging techniques have included intravenous urography, cystography, lymphangiography, arteriography, bimanual examination, and transurethral biopsy, all of which are recognized to be associated with errors approaching 50% in this patient category (13–17). Although not unassociated with false negative studies, ultrasonography has

been shown to improve the estimation of local tumor involvement (4, 14, 15, 18–21). Small, superficial, noninfiltrating bladder tumors are difficult to visualize ultrasonically, and direct endoscopic visualization continues to be the most accurate diagnostic modality in the assessment of patients with this condition. Larger bladder tumors appear ultrasonically as echogenic masses projecting into the lumen of the echo-free urinary bladder. These areas are fixed to the wall and, unlike blood clots or stones, do not alter their location with changes in patient position (Figs. 10.7 to 10.9). Although fixed to the bladder wall, ureteroceles can be differentiated from tumors by their lack of echogenicity and identification of their thin wall (Fig. 10.10). Superficial and noninvasive tumors have a well-defined base. It is important to be able to distinguish bladder tumors from reverberation patterns, which can usually be eliminated by altering the angle of the transducer and which are usually parallel to the bladder wall (Fig. 10.11). Superficial bladder tumors will not cause fixation or distortion of the bladder wall. If multiple scans are obtained during the filling phase, nor-

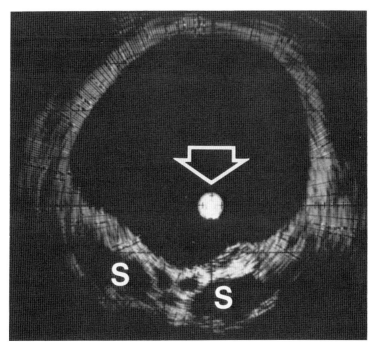

Figure 10.7. Transurethral sonogram of normal bladder. Seminal vesicles (*S*) are visualized posteriorly. Transducer is present in center of bladder (*arrow*).

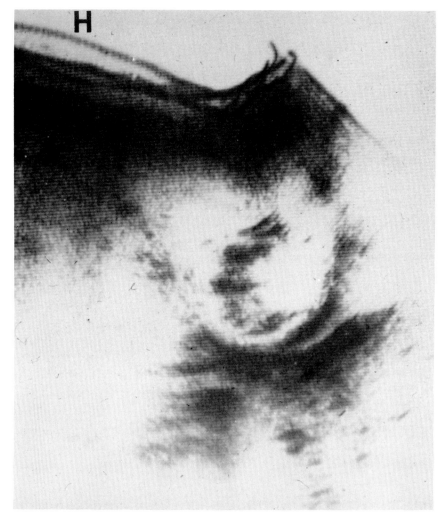

Figure 10.8. Transabdominal (longitudinal) gray-scale sonogram demonstrating blood clots in the bladder. The clots are not fixed to the bladder wall and change location with alteration in patient position. *H*, head.

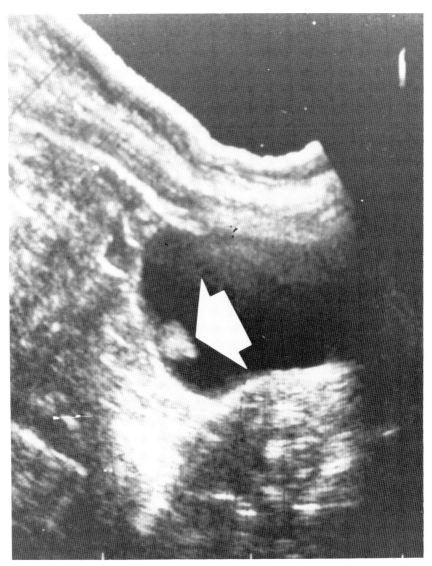

Figure 10.9. Transabdominal (longitudinal) gray-scale sonogram of bladder demonstrating superficial tumor located on dome (*arrow*). The bladder wall is free of distortion and is not fixed.

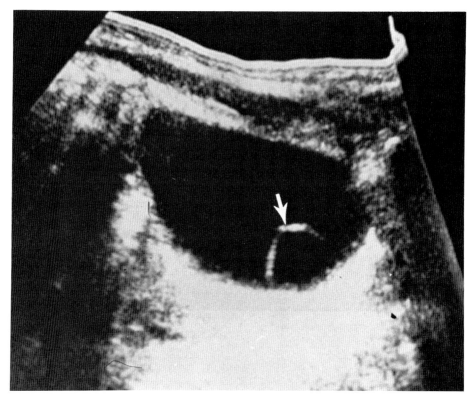

Figure 10.10. Transabdominal sonogram demonstrating a walled ureterocele (*arrow*) projecting into the bladder lumen.

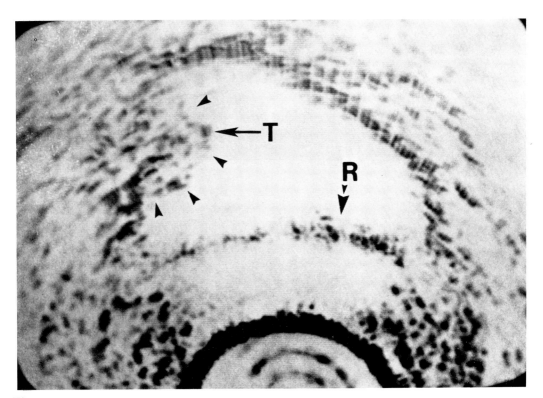

Figure 10.11. Transrectal gray-scale sonogram of bladder demonstrating tumor involvement of wall. Depth of invasion cannot be detected. *T*, tumor; *R*, reverberation echo.

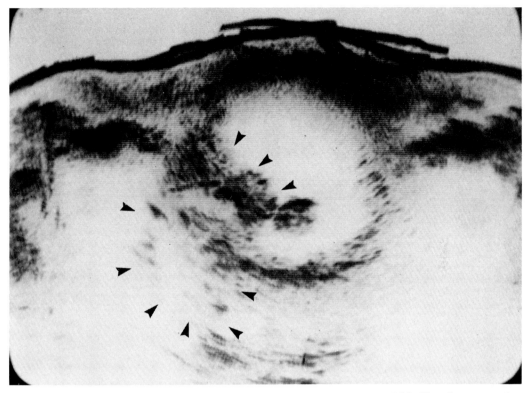

Figure 10.12. Transabdominal (transverse) gray-scale sonogram of bladder demonstrating tumor (*arrows*) distorting the bladder wall and invading the perivesicle space.

mal contour will be preserved and movement of the bladder wall with increasing intraluminal volume will be appreciated.

Infiltrative tumors tend to have a broader base that can be visualized ultrasonically (Figs. 10.11 to 10.15). Often the bladder wall will be fixed and the natural contour distorted when the bladder is full. Tumors that have completely extended through the bladder wall can be identified by the presence of an extravesical mass. With extensive extravesical invasion, the bladder wall becomes fixed and is often markedly distorted.

Recent studies report that transurethral scanning is more accurate in staging bladder tumors than either transabdominal or transrectal scanning (6, 7, 9). We have had similar experience. Transurethral scanning offers the potential to differentiate stages B and B2 tumors and tumors with only minimal extravesical involvement from those with muscle involvement, which is a great advantage (Figs. 10.16 and 10.17). This differentiation cannot be reliably made with either transrectal or transabdominal techniques alone.

Ultrasonography has been found to be of value in the assessment of bladder tumor patients following radiation therapy. Preoperative radiation therapy is becoming increasingly utilized as a means of diminishing the extent of the tumor involvement in patients with high grade bladder malignancies (18). Ultrasound is a useful noninvasive method of assessing response to treatment and assessing tumor staging prior to surgery so that appropriate therapy may be instituted (Fig. 10.18, *A* and *B*). If extravesical tumor involvement persists following an appropriate course of preoperative radiotherapy, extensive operative procedures could be avoided in patients who would not benefit from such treatment. Computed tomography gives similar information to that provided by ultrasonography. Extension of tumor into the perivesical fat is more obvious on computed tomography (CT), and CT is also superior to ultrasonography in demonstrating metastatic involvement of pelvic

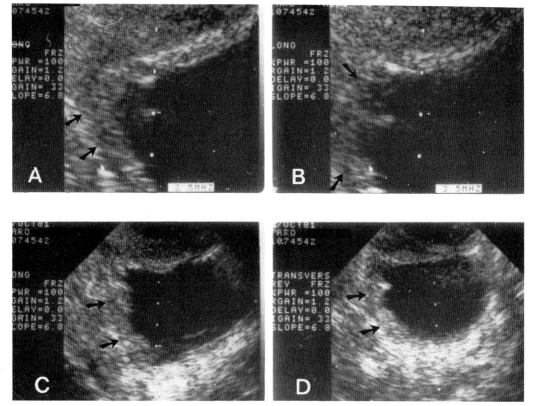

Figure 10.13. Irregular plaque-like bladder carcinoma. Four scans at different levels show irregular thickening of the right wall of the bladder (*arrows*). There is no evidence of extension of tumor beyond the bladder wall into the perivesical fat.

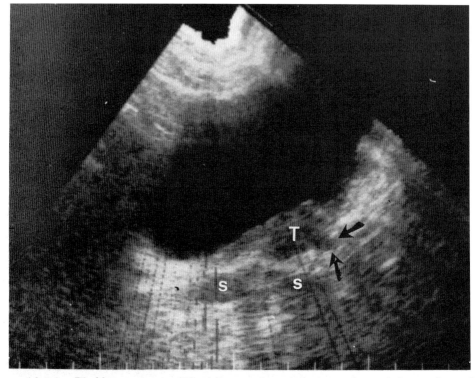

Figure 10.14. Bladder carcinoma (*T*) with extension of the tumor beyond the confines of the bladder wall into the perivesical fat (*arrows*). This indicates that the tumor is at least a stage C. *S*, seminal vesicles.

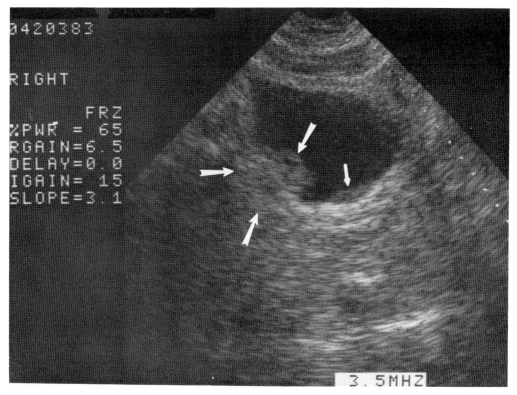

Figure 10.15.   Two bladder carcinomas. A small one posterially on the left (*small arrow*) does not extend beyond the bladder wall, but the larger one on the right side does extend into the perivesical fat (*large arrows*), indicating that this is a stage C tumor.

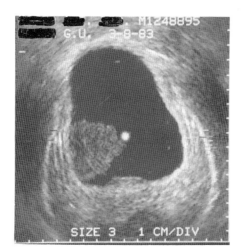

Figure 10.16.   Transurethral scan demonstrating superficial bladder tumor. Bladder wall is preserved. No invasion of lamina propria was detected histologically following resection.

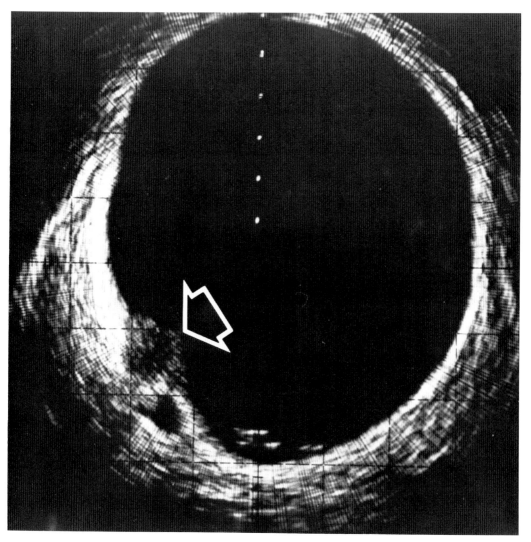

Figure 10.17. Transurethral scan demonstrating bladder tumor invasive into but not through muscle.

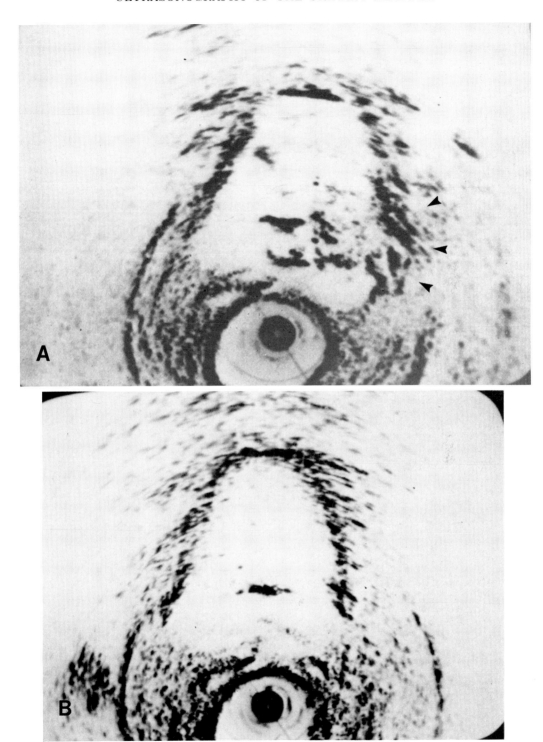

Figure 10.18.   Transrectal gray-scale sonogram in patient with invasive bladder tumor treated with preoperative irradiation. *A*, Preradiation scan demonstrating large tumor on left lateral wall of bladder invading perivesicle space (*arrows*). *B*, Postradiation scan showing no evidence of tumor. Cystectomy specimen was negative for tumor.

and abdominal lymph nodes. One must be aware that benign conditions, such as cystitis (22) and endometriosis (23), can at times have an ultrasonic appearance similar to that of bladder neoplasms.

BLADDER DIVERTICULA

Bladder diverticula are usually associated with diseases resulting in bladder outlet obstruction (benign prostatic hyperplasia) or neurogenic conditions resulting in abnormalities in bladder function. Diverticula resulting from these processes do not possess muscular coatings and can often be differentiated from the thickened and irregular. Diverticula greater than 2 cm in diameter can usually be seen ultrasonically, and with multiple scans often the narrow communication between a diverticulum and the bladder can be demonstrated (Fig. 10.19). Tumors or stones will occasionally be seen in these structures and should be sought. Postvoiding

scans are helpful since often diverticula will not empty and occasionally will actually increase in size. Diagnosis should be confirmed by cystography or cytoscopy, which are necessary procedures in the evaluation of patients with conditions that lead to diverticula formation. Pelvic ultrasonography is also of value in detecting the presence of urachal remnants (24) (Fig. 10.20), urethral diverticula (25), and bladder duplication (26).

BLADDER CALCULI

Bladder stones are usually seen in association with bladder outlet obstruction, chronic indwelling urinary catheters, and neurogenic diseases resulting in bladder dysfunction. Like stones in the kidney, bladder stones are strongly echogenic and are highly reflective of the ultrasonic beam. Due to their extreme density, echo shadows are often produced because of the inability of the sound waves to penetrate the stone (Fig. 10.21, A and B).

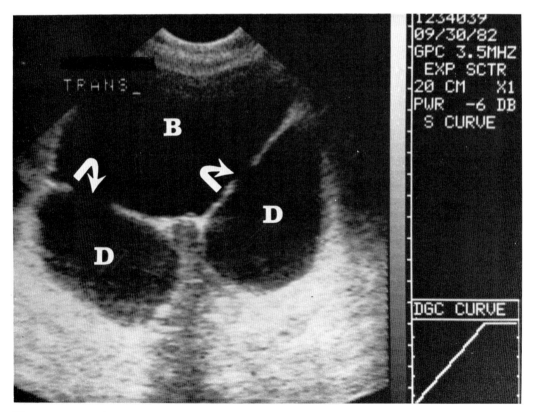

Figure 10.19.   Transverse scan showing two large diverticula (D). Note large diverticular orifices (*curved arrows*). B, bladder.

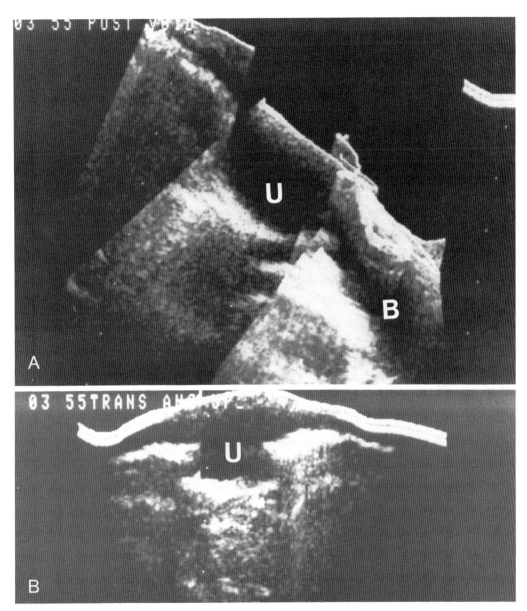

Figure 10.20. *A*, Transabdominal (longitudinal) sonogram demonstrating normal bladder (*B*) and urachal cyst (*U*) superior to the bladder. *B*, Transverse view shows that the urachal cyst invades the abdominal wall and intraperitoneal area.

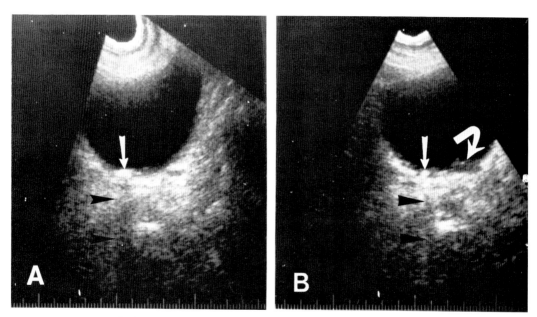

Figure 10.21.   *A* and *B*, Two scans of the bladder showing calculi (*straight arrows*) with posterior acoustic shadowing (*arrowheads*). There is a coexisting small bladder carcinoma (*curved arrow*).

MEASUREMENT OF BLADDER VOLUME AND RESIDUAL URINE

Several ultrasonic techniques have been devised for estimating bladder volume (27–30). Simple measurements of anterior and posterior diameters have shown poor correlation with true bladder volume, and other techniques have been developed utilizing sequential scans and planimetry (31). Using these techniques, bladder volume estimates have approached an accuracy of ± 20%. At times, an unexpected finding on an abdominal scan will be a large distended bladder in a patient with a mass and minimal or no voiding symptoms. Following catheterization and drainage, disappearance of the mass can be easily confirmed by repeat scan.

The presence of residual urine often indicates bladder dysfunction and decompensation, and its determination is an important part of the examination of patients with urinary tract disorders. When catheterization is not desirable, such as in children or in patients having 24-hour urinary collections for measurement of renal function, ultrasonic scans can be used to estimate the amount of residual urine. Residual urine can be estimated by obtaining scans prior to and after voiding. The presence of residual urine can easily be seen and the volume estimated by appropriate measurements with a planimeter. One must be careful, however, since the accuracy of measurement is poor with small bladder volumes; however, the study is often qualitatively helpful.

EXTRINSIC MASSES

Diseases of structures adjacent to the bladder will at times deform it and cause distortion and fixation of its walls. Cervical, colon, and prostatic carcinomas are common malignancies that frequently will extend locally into the bladder musculature (Figs. 10.22 to 10.24). Although an intraluminal mass may not be present, often the involved wall will be fixed and associated with the mass produced by the primary tumor. As is seen with primary malignancies of the bladder, scans obtained following surgery and/or radiotherapy are useful in the assessment of tumor response and in the detection of tumor recurrence. It is often very helpful to know the extent of bladder involvement prior to initiating surgical exploration and/or radiotherapy. Other perivesical benign processes or diseases that may distort the bladder include Müllerian duct remnants, abscesses, urinary extravasation, uterine fibroids, and ovarian cysts (Fig. 10.25, *A* and *B*). Ultrasound can also be helpful in differentiating a distended bladder from another type of pelvic disorder (32).

SUPRAPUBIC ASPIRATION

The techniques employed in percutaneous aspiration of the urinary bladder are similar to those used in renal cyst aspiration (Chapter 16). The technique is particularly valuable in children when it may be difficult to palpate the full bladder (33). Utilizing these techniques, the presence of urine in the bladder can be confirmed; with utilization of an ultrasonic aspiration transducer, a sterile urine specimen can be obtained (Fig. 10.26).

URODYNAMIC STUDIES

Ultrasonic techniques only have had limited application in studying the functional aspects of the lower urinary tract (34, 35). Bladder shape has been shown to vary with alterations in patient position and changes in amount of contained urine. Changes in bladder shape have also been shown to vary from day to day in the same individual and can be influenced by changes in uterine and rectal size. The value of these techniques in estimating the presence of residual urine has already been discussed. A more detailed review of the use of ultrasonography in the assessment of bladder function is presented in Chapter 19.

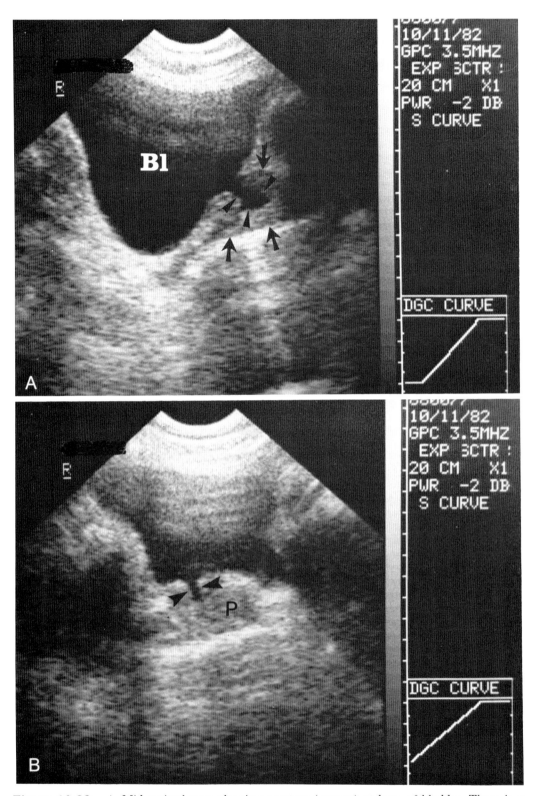

Figure 10.22. *A*, Mid-sagittal scan showing prostate (*arrows*) at base of bladder. There is a fluid-filled defect in the prostate (*arrowheads*) following previous prostatectomy. *B*, Transverse scan, angled caudally, showing postprostatectomy defect at urethral orifice (*arrowheads*). Note numerous reverberation echoes anteriorly in the bladder.

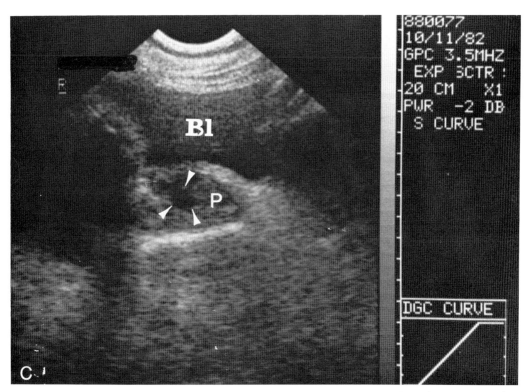

Figure 10.22.   *C*, Scan in same plane as *B* but slightly caudally, showing dilated prostatic urethra (*arrowheads*). *Bl*, bladder; *P*, prostate.

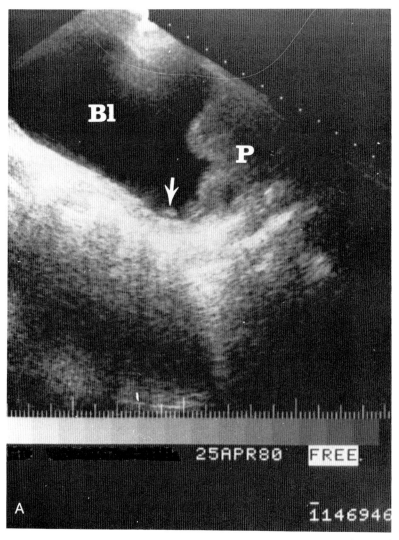

Figure 10.23. *A*, Sagittal scan showing dilated bladder (*Bl*) with enlarged irregular prostatic carcinoma (*P*). Note metastatic lesion in bladder wall (*arrow*).

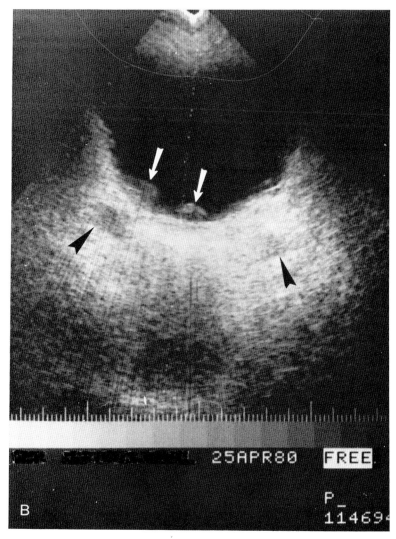

Figure 10.23. *B*, Transverse scan showing two small metastases on bladder wall from the prostatic carcinoma (*arrows*). The ureters (*arrowheads*) are dilated due to obstruction by the bladder carcinoma.

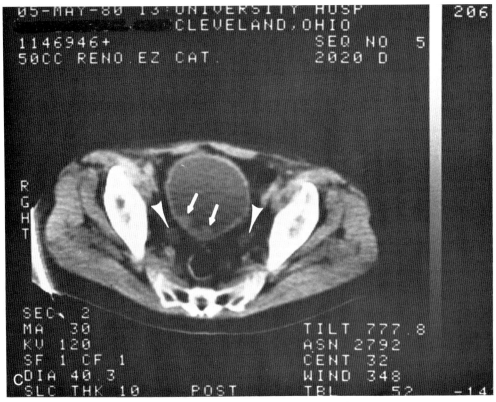

Figure 10.23. *C*, CT scan showing metastatic lesions in bladder wall (*arrows*). The dilated ureters (*arrowheads*) are also seen on the CT scan.

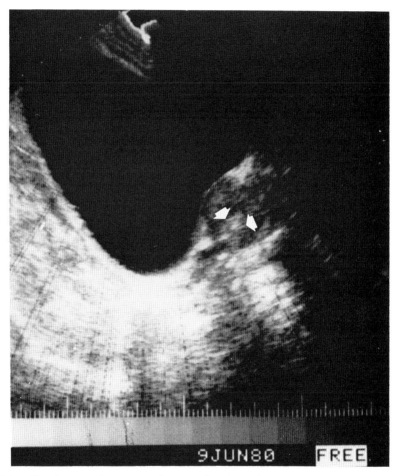

Figure 10.24.   Carcinoma of prostate. A somewhat irregular echogenic focus representing the carcinoma is seen within the prostate (*arrows*) on this sagittal transabdominal scan.

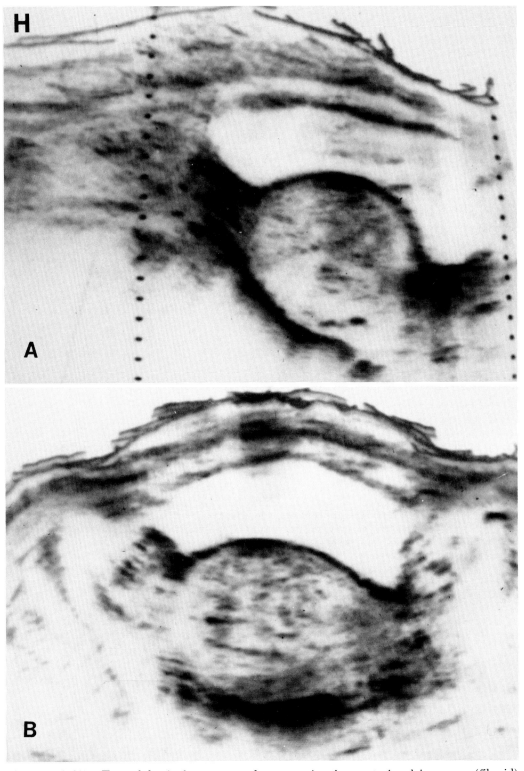

Figure 10.25. Transabdominal sonogram demonstrating large uterine leiomyoma (fibroid) posterior to bladder. *A*, Longitudinal scan. *H*, head. *B*, Transverse scan.

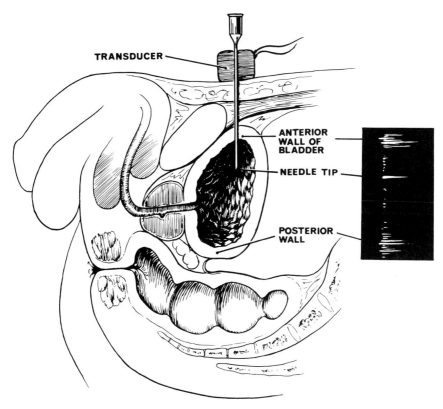

Figure 10.26. Anatomical drawing demonstrating use of aspiration transducer and A-mode for percutaneous aspiration of urinary bladder.

References

1. Schmidt JD, Weinstein SH: Pitfalls in clinical staging of bladder tumors. *Urol Clin North Am* 3:107, 1976.
2. Watanabe H, Kaiho H, Tanaka M, Terasawa Y: Diagnostic application of ultrasonography to the prostate. *Invest Urol* 8:548, 1971.
3. Watanabe H, Igari D, Tanahasi Y, Harada K, Saitoh M: Development and application of new equipment for transrectal ultrasonography. *J Clin Ultrasound* 2:91, 1974.
4. Resnick MI, Willard JW, Boyce WH: Recent progress in ultrasonography of the bladder and prostate. *J Urol* 117:444, 1977.
5. Hallemans E, Declercq G, Denis L: Transrectal ultrasonotomography. *Eur Urol* 3:37, 1977.
6. Gammelgaard J, Holm HH: Transurethral and transrectal ultrasonic scanning in Urology. *J Urol* 124:863, 1980.
7. Nakamura S, Niijima T: Transurethral real-time scanner. *J Urol* 125:781, 1981.
8. von Micksy LI: Gynecologic ultrasonography. In King DL: *Diagnostic Ultrasound*. St Louis, CV Mosby, 1974, p 207.
9. Holm HH, Northeved A: A transurethral ultrasonic scanner. *J Urol* 111:238, 1974.
10. Kremer H, Dobrinski W, Mikyska M, Baumgartner M, Zollner N: Ultrasonic in vivo and in vitro studies on the nature of the ureteral jet phenomenon. *Radiology* 142:175, 1982.
11. Dubbins PA, Kurtz AB, Darby J, Goldberg BB: Ureteric jet effect: the echographic appearance of urine entering the bladder. *Radiology* 140:513, 1981.
12. Wenzel WW, Carson PL, Johnson FB: Prostatic localization using ultrasound B-mode in scanning. In White D: *Ultrasound in Medicine*. New York, Plenum Press, 1975, p 149.
13. Schmidt JD, Weinstein SH: Pitfalls in clinical staging of bladder tumors. *Urol Clin North Am* 3:107, 1976.
14. Kyle KF, Deane RF, Morley P, Barrett E: Ultrasonography of the urinary tract. *Br J Urol* 43:709, 1971.
15. McLaughlin IS, Morley P, Deane RF, Barrett E, Graham AG, Kyle KF: Ultrasound in the staging of bladder tumors. *Br J Urol* 47:51, 1975.
16. Wittenberger AR, Murphy GP: Correlation of B-scan ultrasonic laminography with bilateral selective hypogastric arteriography and lymphography in bladder tumors. *Vasc Surg* 8:169, 1974.
17. Whitmore WF: Special article: summary of all phases of bladder carcinoma. *J Urol* 119:77, 1978.
18. Bree RL, Silver TM: Sonography of bladder and perivesical abnormalities. *AJR* 136:1101, 1981.
19. Cronan JJ, Simeone JF, Pfister RC, Newhouse JH, Ferrucci JT: Cystosonography in the detec-

tion of bladder tumors: a prospective and retrospective study. *J Ultrasound Med* 1:237, 1982.

20. Itzchak Y, Singer D, Fischelovitch Y: Ultrasonographic assessment of bladder tumors. I. Tumor detection. *J Urol* 126:31, 1981.

21. Singer D, Itzchak Y, Fischelovitch Y: Ultrasonographic assessment of bladder tumors. II. Clinical staging. *J Urol* 126:34, 1981.

22. Rifkin MD, Kurtz AB, Pasto ME, Goldberg BB: Unusual presentations of cystitis. *J Ultrasound Med* 2:25, 1983.

23. Goodman JD, Macchia RJ, Macasaet MA, Schneider M: Endometriosis of the urinary bladder: sonographic findings. *AJR* 135:625, 1980.

24. Sanders RC, Oh KS, Dorst JP: B-scan ultrasound: positive and negative contrast material evaluation of congenital urachal anomaly. *AJR* 120:448, 1974.

25. Lee TG, Keller FS: Urethral diverticulum: diagnosis by ultrasound. *AJR* 128:690, 1977.

26. Richman TS, Taylor KJW: Sonographic demonstration of bladder duplication. *AJR* 139:604, 1982.

27. McDonald DS: Ultrasound of the urinary tract. *Curr Prob Diag Radiol* 7:43, 1977.

28. Pedersen JF, Bartrum RJ, Grytter C: Residual urine determination by ultrasonic scanning. *AJR* 125:474, 1975.

29. Harrison NW, Parks C, Sherwood T: Ultrasound assessment of residual urine in children. *Br J Urol* 47:805, 1975.

30. Orgaz RE, Gomez AZ, Ramirez CT, Torres JLM: Applications of bladder ultrasonography. I. Bladder content and residue. *J Urol* 125:174, 1981.

31. Holm HH, Kristensen JK, Rasmussen SN, Pedersen JF, Hancke S: *Abdominal Ultrasound.* Baltimore, University Park Press, 1976, p 158.

32. Lee TG, Reed TA: Ultrasonic diagnosis of the bladder as a symptomatic pelvic mass. *J Urol* 144:283, 1977.

33. Goldberg BB, Meyer H: Ultrasonically guided suprapubic urinary bladder aspiration. *Pediatrics* 51:70, 1973.

34. Holmes JH: Ultrasonic studies of the bladder. *J Urol* 97:654, 1967.

35. Holmes JH: Ultrasonic studies of bladder filling and contour. In Hinman F: *Hydrodynamics of Micturition.* Springfield, IL, Charles C Thomas, 1971, p 303.

CHAPTER 11

Disorders of the Prostate

KAZUYA HARADA, M.D.

In the diagnosis and the treatment of prostatic diseases it is very important for the urologist to estimate the size and shape of the prostate accurately. Rectal palpation and urethrography are commonly used techniques for the clinical examination of the prostate. Neither is adequate to demonstrate the entire prostate because the former is a subjective method which varies from observer to observer, and the latter only shows an indirect effect on the prostatic urethra.

Ultrasonic diagnosis of the prostate was first attempted by Wild and Reid (1), who developed the first transrectal scanner in 1955. Takahashi and Ouchi (2) and Gotoh and Nishi (3) followed with similar transrectal scanners in 1963 and 1965, respectively, but satisfactory images for clinical use were not obtained. The first practical transrectal echogram of the prostate was reported by Watanabe et al. in 1968 (4). Since then, many observations on the morphology of the prostate have made it possible to evaluate prostatic disorders reproducibly, and many reports on the diagnostic applications of transrectal ultrasonography in the examination of the intrapelvic structures have been published (5–19). Recent echogram quality has been improved by the development of gray-scale ultrasonic technology. One can analyze not only the size and shape but also the internal structure and pathological changes within the prostate (20–23). More recently, transrectal longitudinal scanning using an electronic linear probe has been reported by Sekine et al. (24). By this new method one can obtain real-time longitudinal echograms of the prostate and observe the movement of the bladder neck and prostatic urethra during micturition.

TECHNICAL CONSIDERATIONS

Transabdominal Scanning

Conventional B-mode scanning via the abdominal wall to examine the prostate (25–27) has not been satisfactory because the technique is difficult and insufficient information is obtained. The prostate is located deep in the pelvis, and a suprapubic transducer has to be angled caudally through the bladder to see behind the pubic symphysis. Transabdominal echograms can barely visualize the whole prostate and failed to show much architecture within the prostate except stones. However, transabdominal real-time scanning is adequate for displaying the size and the shape of the prostate (Fig. 11.1).

Transrectal Scanning

Both a chair type scanner (Fig. 11.2) with the patient in sitting position and a pistol type scanner (Fig. 11.3) when the patient is in the lithotomy or lateral decubitus position are available for this method. In the sitting position the prostate is stable on the pelvic floor due to abdominal pressure and is not influenced by respiration or insertion of the probe (Fig. 11.4). When the patient is in the lithotomy position the prostate is movable and shows movement

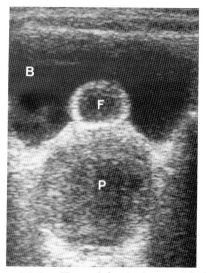

Figure 11.1. Transabdominal scan with electronic linear probe. *B*, urinary bladder; *F*, Foley catheter; *P*, prostate.

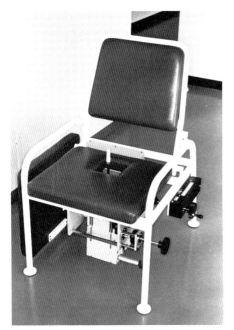

Figure 11.2. A special chair equipped with transrectal scanner.

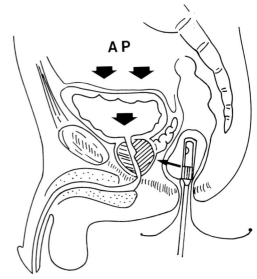

Figure 11.4. Transrectal scan in sitting position. *AP*, abdominal pressure.

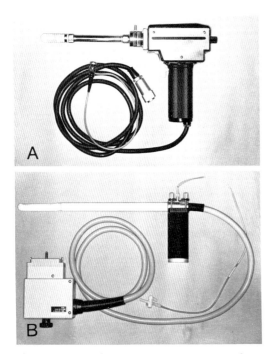

Figure 11.3. A pistol type apparatus used for transrectal scan. *A*, Radial scanner. *B*, Electronic linear probe.

with respiration (Fig. 11.5). Consequently, the sitting position is preferred for examining the prostate with ultrasound.

On the day of the examination, bowel preparation is not usually necessary, if the patient has defecated earlier. The patient is instructed to drink plenty of water prior to the examination and to retain urine in the urinary bladder. Prior to insertion of the probe into the rectum, the tip of the probe is covered with a rubber condom, the air in the condom is removed completely, and the surface of the balloon is coated with jelly for smooth probe insertion. The top of the probe protrudes 2 to 3 cm above the seat level. With the patient seated in the chair, the probe is slowly and carefully inserted into the anus. Elderly patients examined for detection of benign prostatic hyperplasia and prostatic cancer are almost free of pain and disagreeable sensations when the probe is inserted. With the probe inserted 7 to 9 cm into the rectum, the balloon is inflated with 50 to 70 ml of water. Scanning is usually carried out in 0.5-cm increments from the base of the bladder and the seminal vesicle toward the apex of the prostate.

Transurethral Scanning

Transurethral ultrasonography is not satisfactory for the screening of prostatic diseases because the procedure requires general or spinal

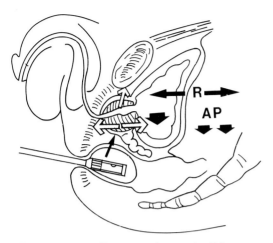

Figure 11.5. Transrectal scan in lithotomy position. *AP*, abdominal pressure; *R*, respiratory movement.

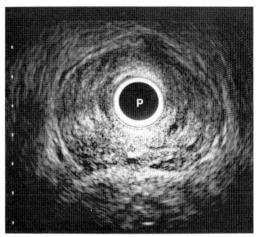

Figure 11.6. Transurethral scan of the prostate in benign prostatic hyperplasia. *P*, probe.

anesthesia or appropriate analgesics, and mucosal injuries are often caused by the rotating tip of the probe. The equipment consists of a pistol-shaped scanner and an outer sheath with an obturator. Prostatic echograms obtained with a transurethral scan visualize far structures and the capsule of the prostate clearly, but the areas in the near acoustic field around the transducer are visualized poorly (Fig. 11.6). Accordingly, the role of this technique is not expected to be significant in the early detection of prostatic cancer.

NORMAL PROSTATE

The normal prostate is usually visualized 3 to 6 cm from the anus with a transrectal scan. A typical echogram of a normal prostate shows a symmetrical crescentic or semilunar shape (Fig. 11.7). The cross-sectional shape of the normal prostate is influenced by the balloon pressure on the probe. Therefore, the anteroposterior diameter of the normal prostate is slightly shortened and the rectal aspect of the prostate is shown as concave and as a continuous regular line.

Generally, the echoes within the prostate may be divided into two zones. An internal zone consists of periurethral glandular tissue and muscle, and an external zone is formed by the true prostate. Toward the bladder base, the internal portion of the normal prostate shows low echo levels due to much muscle content. Additionally, this segment of the prostate is often

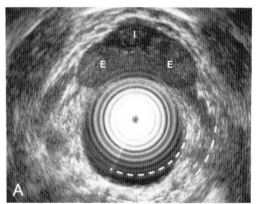

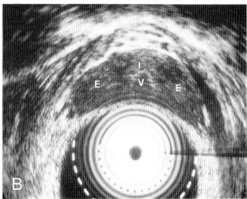

Figure 11.7. Transrectal radial scan of normal prostate. *A*, Transverse echogram in the upper segment. *B*, Transverse echogram at the level of the verumontanum. *I*, internal zone; *E*, external zone; *V*, verumontanum.

surrounded by a weakly reflective layer which is considered to be the muscle layers continuing from the bladder. In the lower segment of the prostate, the periurethral echopenic area becomes dominant, and the annular dark layer disappears. The peripheral glandular tissue occupies the bulk of the parenchyma of the normal prostate. This area usually displays fine even echoes, but even in normal cases, unusual echo patterns can be seen. Fine dotted echoes, diffuse and increased reflections, and strong echoes with shadowing (stone echoes) are occasionally recognized. The ejaculatory ducts and prostatic utricle often appear as a small oval area of decreased reflections in the median region of the external zone in the upper segment of normal or early hyperplastic glands (Fig. 11.8).

Voiding echograms obtained with transrectal scans allow the visualization of transverse and longitudinal sections of the prostatic urethra during micturition. In normal patients transverse sections of the prostatic urethra are obtained with the radial scan (Fig. 11.9), and the total length of prostatic urethra is shown with a longitudinal scan (Fig. 11.10).

BENIGN PROSTATIC HYPERPLASIA

The prostate increases in size in relation to aging. Over 50 years of age, the prostate occasionally develops atrophy, but in the majority of men hyperplasia of the periurethral glands, i.e., benign prostatic hyperplasia (BPH), occurs.

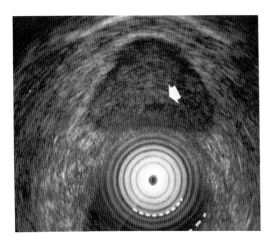

Figure 11.8. Transrectal radial scan of early benign prostatic hyperplasia shows a small oval spot with low echo density due to ejaculatory ducts and prostatic utricle (*arrow*).

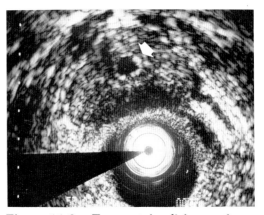

Figure 11.9. Transrectal radial scan of normal prostate during micturition shows a round cross-section of urethra (*arrow*).

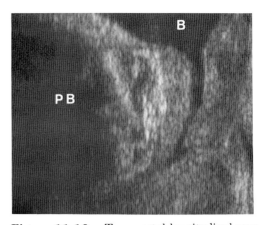

Figure 11.10. Transrectal longitudinal scan of normal prostate during micturition. *PB,* pubic bone; *B,* urinary bladder.

However, BPH varies from one patient to another. For instance, some men remain asymptomatic throughout their lives despite an enlarged prostate, whereas others have severe dysuria with small glands. There is no correlation between the size of the prostate and the severity of the symptoms in BPH.

The shape of the hyperplastic prostate changes according to the severity of the disorder. In slight to moderate-sized glands, a cross-section shows a kidney or semilunar shape; with severe BPH the cross-section becomes more circular (Fig. 11.11). When a typical hyperplastic gland is scanned from the level of the bladder caudally (Fig. 11.12), the protruded internal zone surrounded by the bladder wall appears in

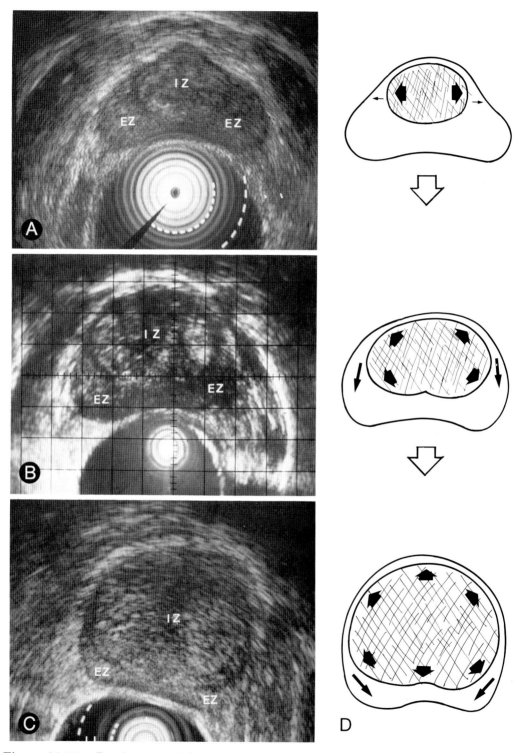

Figure 11.11.   Development of the internal zone in benign prostatic hyperplasia. *A*, Prostatic echogram in early BPH. *B*, Prostatic echogram in typical BPH. *C*, Prostatic echogram in advanced BPH. *D*, Change of the internal zone (*IZ*) and the external zone (*EZ*).

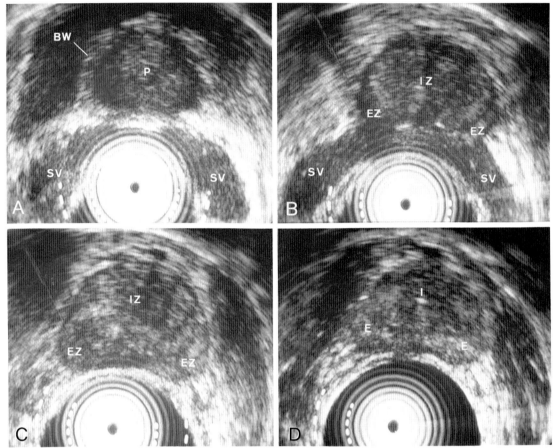

Figure 11.12. Cross-sectional changes in a typical BPH. *A*, At the level of the bladder. *B*, At the level of the upper segment. *C*, At the level of the middle segment. *D*, At the level of the lower segment. *BW*, bladder wall; *P*, prostate; *IZ*, internal zone; *EZ*, external zone; *SV*, seminal vesicle.

the bladder cavity initially. A circular transverse upper section shows a prostate mostly occupied by the internal zone with boomerang-shaped seminal vesicles posteriorly. In the middle to lower segment a transverse section shows a prostate with semilunar or kidney shape with the external zone increasing. A cross-section of the hyperplastic prostate is overall symmetrical, but it may become asymmetrical in the upper segment near the bladder neck if there is a marked difference in growth between the right and left lobes of the adenoma (Fig. 11.13). There is a similarity in shape between adjacent sections, and the rectal aspect is concave—a differentiating point between BPH and cancer. The margin in BPH is usually well defined and smooth as in the normal subject; however, capsular echoes are poorly seen when the direction of the beam is tangential to the prostate.

Reflections from the internal zone in BPH

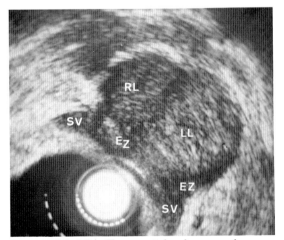

Figure 11.13. Transrectal echogram shows asymmetrical enlargement of the internal zone. *RL*, right lobe; *LL*, left lobe; *EZ*, external zone; *SV*, seminal vesicle.

are somewhat rough and uneven. When nodules (Fig. 11.14), stones, inflammation, infarction, and/or dilatation of the ducts and acini exist, the transverse scan of the hyperplastic prostate shows complex echoes. Prostatic calculi are recognized on the echogram in most cases of BPH (Fig. 11.15). Stone echoes showing strong reflections are considered to originate from the surface of the round stone and the calcified corpora amylacea (28). The stone echo pattern of the hyperplastic prostate is often shown as a link (Fig. 11.16) or as a mass (Fig. 11.17) on the course of the prostatic duct near the boundary between the internal and external zone.

Voiding echograms using a radial scan technique of hyperplastic prostates reveal deformation or displacement of the urethra corresponding to the severity of the disorder (Fig. 11.18). Significantly less satisfactory findings may be obtained with longitudinal scans except after transurethral resection of the prostate (TURP).

Prostatic echography is also very useful for the evaluation of treatment of BPH. The resected area following TURP can be accurately assessed with transrectal (Fig. 11.19) and trans-

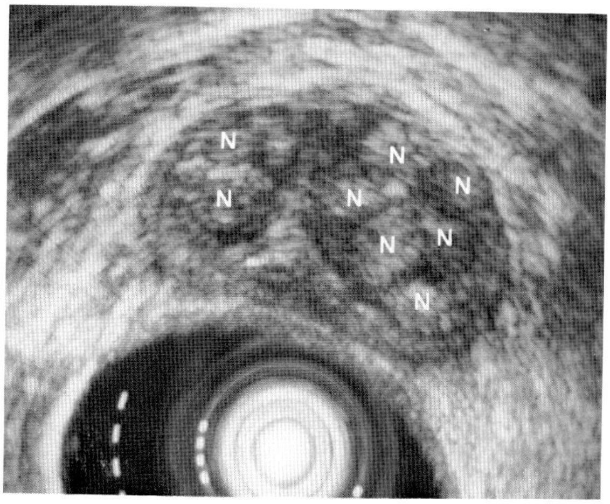

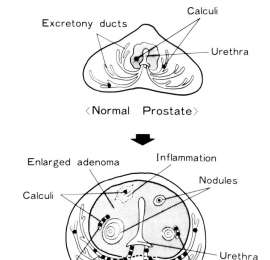

Figure 11.14. Transrectal echogram shows asymmetrical enlargement of lobes with multiple nodules (*N*).

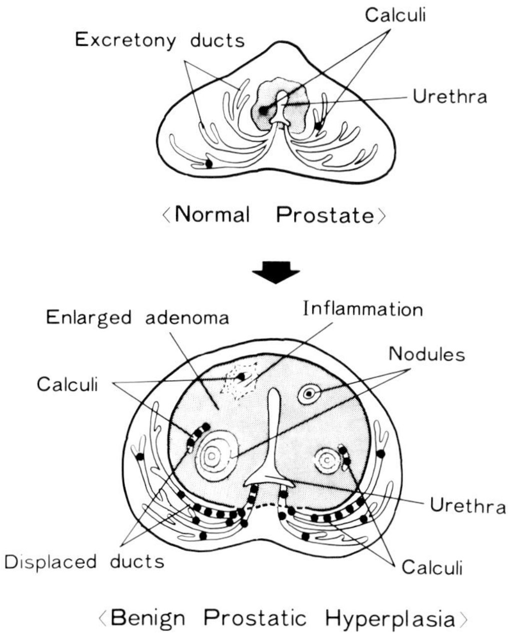

Calculi

Excretony ducts

Urethra

〈 Normal Prostate 〉

Enlarged adenoma   Inflammation

Calculi   Nodules

Urethra

Displaced ducts   Calculi

〈 Benign Prostatic Hyperplasia 〉

Figure 11.15. Stone formation in normal subjects with benign prostatic hyperplasia.

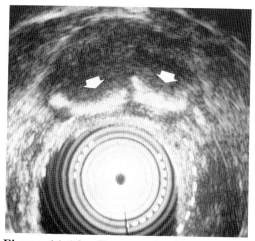

Figure 11.16. Transrectal echogram of benign prostatic hyperplasia shows stone echoes in an arc (*arrows*).

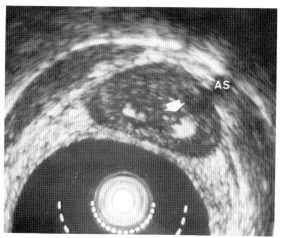

Figure 11.17. Transrectal echogram of benign prostatic hyperplasia shows a mass of stone echoes (*arrow*). *AS*, acoustic shadow.

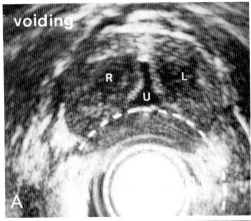

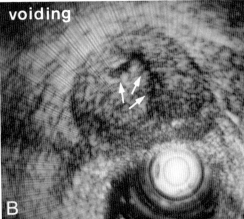

Figure 11.18. Voiding echogram of benign prostatic hyperplasia by transrectal radial scan. *A,* Cross-section of the urethra (*U*) compressed symmetrically by bilateral lobes. *B,* Cross-section of the urethra (*arrows*) deformed markedly. *R,* right lobe; *L,* left lobe.

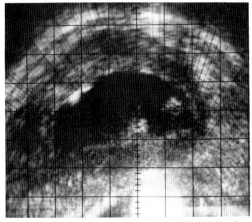

Figure 11.19. Transrectal radial scan after transurethral prostatic resection shows the resected area clearly.

urethral scans during and after surgery. In cryosurgery, the maximum freezing effect can be assessed safely by ultrasonic monitoring of ice ball formation (29). Effects of antiandrogen therapy can be monitored objectively by measuring prostatic volume before and after the administration of these agents.

PROSTATIC CARCINOMA

According to autopsy studies, prostatic carcinoma is found in 12 to 46% of men over 50 years of age, and the incidence increases with the age (30–33). In the United States, prostatic carcinoma is the second most common cause of cancer death in men; therefore, it is important to establish the diagnosis early, stage the disease precisely, and evaluate the response to therapy accurately. Prostatic cancers seldom begin to manifest clinical symptoms until the tumor infiltrates locally and distant metastases occur.

Ultrasonic findings in the advanced stage can be characterized by "irregularity." The primary site of the cancer is almost always in the external zone. If the cancer develops from the median region of the external zone, it pushes the internal zone forward to lengthen the anteroposterior diameter (Fig. 11.20). If the cancer develops from the lateral region of the external zone, an asymmetrical transverse shape develops (Fig. 11.21). In either case the cancer growth and infiltration are not uniform so that the prostatic echogram shows a marked deformity and textural asymmetry. When extracapsular invasion exists, there is a disruption of the capsular echoes, an irregularity of the boundary, prostatic deformity, and an irregular protrusion of the prostate into the bladder cavity (Fig. 11.22).

The interior echoes from the cancer have no characteristic pattern. In some cases the echoes are decreased initially, and, following initiation of hormone therapy, they gradually increase with associated contraction of the prostate (Fig. 11.23). Calcifications in the prostate are seen pathologically and roentgenographically in many patients with prostate cancer. It has been suggested that they form because cancer infiltration results in obstructed prostatic ducts. The calcifications in cancer on the echogram show an irregular distribution, and they are often accompanied with diffuse increased echoes which probably result from inflammatory changes around stones. With cancer the internal zone is poorly visualized, but if the cancer is early or is associated with adenomatous hyperplasia, the internal zone may be visualized often

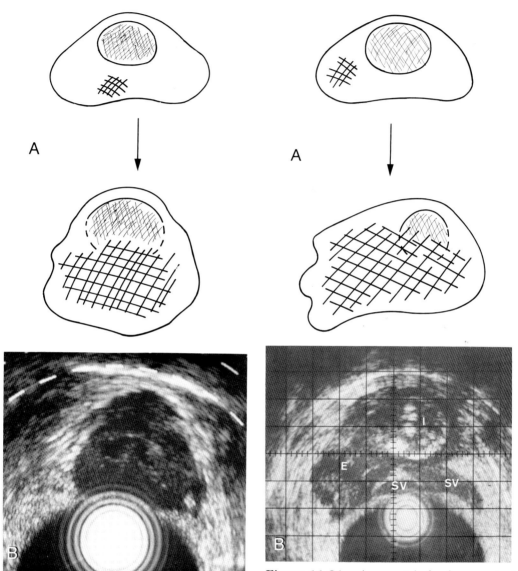

Figure 11.20. Anteroposterior enlargement of the cross-section in prostatic cancer. A, Cancer growth originated from the median region. B, Prostatic echogram of cancer with elongation of the anteroposterior diameter.

Figure 11.21. Asymmetrical enlargement of the cross-section in prostatic cancer. A, Cancer growth originated from the lateral region. B, Prostatic echogram of cancer with asymmetrical enlargement of the cross-section. I, internal zone; E, external zone; SV, seminal vesicle.

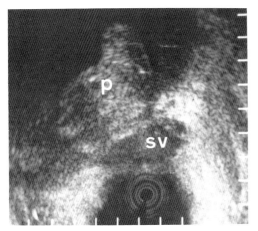

Figure 11.22. Transrectal echogram shows an irregular protrusion of the prostate into bladder cavity and deformed seminal vesicles. *P*, prostate; *SV*, seminal vesicle.

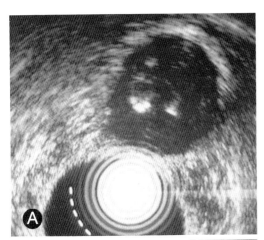

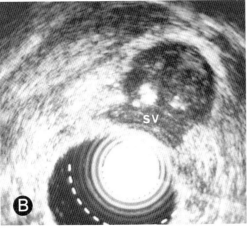

Figure 11.23. Therapeutic effect following hormone therapy for treatment of prostatic can-

surrounded by an asymmetrical external zone (Fig. 11.24).

Ultrasonic changes after hormone therapy for prostatic cancer are as follows: (*a*) size contraction, (*b*) recovery of symmetry, (*c*) a recovery of the outline and continuity of the capsular echo, and (*d*) an increase of the interior echoes. When prostatic volume is measured ultrasonically following initiation of hormone therapy, a sharp decrease in size is usually observed within a month; thereafter, the contraction rate diminishes gradually. In the case of hormone-resistant cancer, the amount of contraction is small or an increase in prostatic volume is observed.

PROSTATITIS

Prostatitis can be divided into acute and chronic. The two conditions have considerable clinical and ultrasonic differences. Acute prostatitis can be easily diagnosed clinically. The prostatic echograms in acute prostatitis (Fig. 11.25) have the following features: (*a*) enlarged and deformed outline, (*b*) indefinite boundary, (*c*) abnormal patterns (stone echoes, fine dotted

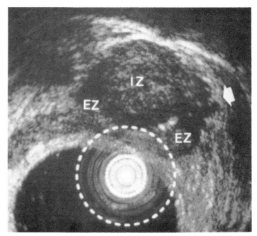

Figure 11.24. Transrectal echogram of cancer associated with benign prostatic hyperplasia shows asymmetrical external zone (*EZ*). *Arrow*, extracapsular invasion; *IZ*, internal zone.

cer. *A*, Prostatic echogram before treatment shows an oval shape with the anteroposterior diameter elongated and marked decrease of internal echoes except for stone echoes. *B*, Prostatic echogram after treatment shows contraction of the cross-section making it possible to distinguish the seminal vesicle (*SV*) from the prostate.

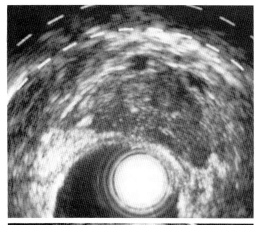

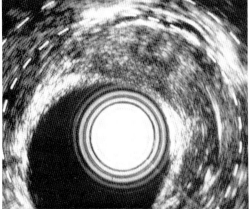

Figure 11.25. Acute prostatitis. *Top*, Prostatic echogram before treatment. *Bottom*, Prostatic echogram after treatment.

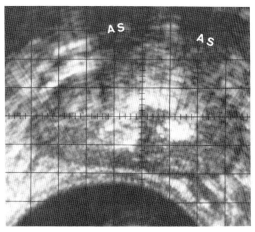

Figure 11.26. Stone echoes of chronic prostatitis are shown in both the internal and external zones. *AS*, acoustic shadow.

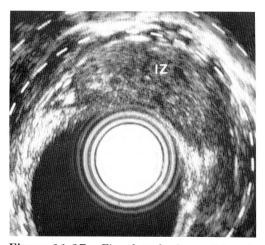

Figure 11.27. Fine dotted echoes of chronic prostatitis are shown on the posterior site of the external zone. *IZ*, internal zone.

echoes, diffuse increased echoes, and decreased echoes). After treatment, recovery in the shape, size, and boundary is observed on the echogram, but many abnormal patterns remain.

Prostatic echograms in chronic prostatitis have the following features: (*a*) rarely is there enlargement and deformity of the transverse shape, (*b*) the prostatic boundary is well defined, and (*c*) abnormal patterns of stone echoes, fine dotted echoes, and diffuse increased pattern exist independently or in combination. Stone echoes (Fig. 11.26) are often recognized posterior to the urethra or along the prostatic ducts in the peripheral zone. If associated with urethritis, stone echoes may be shown around the urethra in the internal zone. Fine dotted echoes (Fig. 11.27), probably from the corpora amylacea, are seen on the posterior aspect of the external zone. A diffuse increased echo pattern may be recognized (Fig. 11.28).

CYSTS IN THE PROSTATE

Prostatic cysts (Fig. 11.29) are very rare and can be overlooked because of lack of clinical symptoms. They can be easily detected with ultrasound. It is believed that prostatic cysts lie either to the right or left. Müllerian duct cysts (Fig. 11.30), i.e., abnormal dilatation of the prostatic utricle, lie centrally posterior to the urethra.

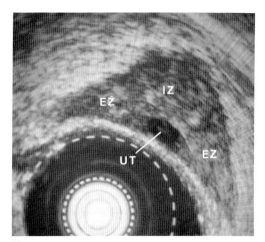

Figure 11.30. Transrectal echogram in small BPH prostate shows a Müllerian duct cyst. *EZ*, external zone; *IZ*, internal zone; *UT*, utricle.

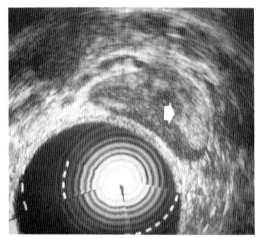

Figure 11.28. Diffuse increased pattern of chronic prostatitis (*arrow*).

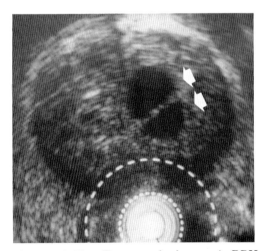

Figure 11.29. Transrectal echogram in BPH prostate shows a cyst with the septum in enlarged adenoma.

References

1. Wild JJ, Reid JM: Progress in techniques of soft tissue examination by 15 MC pulsed ultrasound. In Kelly E: *Ultrasound in Biology and Medicine.* Washington, DC, American Institute of Biological Science, 1975, p 30.
2. Takahashi H, Ouchi T: The ultrasonic diagnosis in the field of urology (the 1st report). *Proc Jpn Soc Ultrasonics Med* 3:7, 1963.
3. Gotoh K, Nishi M: Ultrasonic diagnosis of prostatic cancer. *Acta Urol Jpn* 11:87, 1965.
4. Watanabe H, Katoh H, Katoh T, Morita M, Tanaka M, Terasawa Y: Diagnostic application of the ultrasonotomography for the prostate. *Jpn J Urol* 59:273, 1968.
5. Watanabe H, Kaiho H, Tanaka M, Terasawa Y: Diagnostic application of ultrasonotomography to the prostate. *Invest Urol* 8:548, 1971.
6. Watanabe H, Igari D, Tanahashi Y, Harada K, Saitoh M: Development and application of new equipment for transrectal ultrasonography. *J Clin Ultrasound* 2:91, 1974.
7. Watanabe H, Igari D, Tanahashi Y, Harada K, Saitoh M: Measurements of size and weight of prostate by means of transrectal ultrasonotomography. *Tohoku J Exp Med* 114:277, 1974.
8. Watanabe H, Igari D, Tanahashi Y, Harada K, Saitoh M: Transrectal ultrasonotomography of the prostate. *J Urol* 114:734, 1975.
9. Watanabe H, Igari D, Tanahashi Y, Harada K, Saitoh M: An evaluation of the function of new special equipment for transrectal ultrasonotomography. *Tohoku J Exp Med* 118:387, 1976.
10. Watanabe H, Saitoh M, Mishina T, Igari D, Tanahashi Y, Harada K, Hisamichi S: Mass screening program for prostatic diseases with transrectal ultrasonotomography. *J Urol* 117:746, 1977.
11. King WW, Wilkiemeyer RM, Boyce WH, McKinney WM: Current status of prostatic echography. *JAMA* 226:444, 1973.

12. Boyce WH, McKinney WM, Resnick MI, Willard JW: Ultrasonography as an aid in the diagnosis and management of surgical diseases of the pelvis; special emphasis on the genitourinary system. *Ann Surg* 184:477, 1976.

13. Resnick MI, Willard JW, Boyce WH: Recent progress in ultrasonography of the bladder and prostate. *J Urol* 117:444, 1977.

14. Resnick MI, Willard JW, Boyce WH: Ultrasonic evaluation of the prostatic nodule. *J Urol* 120:86, 1978.

15. Resnick MI, Willard JW, Boyce WH: Transrectal ultrasonography in the evaluation of patients with prostatic carcinoma. *J Urol* 124:482, 1980.

16. Tanahashi Y, Yatanabe H, Igari D, Harada K, Saitoh M: Volume estimation of the seminal vesicles by means of transrectal ultrasonotomography: a preliminary report. *Br J Urol* 47:695, 1975.

17. Hallemans E, Declercq G, Denis L: Transrectal ultrasono-tomography. *Eur Urol* 3:37, 1977.

18. Harada K, Igari D, Tanahashi Y, Watanabe H, Saitoh M, Mishina T: Staging of bladder tumors by means of transrectal ultrasonography. *J Clin Ultrasound* 5:388, 1977.

19. Taylor WB, Hunt JW, Foster FS, Blend R, Worthington A: A high-resolution transrectal ultrasonographic system. *Ultrasound Med Biol* 5:129, 1979.

20. Harada K, Igari D, Tanahashi Y: Gray scale transrectal ultrasonography of the prostate. *J Clin Ultrasound* 7:45, 1979.

21. Harada K, Tanahashi Y, Igari D, Numata I, Orikasa S: Clinical evaluation of inside echo patterns in gray scale prostatic echography. *J Urol* 124:216, 1980.

22. Peeling WB, Griffiths GJ, Evans KT, Roberts EE: Diagnosis and staging of prostatic cancer by transrectal ultrasonography: a preliminary study. *Br J Urol* 51:565, 1979.

23. Gammelgaard J, Holm HH: Transurethral and transrectal ultrasonic scanning in urology. *J Urol* 124:863, 1980.

24. Sekine H, Oka K, Takehara Y: Transrectal longitudinal ultrasonotomography of the prostate by electronic linear scanning. *J Urol* 127:62, 1982.

25. Miller SS, Garvie WHH: The evaluation of prostate size by ultrasonic scanning: a preliminary report. *Br J Urol* 45:189, 1973.

26. Hennerberry M, Cater MF, Neiman HL: Estimation of prostatic size by suprapubic ultrasonography. *J Urol* 121:615, 1979.

27. Jimenez-Cruz JF, Mayato T, Lovaco F, Garcia J, Navio S, Romero-Aquirre C: Transabdominal sonography of seminal vesicles. *J Urol* 127:260, 1982.

28. Harada K, Tanahashi Y, Numata I, Kanbe K, Chiba Y, Toyota S: Evaluation of the stone echo pattern in the excised prostate (the 1st report). *Proc Jpn Soc Ultrasonics Med* 3:675, 1982.

29. Tanahashi Y: Monitoring of cryosurgery. In Watanabe H, Holmes JH, Holm HH, Goldberg BB: *Diagnostic Ultrasound in Urology and Nephrology.* Tokyo, Igaku-Shoin, 1981, p 183.

30. Andrews GS: Latent carcinoma of the prostate. *J Clin Pathol* 2:197, 1949.

31. Baron E, Angrist A: Incidence of occult carcinoma of the prostate after 50 years of age. *Arch Pathol* 32:787, 1941.

32. Moor RA: The morphology of small prostatic carcinoma. *J Urol* 33:224, 1935.

33. Rich AR: On the frequency of occurrence of occult carcinoma of prostate. *J Urol* 33:215, 1935.

CHAPTER **12**

Scrotal Ultrasonography*

WILLIAM SCHEIBLE, M.D.

Clinical evaluation of intrascrotal pathology is considered to be relatively straightforward. In the past, the urologist has not relied upon imaging tests to establish a diagnosis. Recent experience with radioisotope scanning and, more importantly, gray-scale ultrasonography has shown that adjunctive diagnostic procedures can be extremely helpful in troublesome cases and can even detect subclinical disease. The most significant contribution of ultrasonic imaging of the scrotum is its reliability in distinguishing conditions that arise within the testis from those that originate in the paratesticular tissues. Testicular lesions are potentially malignant, and treatment is generally considered to be surgical. Extratesticular disorders are seldom neoplastic, and most can be managed conservatively. In the presence of hydrocele, edematous or indurated soft tissues, or severe pain, palpation of the testis can be quite difficult. Ultrasonography, unique among imaging modalities, is capable of depicting testicular parenchyma and confirming its integrity or identifying alterations thereof.

INSTRUMENTATION AND TECHNIQUE

Early ultrasonographic investigations of scrotal pathology utilized articulated arm B-scanners with bi-stable or primitive gray-scale image recording (1–3). Although examinations of diagnostic quality were possible with these systems, the technique failed to gain widespread physician acceptance. A major problem with contact B-scanning of the scrotal contents is the difficulty in immobilizing the testis. Consequently, reproducibility of scan planes and precise lesion localization become quite difficult, and contact scanning requires considerable technical expertise. Nonetheless, contact scanning can be useful in cases of massive scrotal

enlargement where many real-time scanners might fail to provide sufficient field of view or depth of penetration (Fig. 12.1).

Improvements in gray-scale image processing led to further advances in scrotal ultrasonography (4, 5). Reliable separation of testicular from extratesticular disorders became possible. The advent of high resolution real-time ultrasonographic units has marked the most recent advance in imaging of the scrotal contents (6, 7). A complete survey of the scrotum can be accomplished in a matter of a few minutes. Moreover, real-time scanning allows instantaneous visual identification of areas of interest, and the practical limitations of contact scanning are minimized. Most real-time systems incorporate transducers of relatively high frequency (5 MHz and above). This is desirable in scrotal imaging because ultrasonic resolution is greater the higher the frequency of the sound wave. The poorer depth of penetration with high frequency transducers is ordinarily not a problem with the superficially located scrotal contents. Recently, experience with direct immersion water bath scanning of the testes has been reported (8, 9). The technique overcomes some of the problems of inadequate referencing of scan planes that result from the mobility of the testes.

Examination of the scrotum with real-time instruments is an easy task and need not be made unnecessarily cumbersome. Mineral oil or acoustic gel can be used as a coupling agent. The hemiscrotum is supported by one hand of the examiner while the other manipulates the transducer assembly. It is sometimes helpful to interpose a water delay between the transducer and the scrotal surface to optimize beam focusing geometry and to allow better visualization of very superficial areas. A surgical glove filled with water can be used for this purpose.

It is preferable to begin scanning the presumed normal testis for proper assignment of gray-scale and adjustment of gain settings. The normal side is then used as a reference organ for

* The author would like to acknowledge the assistance of Ms. Elizabeth Novak and Laura Martin in the preparation of this manuscript.

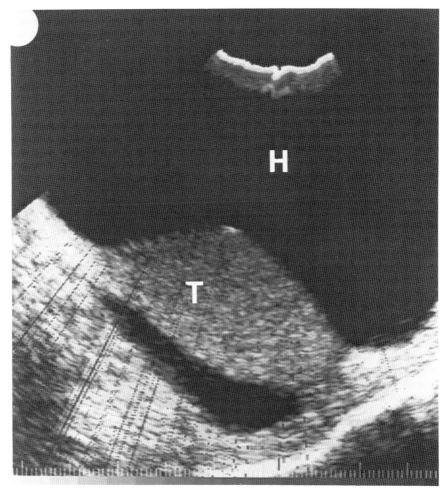

Figure 12.1.   Contact B-scan in case of massive scrotal enlargement due to hydrocele (*H*). The testis (*T*) is displaced posteriorly, but normal glandular texture is demonstrated.

the sometimes subtle pathology in the contralateral testis. Real-time examinations allow the choice of a variety of scan planes, although a longitudinal section is generally the most helpful.

NORMAL ANATOMY

The normal adult testis is ovoid and measures approximately $4 \times 3 \times 3$ cm, with the longitudinal axis being the longest dimension. The parenchyma of the testis is divided into lobules, but this architecture is not discerned on sonograms. The texture of the testis is homogeneous and granular on sonograms, with uniform echoes of mid-amplitude intensity (Fig. 12.2). An adherent fibrous capsule, the tunica albuginea,

invests the testis, and an infolding of this structure forms the mediastinum testis (8). This is sometimes recognizable on sonograms as a thin linear reflection immediately beneath the capsule (Fig. 12.3).

The anterior and lateral aspects of the testis are covered by the visceral layer of the tunica vaginalis, the parietal layer of which reflects off the inner scrotal wall. Between these two layers, which form an isolated sac of peritoneum, a small amount of fluid is generally present (Fig. 12.4). Posteriorly, each testis is attached to the epididymis and peritesticular tissues.

The epididymis is a worm-like appendage that extends alongside the testis from the upper pole, where it is termed the globus major, to the

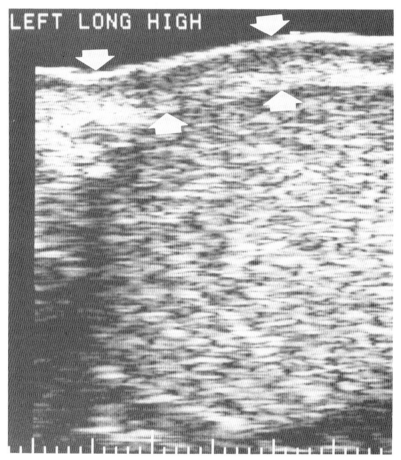

Figure 12.2.   Normal testis. A longitudinal section through the upper pole shows the homogeneous mid-amplitude reflections of testicular parenchyma. The scrotal wall (*arrows*) is identified separately.

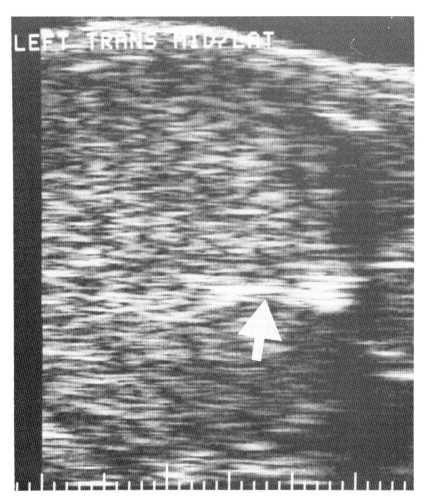

Figure 12.3. Normal testis. A transverse section shows the uniform granularity of testis parenchyma. The mediastinum testis (*arrow*) is an intense linear reflection within the gland.

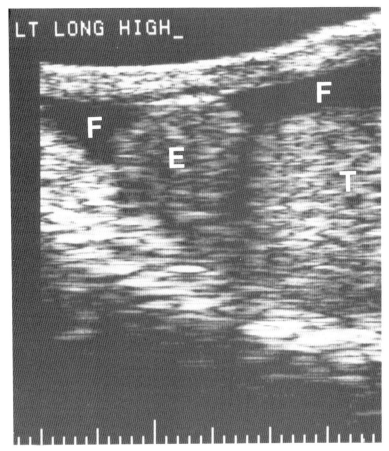

Figure 12.4. Normal testis and epididymis. This longitudinal section illustrates the small amount of fluid (*F*) that is typically seen within the tunica vaginalis at the upper end of the testis. *E*, epididymis; *T*, testis.

inferior pole, where it is called the globus minor. The epididymis courses along the posterolateral aspect of the testis, then gives rise to the vas deferens, which ascends up the posteromedial aspect. The vas deferens is not routinely identified as a separate structure on ultrasonograms. Normally the epididymis displays a somewhat coarser and more echogenic appearance when compared with the homogeneous nature of the adjacent testis (Fig. 12.5).

The spermatic cord is composed of the arteries and veins of the testis, its lymphatics and nerves, and the vas deferens. Individually, these structures are below the threshold of ultrasonic resolution. Similarly, the several layers of the scrotal wall are not recognizable.

INDICATIONS FOR SCROTAL ULTRASONOGRAPHY

The clinical utility of scrotal ultrasonography is now fairly well established (10–13). Probably the most significant contribution of the technique is the reliable distinction between disorders that arise within the testis from those originating elsewhere in the scrotum. Ultrasonography is most helpful in evaluating the causes of chronic symptoms and scrotal enlargement, although acute conditions can also be investigated with some success (14). Certain ultrasonographic criteria have been advanced for differentiating among lesions that are demonstrably intratesticular in location (15). Further experience is necessary to confirm the validity of these observations.

EXTRATESTICULAR DISORDERS

Epididymitis versus Torsion

Acute epididymitis and testicular torsion are relatively frequent disorders affecting the scrotal contents. Epididymitis can usually be treated

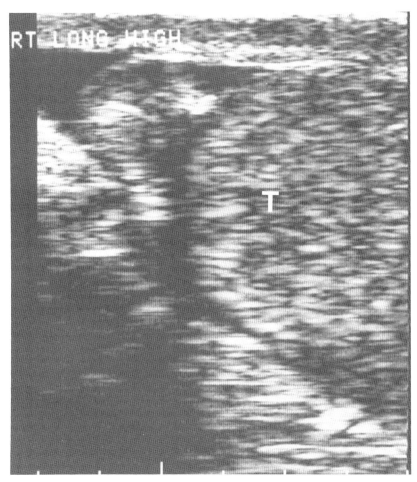

Figure 12.5. Normal epididymis. The globus major portion of the epididymis caps the cephalic pole of the testis. The texture of the epididymis is slightly irregular, and more echogenic than the testis (*T*).

conservatively with antibiotics and analgesia. It is commonly the result of nonspecific infectious agents, and in older men it is often related to instrumentation or prostatitis. Torsion of the spermatic cord is usually encountered in adolescent males. It is a urological emergency and demands immediate surgery because testicular salvage is rarely possible if the process exceeds 24 hours duration (16). Although epididymitis is frequently associated with leukocytosis and an abnormal urinalysis, and torsion is usually of a more sudden onset, often during sleep, the clinical distinction between the two entities is not always straightforward. Radionuclide scanning and ultrasonography can be useful adjuncts in the diagnosis of these acute disorders of the scrotum (17–19).

The sonographic features of acute epididymitis are variable, but a frequent observation is enlargement due to inflammatory edema (Fig. 12.6). The echogenicity of the epididymis is sometimes accentuated and results in intense reflectivity (Fig. 12.7). In uncomplicated cases, the testis is not involved; documentation of focal hypoechoic areas in the adjacent testicular parenchyma justifies the diagnosis of epididymoorchitis (Fig. 12.8). Reactive hydroceles are commonly observed with epididymitis. These are often quite complex with multiple areas of septation probably due to fibrin strands and inflammatory debris (Fig. 12.9).

Radionuclide scanning during the acute phase also exhibits rather typical features (20). Dynamic vascular imaging with technetium[99m] pertechnetate shows relative hyperemia in the epididymal area of the involved side (Fig. 12.10). This is in contrast to the appearance of acute testicular torsion, which, because it is an

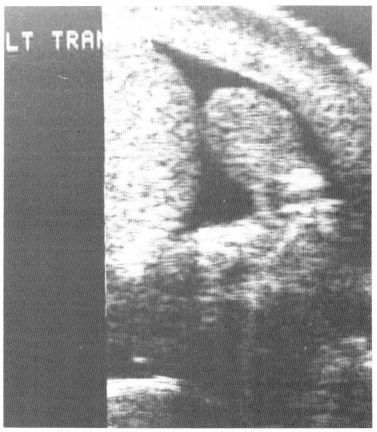

Figure 12.6. Acute epididymitis. The posterolaterally situated epididymis (transverse section) is enlarged and slightly less echogenic than normal. The scrotal wall is also slightly thickened.

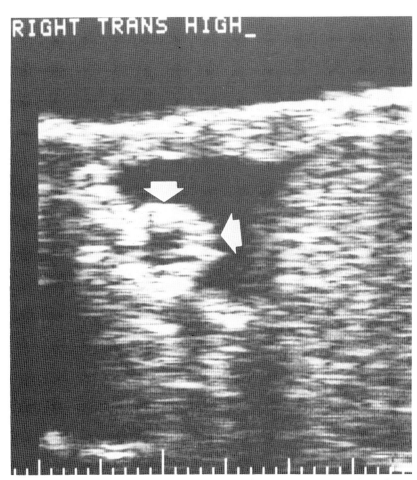

Figure 12.7. Acute epididymitis. In this case the globus major is intensely reflective (*arrows*) presumably secondary to inflammatory exudate. The adjacent testis remains normal.

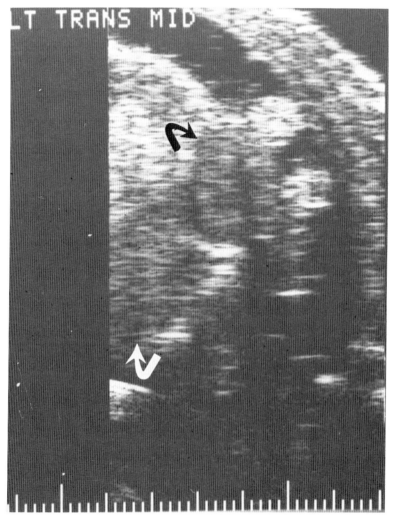

Figure 12.8.   Epididymo-orchitis. The margins of the inflamed epididymis are indistinct, and the neighboring testis exhibits an irregular pattern with focal hypoechoic areas (*arrows*).

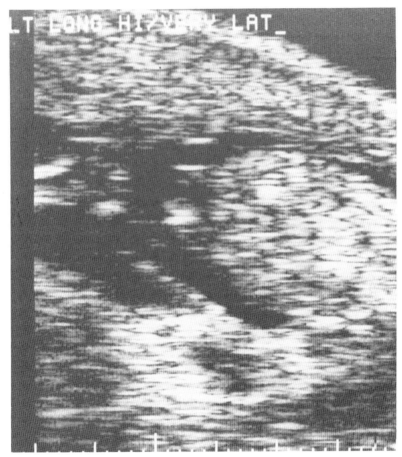

Figure 12.9. Reactive hydrocele. Several thin strands and septations are present within a small hydrocele in this case of acute epididymitis.

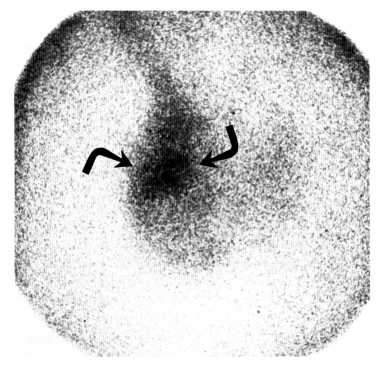

Figure 12.10.   Acute epididymitis. A technetium[99m] pertechnetate scan obtained at 1 minute shows increased uptake in the region of the involved right epididymis (*arrows*). (Case courtesy of Kathryn Witztum, M.D., San Diego, CA.)

ischemic process, interrupts the blood supply to the testis (21, 22). Little or no radiopharmaceutical accumulates on the affected side (Fig. 12.11).

Sonography can also be helpful in cases of torsion of the spermatic cord. Doppler technology has been used with some success, for the same reason that radioisotope imaging is successful. No Doppler signal will be returned when the probe is placed over the affected ischemic side (23, 24). Sonographic B-scanning has also been used in cases of testicular torsion (14, 25). Early in the process, the testis is enlarged and often becomes somewhat hypoechoic when compared to the other side (Fig. 12.12).

Undiagnosed testicular torsion (missed torsion) results in infarction and hemorrhagic necrosis of the testis. Although the involved testis is no longer salvageable, it is important to establish this diagnosis because the anatomical defect that predisposes to the condition is frequently bilateral. Current urological practice advocates prophylactic repair of the "bell-clapper" deformity or other abnormalities of suspension at the time of orchiectomy for the affected side.

Sonography and radionuclide imaging can be used to clarify the situation in cases of missed torsion (26). Sonography depicts the pathoanatomy; hemorrhage and necrosis produce a disorganized testicular parenchyma with areas of cystic change often a prominent feature (Fig. 12.13). Radioisotope scans show a classic "doughnut" sign of peripheral uptake around a photon-deficient center (Fig. 12.14). For both tests, these same findings can also be observed in testicular abscess or tumor (27). Correlation with the clinical setting should allow an appropriate diagnosis to be made.

For acute presentations of scrotal pain, when the distinction between epididymitis and torsion is not clear-cut, one could recommend sonography if epididymitis seems more likely and nuclear medicine techniques for those cases thought to be torsion. It is important to recognize that testicular neoplasms can present as an episode of clinical epididymitis. It is helpful, therefore, to confirm resolution of presumed epididymitis with a follow-up sonogram to demonstrate integrity of the testis. Any persistent abnormality within the testis should be looked

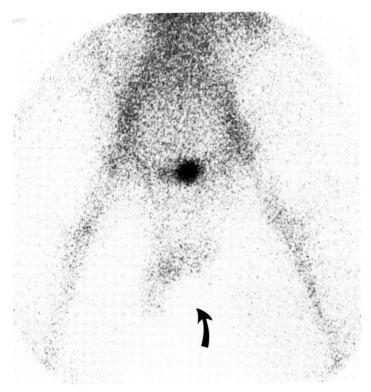

Figure 12.11.   Testicular torsion. A 5-minute scan from a technetium^{99m} pertechnetate study shows absent accumulation of radiopharmaceutical in the torsed left testicle (*arrow*). (Case courtesy of Kathryn Witztum, M.D., San Diego, CA.)

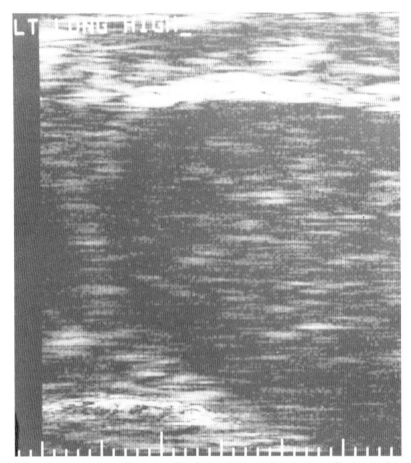

Figure 12.12. Acute torsion. The overall echogenicity of the testis is diminished (cf. Fig. 12.2).

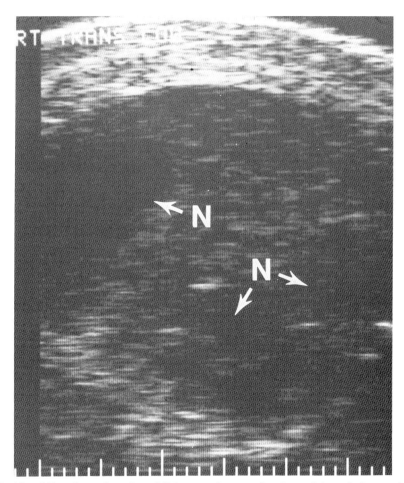

Figure 12.13. Missed torsion. In addition to decreased echogenicity of the testis, areas of hemorrhagic necrosis (*N*) produce focal cystic lesions.

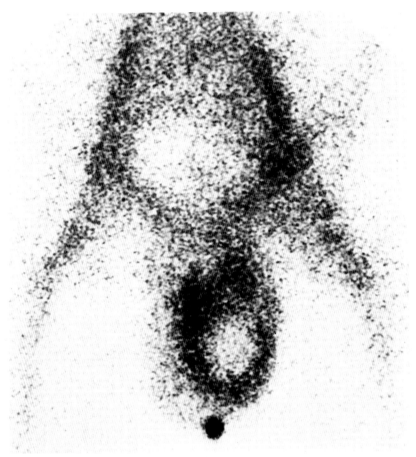

Figure 12.14. Missed torsion. Static imaging with technetium[99m] pertechnetate shows enhanced peripheral uptake around the "cold" infarcted testis.

upon as suspicious for indolent testicular abscess or occult malignancy. Rarely, an adherent postinflammatory mass arising from the epididymis can masquerade as an intratesticular lesion (28).

Paratesticular Masses

A varicocele is simply a collection of dilated veins in the pampiniform plexus immediately cephalad and slightly posterior to the testis. This anomaly is more frequent on the left and is thought to be a leading cause of male infertility. In middle-aged men, in particular, the recent onset of varicocele should prompt an investigation into the possibility of venous compression by an intra-abdominal mass, such as retroperitoneal node enlargement or renal carcinoma. The appearance of varicocele on high resolution ultrasonograms is predictable. The tortuous, ectatic veins are noted as a mass of tubular fluid-filled structures above and sometimes behind the testicle (Fig. 12.15). Occasionally, these veins can be made more prominent by asking the patient to stand and then rescanning the involved side.

Spermatoceles are collections of cloudy fluid containing nonviable sperm. These lesions are usually single and seldom exceed 2 to 3 cm in diameter. They typically arise in the region of the efferent ductules near the head of the epididymis (Fig. 12.16). Their extratesticular location is usually easy to establish on palpation. Spermatoceles seldom become infected, and excision is usually done only for cosmetic reasons.

Loculated hydroceles can occur anywhere along the course of the once patent processus vaginalis. Because they are fluid filled, they are

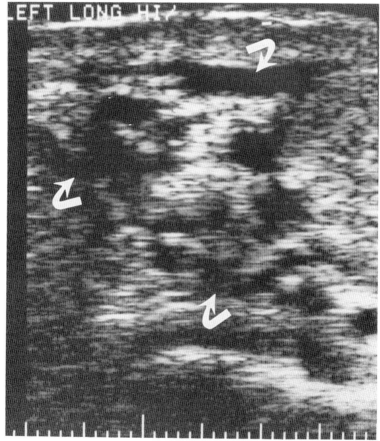

Figure 12.15. Varicocele. Above the testis, a mass of dilated veins in the pampiniform plexus is seen as a collection of fluid-filled structures (*arrows*).

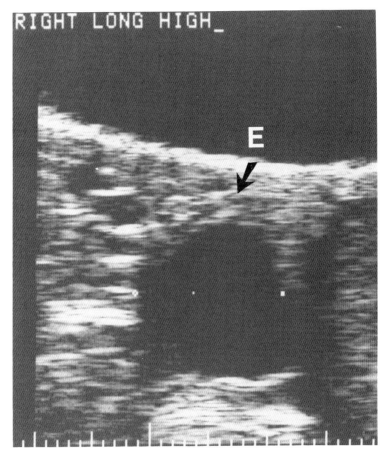

Figure 12.16. Spermatocele. A cystic mass is clearly separable from the upper pole of the testis. The head of the epididymis (*E*) is draped over the spermatocele.

indistinguishable from spermatoceles on ultra-sonograms (Fig. 12.17). This is not a significant limitation of the method since the treatment is the same and tends to be conservative.

Occasionally, small cysts are detected in the epididymis, but these are seldom clinically apparent. The epididymis itself can sometimes present as a discrete mass in cases where a history of chronic or repeated bouts of inflammatory disease is elicited (Fig. 12.18). The ultrasonic features of epididymal enlargement and coarsened texture, often with apparent calcification, are also supportive of chronic inflammatory changes.

Primary neoplasms of the epididymis and adnexal structures of the scrotum are very rare. If a solid-appearing extratesticular mass cannot be explained on the basis of previous infection or trauma, one might then consider the possibility of neoplasm.

Hydrocele

A hydrocele is a collection of excessive fluid between the visceral and parietal layers of the tunica vaginalis. This space exists anterior and to both sides of the testis, so in the presence of a large hydrocele, the testis is compressed into the posterior aspect of the scrotum. Hydroceles that occur in response to inflammation or trauma are sometimes termed "complicated" because they contain inflammatory cells or blood. Simple hydroceles are commonly idiopathic in origin but may signal an occult underlying malignancy. Scrotal swelling is frequently a result of hydrocele, and physical examination and transillumination readily establish the diagnosis. Chronic hydroceles frequently do not transilluminate, however. In either case, the presence of a large amount of fluid makes palpation of the testis very difficult. One should remember

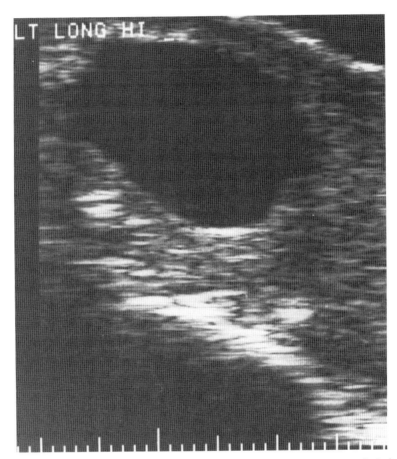

Figure 12.17. Loculated hydrocele. A 2-cm diameter cystic mass presents cephalad to the testis, and its appearance is similar to that of spermatocele (cf. Fig. 12.16).

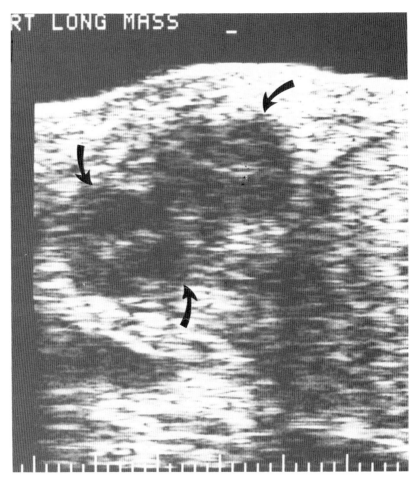

Figure 12.18. Chronic epididymitis. This supratesticular mass (*arrows*) is solid, and a separate epididymis could not be identified. At surgery, the lesion proved to be granulomatous epididymitis.

that approximately 15% of cases of testicular malignancy present to the physician as a hydrocele. Sonography can be extremely helpful, because the accumulated fluid acts as a convenient sonic medium and the testis is easily evaluated. The integrity of the testis can be confirmed, or impalpable lesions can be identified (Fig. 12.19). If the underlying testis can be demonstrated to be normal, treatment, if necessary for relief of symptoms or for cosmetic reasons, is simply aspiration of the fluid collection. Surgical excision is not usually required.

Hernias

Herniation of bowel and/or omentum into the scrotal sac is not unusual. Physical examination is quite reliable in making this diagnosis, but occasionally the findings are inconclusive and ancillary studies are requested. Ultrasonography is most helpful when real-time examination documents peristalsis of fluid-filled loops of bowel (Fig. 12.20). Air in bowel and fat in omentum in the hernia can be troublesome for ultrasonic visualization. Extending the examination to include the inguinal areas is very helpful in these situations (29). Contiguity of the scrotal "mass" with the inguinal canal, coupled with identification of separate and normal testes, should enable correct interpretation.

TESTICULAR DISORDERS
Neoplasms

Although primary malignant tumors of the testis are uncommon, they constitute the third

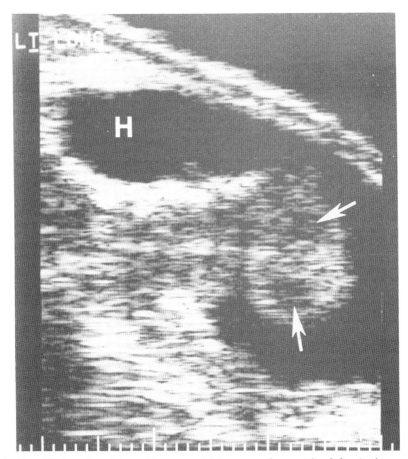

Figure 12.19. Hydrocele with malignancy. This young boy with abdominal neuroblastoma presented with scrotal swelling. The testis was difficult to palpate because of a hydrocele (*H*), but sonography demonstrated focal irregularities of the parenchyma (*arrows*). Autopsy confirmed testicular involvement with neuroblastoma.

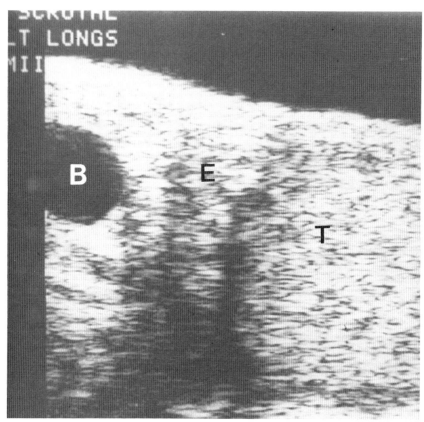

Figure 12.20. Scrotal hernia. A fluid-filled loop of bowel (B) is noted above the epididymis (E) and testis (T). This mass could be reduced at the time of the sonogram, confirming its origin. (Case courtesy of Edward Miller, M.D., Newport Beach, CA.)

leading cause of cancer death in American males between the ages of 15 and 35 (30, 31). Yet these cancers are among the most curable malignancies in humans. Seminoma is extremely radiosensitive. Nonseminomatous germ cell neoplasms usually respond very well to recently developed chemotherapy protocols. Early diagnosis is the key to continued improvement in survival from these lesions, and ultrasonography, by virtue of depicting testicular parenchyma, can contribute significantly to this success.

Almost all testicular malignancies are of germ cell origin; the supporting tissues are rare sites of primary neoplasia. Mixed neoplasms are common, with two or more distinct cell types occurring in one tumor. Many testis cancers are associated with elevations of serum glycoproteins. These substances can be detected with sensitive radioimmunoassays and thus become a helpful

feature in both initial diagnosis and subsequent follow-up of treated disease. Approximately 70% of teratocarcinomas and embryonal cell carcinomas have an increased serum α-fetoprotein (AFP) and 40 to 60% of nonseminomatous germ cell tumors, particularly choriocarcinoma, are associated with elevations of human chorionic gonadotropin (HCG). High titers of both serum markers are frequently present with mixed tumors.

Treatment of primary testicular neoplasia is radical orchiectomy via an inguinal approach. This involves removal of the entire scrotal contents and spermatic cord to the level of the inguinal ring on the side harboring the tumor. Although many lesions are palpable, some men present with extensive metastases to the retroperitoneal lymph nodes yet have normal testes to examination (32, 33). Scrotal ultrasonography affords a unique contribution to these cases (Fig.

12.21). Current urological practice recommends against percutaneous trans-scrotal biopsy of intratesticular neoplasms. The lymphatic drainage of the testes is along well-established pathways that ascend with the gonadal veins to the inferior vena cava on the right and the left renal vein on the left side. The scrotal lymphatics, on the other hand, drain to superficial inguinal nodes, and it is thought that metastatic pathways might thus be altered if the scrotal wall has been transgressed. This would have therapeutic implications because likely sites of disease would be extended.

Seminoma accounts for roughly 40% of testicular malignancies. It has a peak occurrence in the fourth and fifth decades, thus is seen in a slightly older age group than other testis can-

cers. Teratocarcinoma and embryonal carcinoma each represent about 25% of testis tumors and occur most frequently in the third decade of life. Pure choriocarcinoma is rare; it usually exists as a component of mixed germinal tumors (34).

It is not possible to accurately predict histological diagnoses from gray-scale ultrasonographic patterns alone, but it seems that certain trends do exist (35). Seminoma appears very fleshy on inspection and is composed of sheets of cells of relatively uniform make-up. The appearance of seminoma on ultrasonograms tends to mirror this uniformity. When compared with the normal testicular parenchyma, the lesions are hypoechoic, sometimes appearing almost cystic. Attention to proper gain settings will

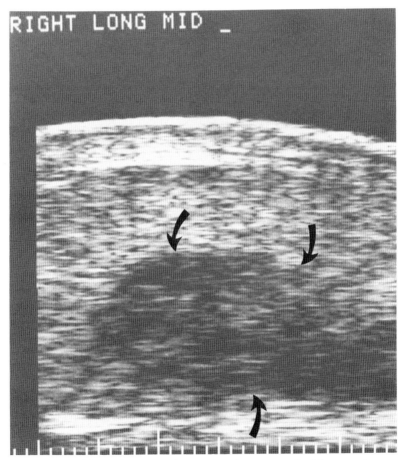

Figure 12.21. Impalpable testis tumor. A young male presented with extensive retroperitoneal lymphadenopathy which proved to be metastatic seminoma. The testes were normal to palpation, but ultrasonography demonstrates a hypoechoic lesion within the posterior aspect of the testis (*arrows*). Surgery confirmed seminoma.

demonstrate the low amplitude signals returned from these masses (Fig. 12.22). Seminomas also tend to be very well demarcated from the surrounding testis and have smooth, clearly defined borders. Conversely, most nonseminomatous neoplasms are irregular tumors, often composed of aggregates of varying cell type. This is particularly so for teratoma/teratocarcinoma, which is likely to undergo internal hemorrhage and contain elements of cartilage and even bone. Sonography of these lesions typically reveals a complex-appearing mass with irregular, poorly defined borders (Fig. 12.23). Intense reflections, presumably from calcified areas, and cystic spaces are commonly observed on ultrasonograms (Fig. 12.24). Sometimes, direct extension of the tumor into the scrotal wall or spermatic cord can be documented, which can potentially alter lymphatic drainage with metastases then presenting in iliac or inguinal nodes.

Synchronous or metachronous testicular neoplasms occur in approximately 2% of cases, so it is always important to survey the contralateral side. Similarly, it is advisable to perform serial ultrasonograms of the remaining testis in anyone who has undergone an orchiectomy for cancer.

Non-germ cell neoplasms arising in the testis are unusual. Although they are rarely malignant, the treatment of such tumors is radical orchiectomy. Experience with these lesions is limited, but it is doubtful that they show any specific ultrasonographic features (36).

Metastases to the testis are also uncommon.

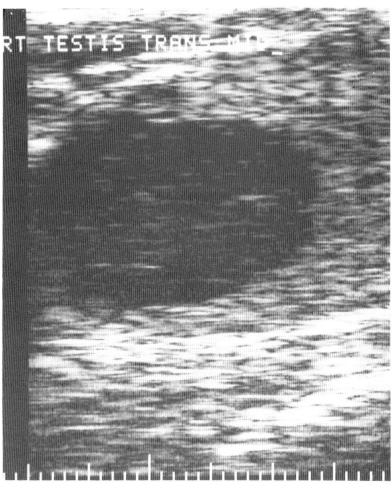

Figure 12.22. Seminoma. This well-demarcated tumor is typical of the sonographic features of seminoma. The lesion is considerably less echogenic than the normal surrounding testis.

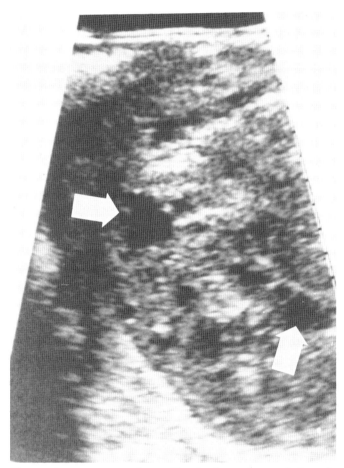

Figure 12.23. Nonseminomatous neoplasm. Nearly the entire testis is replaced by a tumor of markedly irregular texture. Cystic areas (*arrows*) are caused by hemorrhage and necrosis. Surgery confirmed embryonal carcinoma. (Case courtesy of Harvey Neiman, M.D., Chicago, IL.)

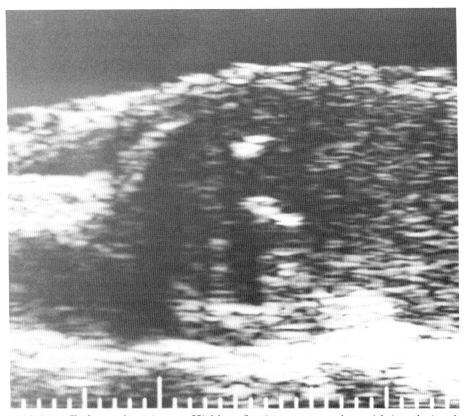

Figure 12.24. Embryonal carcinoma. Highly reflective areas correlate with intralesional calcification. The internal architecture of the tumor is complex, and its demarcation from adjacent testis is poorly defined. (Case courtesy of Edward Miller, M.D., Newport Beach, CA.)

The most frequent sites of primary cancer to metastasize to the testis are lung, prostate, and melanoma (37). On the other hand, non-Hodgkin lymphoma of the testis is not rare. In males over the age of 50, approximately one-half of testicular neoplasms are lymphoma. Lymphoma seldom originates in the testis but is much more likely to be a manifestation of systemic disease, sometimes still occult when the testicular lesion is discovered (38). On scrotal ultrasonograms, lymphoma deposits look extremely homogeneous and are very hypoechoic, reminiscent of the features of lymphomatous lymph nodes in the abdomen and retroperitoneum (Fig. 12.25). The lesions resemble those seen with seminoma, although lymphoma is more likely to be multicentric.

Leukemia in males also involves the testes with some frequency. In fact, the testis, like the central nervous system, is considered to be an "immunologically privileged sanctuary site" that is somehow able to escape the effects of chemotherapy that control the disease elsewhere. The testes thus become a common site of relapse in young men whose disease is otherwise in remission (39, 40). Testicular leukemia shows ultrasonographic features indistinguishable from those of lymphoma or primary tumor such as seminoma. The involved portions are well-circumscribed hypoechoic masses (Fig. 12.26). Sometimes the entire testis is affected, in which case it becomes enlarged.

Infection

The testis can become inflamed in a number of systemic viral infections, particularly mumps and Coxsackie virus. The affected testis in orchitis is swollen because of edema, and this pathoanatomy is depicted on the ultrasonogram. The testis is enlarged, and, although the overall granular texture is maintained, the testis be-

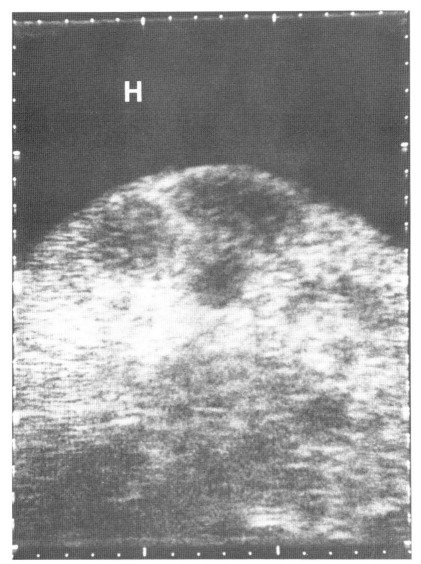

Figure 12.25. Testicular lymphoma. A large anterior hydrocele (*H*) prevented adequate palpation of the testes in this man with diffuse histiocytic lymphoma. Sonography demonstrated multiple
hypoechoic lesions within the testis, typical of the findings seen with lymphoma deposits.

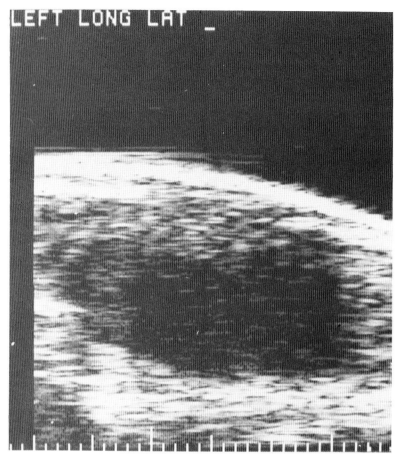

Figure 12.26. Testis leukemia. A strikingly hypoechoic mass occupies the lower portion of the testis in this youngster with acute lymphoblastic leukemia.

comes hypoechoic when contrasted with its normal state (Fig. 12.27). Uncomplicated orchitis seldom progresses to surgical complications such as abscess; infertility is a feared consequence of mumps orchitis, however.

Trauma

The major consequence of blunt trauma to the scrotum is testicular rupture, which is a surgical condition (41). The documentation of rupture is sometimes difficult on clinical findings, and ultrasonography can be very helpful in these situations (42, 43). Extrusion of testicular material beyond the tunica albuginea is diagnostic of rupture on ultrasonograms (Fig. 12.28). There is frequently an associated hematocele.

Severe intratesticular hematomas without frank capsular rupture may require surgical evacuation and even orchiectomy. Lesser injuries can be managed conservatively. The ultra-sonographic spectrum of hematomas varies from totally cystic, when the lesion has undergone liquification and is, therefore, actually a seroma, to exceedingly complex and echogenic, when organization and scarring have occurred (Fig. 12.29). Any testicular mass palpated after an episode of trauma should be sequentially followed with ultrasonography. Frequently it is trauma that first alerts the patient and/or his physician to the existence of a mass, but the mass is sometimes a pre-existing neoplasm rather than a result of trauma. If an intratesticular mass does not resolve or show the temporal changes compatible with hematoma, the possibility of coincidental tumor should be borne in mind.

Undescended Testes

Embryological development of the testes begins in the high retroperitoneum near the site

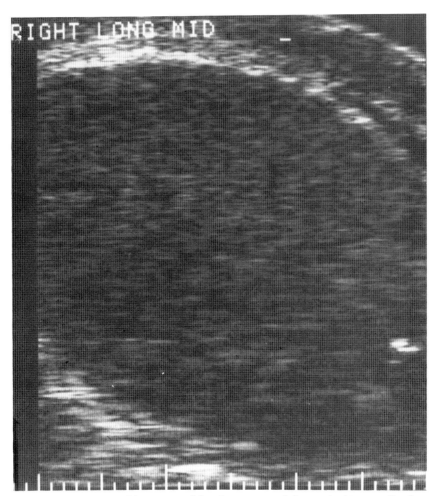

Figure 12.27. Orchitis. In addition to mild enlargement of the testis, its overall echogenicity is diminished (cf. Fig. 12.2).

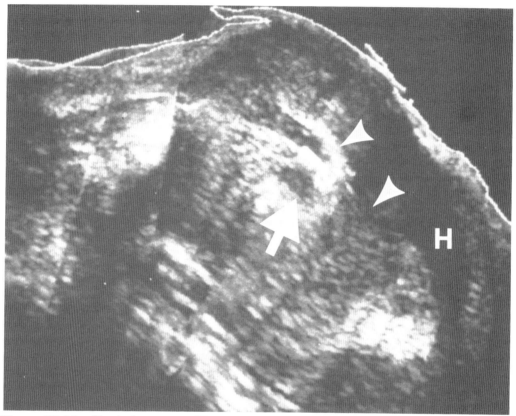

Figure 12.28. Testicular rupture. This contact B-scan shows a portion of testicular substance extending beyond the interrupted tunica (*arrowheads*) in association with a small hematocele (*H*). A small intratesticular hematoma is also present (*arrow*).

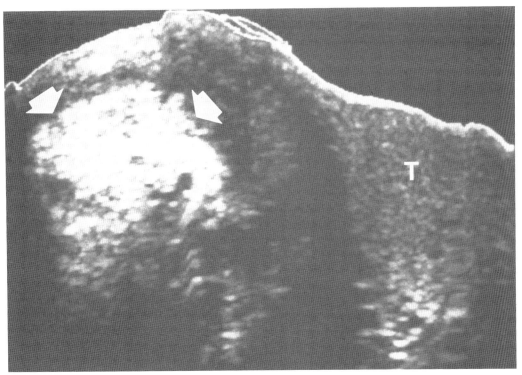

Figure 12.29.   Chronic hematoma. Contact B-scan demonstrates a highly echogenic complex mass essentially replacing the right testis (*arrows*). Note the normal left testis (*T*). Surgery showed an infarcted testis with organized hematoma and fibrosis.

of the fetal kidneys. Descent into the scrotum occurs near term, but about 1% of boys have persistent cryptorchidism beyond the age of 1 year (44). The most frequent location for maldescent is in the inguinal canal, accounting for about 70% of cases. In this location, the testis can sometimes be palpated. Whether or not they are palpable, these testes are candidates for ultrasonographic evaluation because of their superficial location (45). Often they are smaller than testes that have entered the scrotum, but the overall sonographic texture should be nearly the same (Fig. 12.30). Confirmation of an undescended testis in the inguinal region is useful information prior to any planned surgical or hormonal attempt at correction. If the testis cannot be found in the inguinal canal, the like-

lihood of a pelvic or intra-abdominal location must be considered. There is a markedly increased risk of malignancy in these testes, thought to be greater the higher the position of the cryptorchidism. Ultrasonography has achieved some success in detecting abdominal or pelvic testes, and neoplastic masses arising from them have been identified (46, 47). Computed tomography may become the procedure of choice for localization, but venography and arteriography must sometimes be performed (48–52).

SUMMARY

It is clear that ultrasonography can be a useful diagnostic procedure in modern urological practice. Additional physician experience with newer

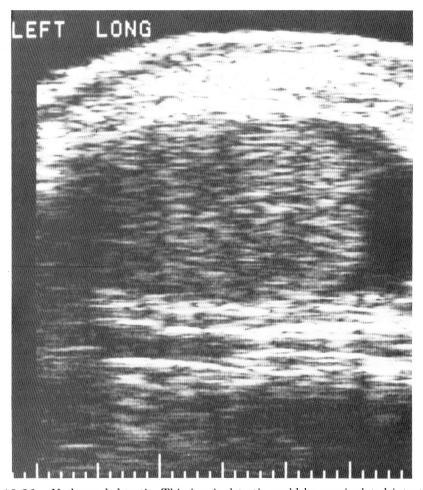

Figure 12.30. Undescended testis. This inguinal testis could be manipulated into the upper scrotum, where it was easily evaluated by sonography. Although smaller than the contralateral testis, its architectural uniformity is preserved.

improved methodology should expand even further its role in scrotal disorders. The separation of testicular from extratesticular pathology is frequently a crucial one to make, and if it could do little else, ultrasound's documented ability in this regard is testimony to the validity of the technique.

References

1. Miskin M, Bain J: B-mode ultrasonic examination of the testes. *J Clin Ultrasound* 2:307–311, 1974.
2. Shawker TH: B-mode ultrasound evaluation of scrotal swellings. *Radiology* 118:417–419, 1976.
3. Miskin M, Buckspan M, Bain J: Ultrasonographic examination of scrotal masses. *J Urol* 117:185–188, 1977.
4. Gottesman JE, Sample WF, Skinner DG, et al: Diagnostic ultrasound in the evaluation of scrotal masses. *J Urol* 118:601–603, 1977.
5. Sample WF, Gottesman JE, Skinner DG, et al: Gray-scale ultrasound of the scrotum. *Radiology* 127:225–228, 1978.
6. Leopold GR, Woo VL, Scheible FW, Nachtsheim D, Gosink BB: High-resolution ultrasonography of scrotal pathology. *Radiology* 131:719–722, 1979.
7. Carroll BA, Gross DM: High-frequency scrotal sonography. *AJR* 140:511–515, 1983.
8. Friedrich M, Claussen CD, Felix R: Immersion ultrasound of testicular pathology. *Radiology* 141:235–237, 1981.
9. Wilson PC, Day DL, Valvo JR, et al: Scrotal ultrasound with an Octoson. *RadioGraphics* 2:24–39, 1982.
10. Phillips GN, Schneider M, Goodman JD, et al: Ultrasonic evaluation of the scrotum. *Urol Radiol* 1:157–163, 1980.
11. Arger PH, Mulhern CB, Coleman BG, et al: Prospective analysis of the value of scrotal ultrasound. *Radiology* 141:763–766, 1981.
12. Richie JR, Birnholz J, Garnick MB: Ultrasonography as a diagnostic adjunct for the evaluation of masses in the scrotum. *Surg Gynecol Obstet* 154:695–698, 1982.
13. Scheible W: Testicular ultrasonography. *Clin Diag Ultrasound*, in press.
14. Bird KI: Emergency testicular scanning. *Clin Diag Ultrasound* 7:55–70, 1981.
15. Blei L, Sihelnik S, Bloom D, et al: Ultrasonographic analysis of chronic intratesticular pathology. *J Ultrasound Med* 2:17–23, 1983.
16. Ransler CW, Allen TD: Torsion of the spermatic cord. *Urol Clin North Am* 9:245–250, 1982.
17. Winston MA, Handler SJ, Pritchard JH: Ultrasonography of the testis—correlation with radiotracer perfusion. *J Nucl Med* 19:615–618, 1978.
18. Smith SP, King LR: Torsion of the testis: techniques of assessment. *Urol Clin North Am* 6:429–443, 1979.
19. Holder LE, Melloul M, Chen D: Current status of radionuclide scrotal imaging. *Semin Nucl Med* 11:232–249, 1981.
20. Holder LE, Martire JR, Holmes ER, et al: Testicular radio-nuclide angiography and static imaging; anatomy, scintigraphic interpretation and clinical indications. *Radiology* 125:739–752, 1977.
21. Stage KH, Schoenvogel R, Lewis S: Testicular scanning: clinical experience with 72 patients. *J Urol* 125:334–337, 1981.
22. Valvo JR, Caldamone AA, O'Mara R, et al: Nuclear imaging in the pediatric acute scrotum. *Am J Dis Child* 136:831–835, 1982.
23. Pedersen JF, Holm HH, Hald T: Torsion of the testis diagnosed by ultrasound. *J Urol* 113:66–68, 1975.
24. Milleret R: Doppler ultrasound diagnosis of testicular cord torsion. *J Clin Ultrasound* 4:425–427, 1976.
25. Bird K, Rosenfield AT, Taylor KJW: Ultrasound in testicular torsion (abstr). Presented at Society of Uroradiology, Palm Beach, Florida, March 1982.
26. Dunn EG, Macchia RJ, Solomon NA: Scintigraphic pattern in missed testicular torsion. *Radiology* 139:175–180, 1981.
27. Vieras F, Kuhn CR: Nonspecificity of the "rim sign" in the scintigraphic diagnosis of missed testicular torsion. *Radiology* 146:519–522, 1983.
28. Dunner PS, Lipsit ER, Nochomovitz LE: Epididymal sperm granuloma simulating a testicular neoplasm. *J Clin Ultrasound* 10:353–355, 1982.
29. Subramanyam BR, Balthazar EJ, Raghavendra BN, et al: Sonographic diagnosis of scrotal hernia. *AJR* 139:535–538, 1982.
30. Boileau MA: Germ-cell tumors of the testis: overview. In Johnson DE, Boileau MA: *Genitourinary Tumors: Fundamental Principles and Surgical Techniques*. New York, Grune & Stratton, 1982.
31. Einhorn LH: *Testicular Tumors: Management and Treatment*. New York, Masson, 1980.
32. Peterson LJ, Catalona WJ, Koehler RE: Ultrasonic localization of a non-palpable testis tumor. *J Urol* 122:843–844, 1979.
33. Glazer HS, Lee JKT, Melson GL, et al: Sonographic detection of occult testicular neoplasms. *AJR* 138:673–675, 1982.
34. Nochomovitz LE, De La Torre FE, Rosai J: Pathology of germ cell tumors of the testis. *Urol Clin North Am* 4:359–578, 1977.
35. Nachtsheim DA, Scheible FW, Gosink B: Ultrasonography of testis tumors. *J Urol* 129:978–981, 1983.
36. Cunningham JJ: Echographic findings in Sertoli cell tumor of the testis. *J Clin Ultrasound* 9:341–342, 1981.
37. Werth V, Yu G, Marshall FF: Nonlymphomatous metastatic tumor to the testis. *J Urol* 127:142–144, 1982.
38. Paladugu RR, Bearman RM, Rappaport H: Malignant lymphoma with primary manifestation in the gonad. *Cancer* 45:561–571, 1980.
39. Rayor RA, Scheible W, Brock WA, et al: High resolution ultrasonography in the diagnosis of testicular relapse in patients with acute lymphoblastic leukemia. *J Urol* 128:602–603, 1982.
40. Upetin AR, King W, Rich P, et al: Ultrasound diagnosis of testicular leukemia. *Radiology* 146:171–172, 1982.
41. Gross M: Rupture of the testicle; the importance of early surgical treatment. *J Urol* 101:196–197, 1969.
42. Albert NE: Testicular ultrasound for trauma. *J*

Urol 124:558–559, 1980.

43. Friedman SG, Rose JG, Winston MA: Ultrasound and nuclear medicine evaluation in acute testicular trauma. *J Urol* 125:748–749, 1981.

44. Frey HL, Rajfer J: Incidence of cryptorchidism. *Urol Clin North Am* 9:327–329, 1982.

45. Medrazo BL, Klugo RC, Parks JA, et al: Ultrasonographic demonstration of undescended testes. *Radiology* 133:181–183, 1979.

46. Mittelstaedt CA, Gosink BB, Leopold GR: Gray scale patterns of pelvic disease in the male. *Radiology* 123:727–732, 1977.

47. Wolverson MK, Houttuin E, Heiberg E, et al: Comparison of computed tomography with high-resolution real-time ultrasound in the localization of the impalpable undescended testis. *Radiology* 145:133–136, 1983.

48. Lee JKT, McClennan BL, Stanley RJ, Sagel SS: Utility of computed tomography in the localization of the undescended testis. *Radiology* 135:121–125, 1980.

49. Wolverson MK, Jagannadharao B, Sundaram M, et al: CT in localization of impalpable cryptorchid testes. *AJR* 134:725–729, 1980.

50. Glickman MG, Weiss RM, Itzchak Y: Testicular venography for undescended testes. *AJR* 129:67–70, 1977.

51. Diamond AB, Meng C-H, Kodross M, et al: Testicular venography in the nonpalpable testis. *AJR* 129:71–75, 1977.

52. Khademi M, Seebode JJ, Falla A: Selective spermatic arteriography for localization of an impalpable undescended testis. *Radiology* 136:627–634, 1980.

CHAPTER 13

Ultrasonography of the Adrenal Gland*

HSU-CHONG YEH, M.D.

Ultrasonographic delineation of the normal adrenal gland and small adrenal lesions is difficult and frequently unsuccessful (1–10) due to the small size of these structures and their high location deep in the rib cage. They are easily obscured by the ribs and spinal transverse processes on posterior scanning and by the ribs, stomach, or bowel gas on anterior scanning. Understanding the anatomy and a proper approach and technique are most important for successful scanning of these small structures (11, 12). High quality gray-scale equipment and a high frequency transducer are not essential (11), but they are certainly helpful. Since many functioning adrenal tumors are small and surgical resection of such tumors may result in permanent cure of serious disease, detection of such small masses is very important. Delineation of large adrenal masses by ultrasonography is usually easy from any approach. However, differential diagnosis of the origin of a huge mass may be difficult.

NORMAL ANATOMY AND SCANNING METHODS

The adrenal glands are flattened structures which consist of an anteromedial ridge and two wings open posterolaterally (11–13) (Fig. 13.1). The two wings have been called "limbs" in description of the computed tomography (CT) findings (14, 15). The term "wing" is more appropriate since it indicates a flat structure. The right gland is somewhat triangular in shape, and the left gland is semilunar (16, 17). Although the glands are 4 to 6 cm long and 2 to 3 cm wide, they are only 0.3 to 0.6 cm in thickness (17), a characteristic feature of a normal gland. They are located anteromedial to the upper pole of the kidneys. Only small portions of the left gland usually extend above the left kidney, and, therefore, it is not really suprarenal in location. A greater portion of the right gland extends above the right kidney. The left adrenal gland extends down to the renal hilar level in 10% of normal individuals (14). The right gland is located immediately posterior to the inferior vena cava, medial to the right lobe of the liver, and lateral to the crus of the diaphragm. The left gland is located lateral or posterolateral to the aorta, posterior to the lesser omental sac superiorly, and posterior to the pancreas inferiorly. Since the lesser omental sac is usually collapsed and located behind the stomach, the superior portion of the left adrenal gland is practically posterior to the stomach. The glands are fixed to the anteromedial aspect of the apices of Gerota's fascia, i.e., at the top of the perirenal space. They are, therefore, not as movable as kidneys. They are usually surrounded by a varying amount of fat; however, little fat may be present between the anteromedial ridge and the inferior vena cava or between the lateral wing of the right gland and liver.

The medial wing is prominent superiorly and small or absent inferiorly and vice versa for the lateral wing. Therefore, a transverse section of the superior portion contains only the anteromedial ridge and the medial wing, and the adrenal gland appears as a single linear or curvilinear structure (Fig. 13.2A). The inferior portion may contain only the anteromedial ridge and the lateral wing; the left adrenal has an "L" shape, and the right gland has a reverse "L" shape. In the middle section, all the structures are present, and the gland has an inverted "Y" shape (11) (Figs. 13.2B and 13.3) or an inverted "V" shape (Fig. 13.4) if the anteromedial ridge is small.

Due to medial location of the glands, they are easily obscured by the rib and transverse process

---

* The author would like to thank Mrs. Gwen Hanley for her excellent secretarial assistance.

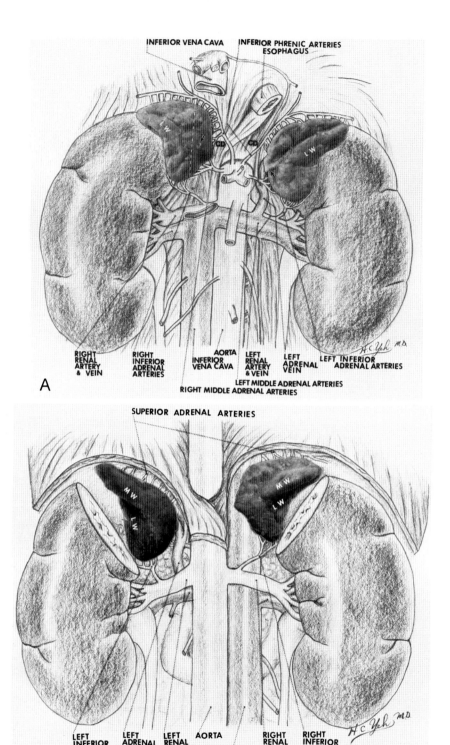

Figure 13.1. Normal anatomy of adrenal glands. Photographs of both adrenal glands are superimposed on the drawings to show their relation to surrounding structures. *A*, Frontal view. Medial part (i.e., medial to dotted line) of right adrenal gland is behind inferior vena cava (part cut out). *Arrows* indicate adrenal veins. *LW*, lateral wing; *CD*, crus of diaphragm. Adrenal glands are anteromedial to the upper pole of the kidneys. *B*, Posterior view. The upper poles of both kidneys are cut and removed to show anteriorly located adrenal glands. *MW*, medial wing. (Reprinted with permission from Yeh (11).)

Figure 13.2. Normal right adrenal gland. *A*, Transverse scan 16 cm above umbilicus shows the superior portion of the right adrenal gland (*arrow*) which is linear shaped. This represents the anteromedial ridge and medial wing. *V*, inferior vena cave; *A*, aorta; *arrowheads*, crus of diaphragm; *K*, kidney; *L*, liver. *B*, Transverse scan 14.5 cm above umbilicus shows middle segment of the right adrenal gland (*arrow*) which is inverted "Y" shaped.

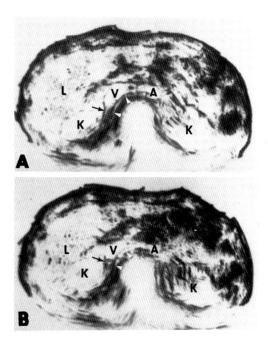

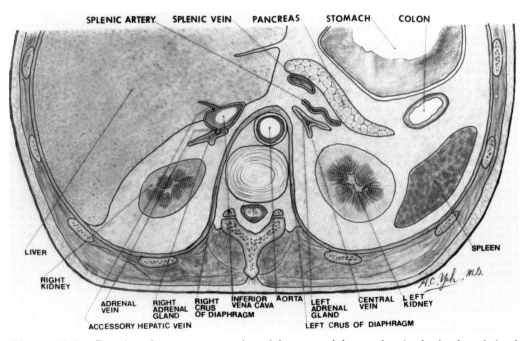

Figure 13.3. Drawing of a transverse section of the upper abdomen showing both adrenal glands and their relation to the surrounding structures. (Reprinted with permission from Mitty and Yeh (13).)

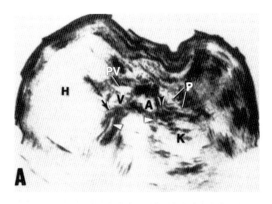

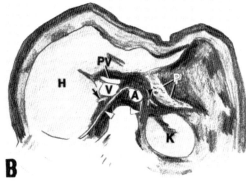

Figure 13.4. Transverse scan (*A*) and drawing of the scan (*B*) showing both adrenal glands. The right gland (*arrow*) is an inverted "V" shape but with a short medial wing. The left adrenal gland (*black arrowhead*) is also an inverted "V" shape. *H*, liver; *V*, inferior vena cava; *P*, pancreas; *PV*, portal vein; *A*, aorta; *white arrowheads*, crus of diaphragm; *K*, kidney. (Reprinted with permission from Mitty and Yeh (13).)

of the spine on posterior scanning. The best approach is an anterior transverse scan in a supine position (11) (Fig. 13.5). For the right gland, using the liver and/or the right kidney as an acoustic window, one can scan from a lateral intercostal space toward the inferior vena cava. On such a scan, the right adrenal gland is confined to a small space surrounded by the inferior vena cava, liver, crus of diaphragm, and the upper pole of the kidney (Fig. 13.3). These structures can usually be delineated by sector scanning through one of the intercostal spaces of the lateral abdominal wall. An anterior linear or linear sector scan can be added to better define the inferior vena cava and right adrenal area. By making a series of closely spaced scans from the level of the renal hilum upward to above the

kidney, the entire adrenal area can be thoroughly examined.

Scanning technique for the left adrenal gland is similar to that for the right adrenal gland except that the spleen and/or left kidney may be used as an acoustic window. The stomach and/or colon gas are sometimes interposed between the adrenal gland and the spleen, and scanning from more posteriorly (i.e., at the posterior axillary line) may be necessary to visualize the adrenal area. Scanning in the semidecubitus position, left side up (11) (Figs. 13.6 and 13.7) may be required.

Anterior longitudinal scanning may show the right adrenal gland, which is located posterior to the inferior vena cava (11). This scan is done with single sweep technique in sustained deep inspiration (Fig. 13.8). The gland assumes a horizontal "Y" or horizontal "V" shape structure (Fig. 13.9*B*). The two wings open inferiorly. The "anterior wing" in this scan actually represents the lateral wing, and the posterior wing represents the medial wing. As one scans more medially, only the anteromedial ridge may be seen. It appears as a single horizontal linear structure (Fig. 13.9*A*). Scanning further medially, a long linear structure may be seen. This represents the crus of the diaphragm. The adrenal gland is at or slightly above the level of the porta hepatis.

The left adrenal gland is only occasionally seen on the anterior longitudinal scan. The features are similar to those of the right gland (11). It is, however, usually obscured by stomach or bowel gas and is not visualized.

A longitudinal oblique scanning technique has been developed by Sample (12) to visualize the adrenal gland in longitudinal coronary section. The plane connecting the long axis of the kidney and aorta (or inferior vena cava for the right adrenal gland) is plotted out of an anterior transverse scan and marked on the skin. The patient lies in the decubitus position. Scanning is done along the skin marks at a predetermined scanning plane. The normal adrenal gland appears as a triangular-shaped structure between the spleen (liver on the right side), aorta, and upper pole of the kidney. Although a high success rate in visualizing the normal gland has been attained, this scanning approach cannot thoroughly examine the adrenal areas, and some small masses are not visualized (11). The visualized portion of the adrenal gland is usually the lateral wing and the anteromedial ridge. The medial wing generally extends posterior to the

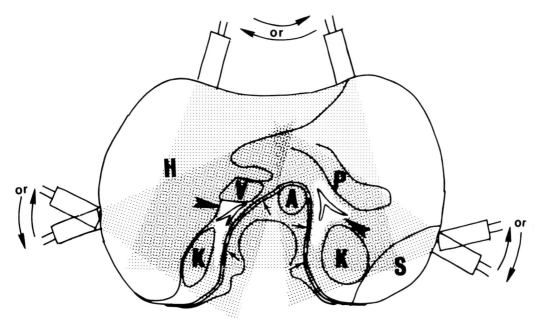

Figure 13.5. Method of scanning adrenal areas (*white areas* indicated by *black arrowheads*). Sector scan is first made from the intercostal space on the lateral or posterolateral aspect of the abdomen. Adrenal gland, kidney (*K*), and crus of diaphragm (*small arrows*) are usually well delineated. A linear sector scan is then obtained across the epigastrium to better delineate the inferior vena cava (*V*) and aorta (*A*). *P*, pancreas; *H*, liver; *S*, spleen. (Reprinted with permission from Yeh (11).)

Figure 13.6. Scanning of left adrenal gland in semidecubitus position. *A*, Transverse scan 13 cm above umbilicus. The left adrenal area is obscured by stomach and bowel gas. *A*, aorta; *L*, liver; *S*, spleen. *B*, The same scan performed in semidecubitus position, left side up. The scanning can be done from more posteriorly using kidney (*K*) and medial portion of spleen as acoustic window. The left adrenal gland (*arrow*) and the tail of the pancreas (*P*) are now clearly seen.

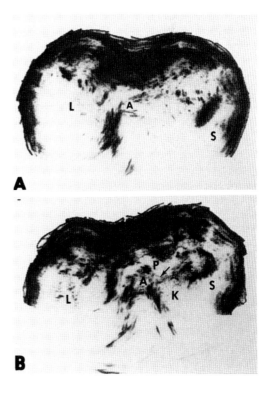

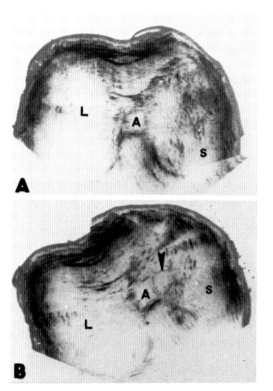

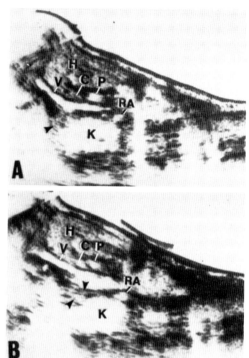

Figure 13.7. Scanning of left adrenal mass (a 2.5-cm aldosteronoma) in semidecubitus position. *A*, Transverse scan 14 cm above umbilicus. The left adrenal area is obscured by stomach and bowel gas. *A*, aorta; *L*, liver; *S*, spleen. *B*, Repeat the same scanning in semidecubitus position, left side up. The left adrenal mass (*arrowhead*) is now clearly seen.

Figure 13.8. Normal right adrenal gland on longitudinal scan. *A*, Anterior longitudinal scan with normal respiration. Poor visualization of the right adrenal gland (*arrowhead*). *P*, portal vein; *C*, caudate lobe; *RA*, right renal artery; *H*, liver; *V*, inferior vena cava. *B*, Same scan during sustained deep inspiration. The adrenal gland (*arrowheads*) becomes well separated from the kidney (*K*) and is clearly seen. (Reprinted with permission from Yeh (11).)

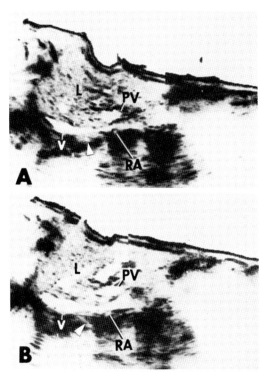

Figure 13.9. Normal right renal adrenal gland on longitudinal scan. *A*, Longitudinal scan 3 cm to the right of midline. The medial portion (i.e., anteromedial ridge) of the right adrenal gland (*white arrowhead*) is seen posterior to the inferior vena cava (*V*). It is above the level of the portal vein (*PV*) because of a large liver (*L*) which causes inferior displacement of the porta hepatis. *RA*, renal artery. *B*, Longitudinal scan 3.5 cm to the right of midline. The adrenal gland (*white arrowhead*) now appears in a horizontal "V" shape which is formed by two wings. (Reprinted with permission from Yeh HC: Ultrasound and CT of the adrenals. *Semin Ultrasound* 3:97–113, 1982.)

scanning plane. Furthermore, some nearby normal structures such as pancreas or stomach may easily be mistaken for an adrenal mass (11, 18). Since the characteristic thin shape of the gland cannot be appreciated on this scan, one may not be certain of the normality of the visualized gland. This scanning method, however, may be used to supplement the findings on anterior transverse scan in certain cases.

Posterior scanning usually does not delineate a normal adrenal gland, and only occasionally may one see a small adrenal mass of less than 2 to 3 cm (11, 19) (Fig. 13.10). The posterior

longitudinal scan, however, is useful in demonstrating the spatial relationship between a large adrenal mass and the kidney.

Real-time scanning may be used for a quick survey of the adrenal areas because it is fast and convenient. A sector scanner may be used to scan through intercostal spaces. However, it is easier to orient surrounding organs such as the kidney or spleen with a linear array (Fig. 13.11). Scanning can be done in a supine or decubitus position with the transducer on the side wall of the upper abdomen, directed toward the aorta or vena cava in a longitudinal, oblique, or transverse plane. One first locates the kidney and then slowly angles the transducer anteromedially to survey the adrenal area. Normal glands and small masses have been delineated by real-time scanning (Fig. 13.10). A high-quality sector scanner is particularly useful for this purpose.

ADRENAL LESIONS

Small adrenal masses (less than 3 cm) are usually round in shape (Figs. 13.12 and 13.13) but occasionally may be oval. They are usually located in one part of the gland, i.e., on the anteromedial ridge or one of the wings. The uninvolved normal part of the gland can also be seen on anterior transverse scan (11) (Figs. 13.14 and 13.15). Therefore, the precise location of the mass in the gland can be determined. The mass is usually poorly echogenic.

A moderate or larger size mass (4 cm or larger) is frequently oval in shape (Fig. 13.16) because it is confined within a flat narrow space, but it may be round and compress the liver or kidney. The mass is typically located anteromedial to the upper pole of the kidney. The uninvolved, normal part of the gland, if present, is rarely seen. The upper pole of the kidney may be displaced laterally or the kidney displaced inferiorly. The posterior wall of the inferior vena cava may be indented or the cava displaced anteriorly. Adrenal masses are hypoechoic, but may contain areas of high level echoes due to necrosis or hemorrhage.

Although a large adrenal mass usually displaces the upper pole of the kidney laterally and/or the whole kidney inferiorly, some large adrenal masses may extend inferiorly anterior to the kidney, causing little inferior displacement of the latter (20) (Fig. 13.17). Hence, the mass may appear almost entirely anterior to the upper and middle portion of the kidney, only a

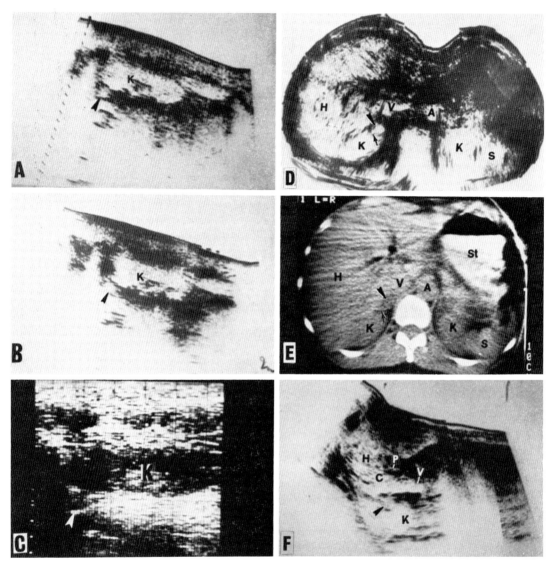

Figure 13.10. A small (1.3 cm) aldosteronoma of the right adrenal gland. *A*, Posterior longitudinal scan. A round mass (*arrowhead*) is located anterior to the upper pole of the right kidney (*R*) and immediately below a rib shadow. A mass of this size can be easily obscured by a rib shadow on a posterior scan. *B*, The same scan in deep inspiration. Note the inferior movement of the kidney, mass, and rib shadow. The movement is greatest for the kidney, as indicated by the wider separation between kidney and rib shadow. However, there is little relative movement between the rib shadow and the mass. *C*, The same scan but with real-time scanning. *D*, Anterior transverse scan. The mass (*arrowhead*) arises from the anteromedial ridge of the inferior portion of the gland. The uninvolved lateral wing is indicated by the *arrow*. *V*, inferior vena cava; *A*, aorta; *S*, spleen; *H*, liver. *E*, CT scan corresponding to *D*. The mass is relatively lucent compared to liver and kidney. *F*, Anterior longitudinal scan. The mass (*arrowhead*) is located behind the inferior vena cava at the level of the portal vein (*P*). *C*, caudate lobe of liver. (*A, B, D, E,* and *F* reprinted with permission from Yeh et al (19). *C* reprinted with permission from Mitty and Yeh (13).)

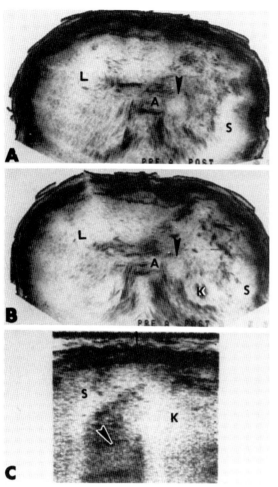

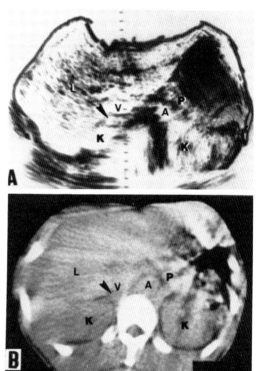

Figure 13.11.   A pheochromocytoma in the left adrenal gland. *A,* Transverse scan 16 cm above umbilicus. A mass (*arrowhead*) is located in the left adrenal gland. *A,* aorta; *S,* spleen; *L,* liver. *B,* Transverse scan 14 cm above umbilicus. The mass (*arrowhead*) is anteromedial to the upper pole of the left kidney (*K*). *C,* Linear array real-time longitudinal scanning along left posterolateral wall of abdomen. The mass (*arrowhead*) is medial to the spleen (*S*). The kidney (*K*) is partly obscured by the rib shadow. However, the kidney was readily recognized during the scanning as it moved with respiration in and out of the rib shadow.

Figure 13.12.   A small aldosteronoma in the right adrenal gland. *A,* Transverse scan 14 cm above umbilicus. A small mass (*arrowhead*) is anteromedial to the upper pole of the right kidney (*K*). *A,* aorta; *V,* inferior vena cava; *L,* liver; *P,* pancreas. *B,* Corresponding CT.

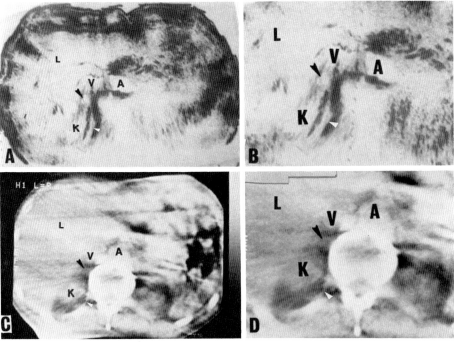

Figure 13.13.   A small right adrenal aldosteronoma in a 70-year old man. *A,* Transverse sonogram 16 cm above the umbilicus. The mass (*black arrowhead*) is seen posterior to the inferior vena cava (*V*) and lateral to the crus of the diaphragm (*white arrowhead*). *K,* kidney; *A,* aorta; *L,* liver. *B,* Close-up view of *A. C,* CT scan corresponding to *A. D,* Close-up view of *C.* Note the low density of the tumor. (Reprinted with permission from Mitty and Yeh (13).)

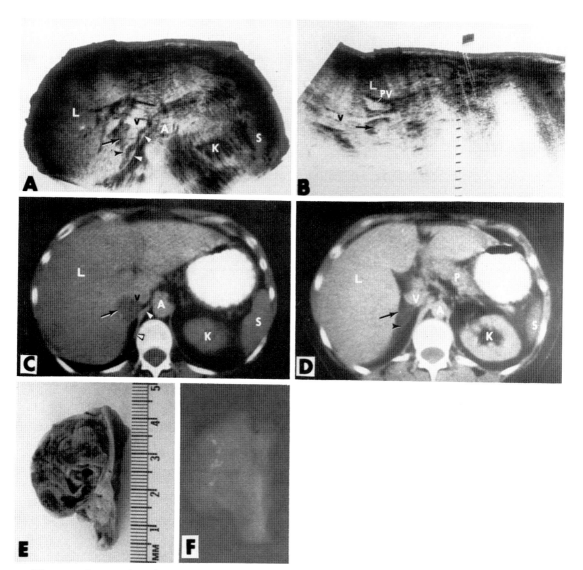

Figure 13.14. An adenoma of right adrenal gland causing Cushing's syndrome. *A*, Transverse scan 15 cm above umbilicus. A 3-cm mass (*arrow*) is located immediately posterior to the inferior vena cava (*V*). The normal medial wing (*black arrowhead*) is also seen. The mass is more echogenic than usual, almost isoechoic to the liver (*L*), due to areas of necrosis, hemorrhage, and calcification. *K*, kidney; *S*, spleen; *A*, aorta. *B*, Longitudinal scan 2 cm to the left of midline. The mass (*arrow*) indents on the posterior wall of the inferior vena cava (*V*). Note the mass is at the level of the portal vein (*PV*). *C*, CT scan slightly above the section in *A*. Note the low density of the mass due to necrosis and high lipid content. Multiple calcifications are also seen. *D*, CT scan slightly below the section in *A*. The medial wing (*arrowhead*) is seen posterior to the mass (*arrow*). *P*, pancreas. *E*, Surgical specimen. The mass is well encapsulated. There are areas of necrosis and hemorrhage. Normal medial wing is seen posteriorly. *F*, Radiography of the specimen shows multiple calcifications.

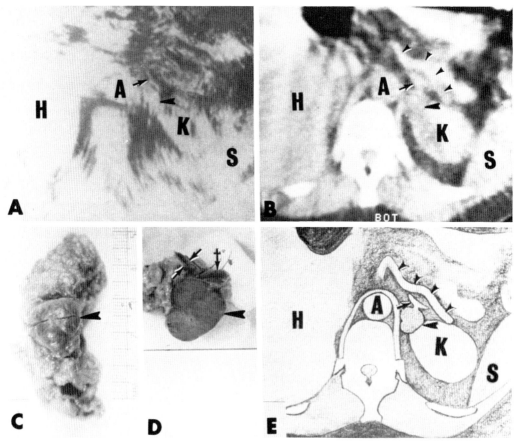

Figure 13.15. Aldosteronoma (1.8 cm) in middle of left adrenal gland. Mass (*large arrowhead*) in posterior edge of medial wing. Anterior ridge (*arrow*) and lateral wing of gland are intact. *A* and *B*, Anterior transverse scan and corresponding CT scan. Splenic artery (*small arrowheads*) is anterior to adrenal gland. *C*, Surgical specimen viewed from posterior. Mass (*arrowhead*) protrudes posteriorly from middle part of gland. Adipose tissue around normal part of gland has not been removed. *D*, Transverse section of specimen corresponding to findings on sonogram and CT scan. Normal adrenal gland (between *arrows*) is thin (3 mm). Lateral wing (*crossed arrow*) of gland appears thicker because tissue has been split open. *E*, Drawing of CT scan. *H*, liver; *A*, aorta; *K*, kidney; *S*, spleen. (Reprinted with permission from Yeh (11).)

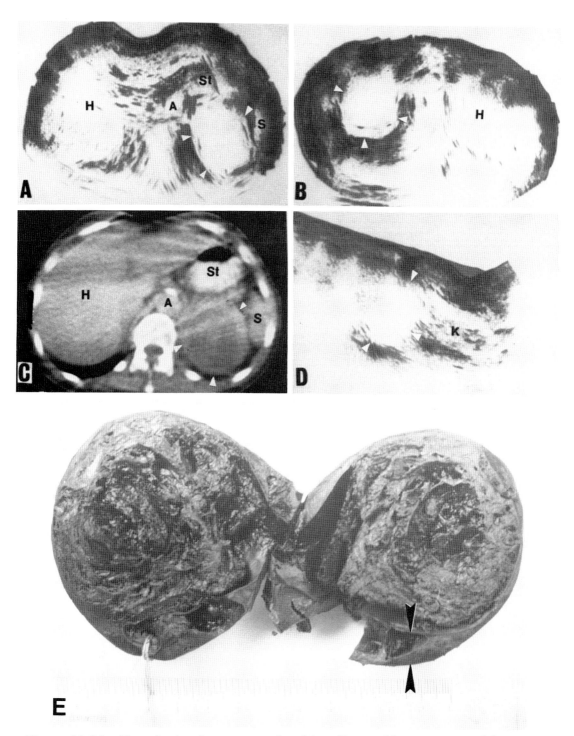

Figure 13.16. Necrotic pheochromocytoma found in a 68-year-old woman screened for unexplained high alkaline phosphatase levels. *A,* Anterior transverse scan 13 cm above the umbilicus. A "cystic" mass (*arrowheads*) is located posterolateral to the aorta (*A*). The wall of the "cyst" is thick but smooth. *St,* stomach; *S,* spleen; *H,* liver. *B,* Posterior transverse scan. The wall of the "cyst" is thickest anteriorly. *C,* CT scan corresponding to *A* confirms a thick-walled "cyst" between aorta and spleen. *D,* Posterior longtudinal scan shows the "cyst" to be located anterosuperior to the kidney, i.e., in the adrenal region. A necrotic or hemorrhagic adrenal tumor was suspected. Clinical investigation showed features of pheochromocytoma. *E,* Surgical specimen confirmed the lesion to be a necrotic (nonliquified) pheochromocytoma with a smooth wall, thickest anteriorly (*arrowheads*). (Reprinted with permission from Yeh et al. (20).)

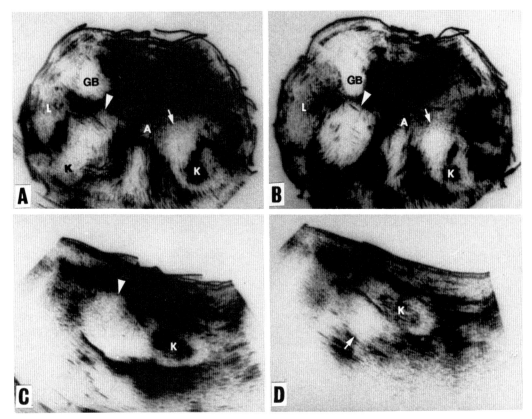

Figure 13.17. Adrenal insufficiency due to metastatic pulmonary carcinoma to both adrenals. *A,* Transverse scan 13 cm above umbilicus. There is a mass in each adrenal gland. *K,* kidney; *A,* aorta; *L,* liver; *GB,* gallbladder; *arrow,* left adrenal mass; *arrowhead,* right adrenal mass. *B,* Transverse scan 14 cm above umbilicus. The main portion of the right adrenal mass (*arrowhead*) is above the right kidney which is not seen in this scan. *C,* Right posterior longitudinal scan. The right adrenal mass (*arrowhead*) is mainly superior to the kidney except the inferior portion which is anterior to the upper pole of the kidney. *D,* Left posterior longitudinal scan. The left adrenal mass (*arrow*) is anterior to the kidney (*K*). (*A* and *B,* reprinted with permission from Mitty and Yeh (13).)

small part may protrude above the upper pole of the kidney. A huge right adrenal mass may markedly indent the liver as well as displacing it upward. It may appear as a large mass occupying most or all of the right lobe of the liver on both anterior longitudinal and transverse scanning (13). A notch between the inferior border of the liver and the mass serves as a clue to the diagnosis of an extrahepatic (or adrenal) mass (Fig. 13.18). A huge left adrenal mass may occupy most of the left upper quadrant of the abdomen, so its origin may be difficult to determine.

Adenomas are usually small, less than 3 cm in size, and may be functional or nonfunctional. A nonfunctional adenoma may be discovered during the work-up for some other purpose. Although a small adrenal mass is less likely to be a primary carcinoma, it cannot be differentiated from a metastatic tumor. In patients with adrenal cortical hyperfunction, a small nodule of 1 cm or smaller may represent an adenoma or a hyperplastic nodule; the latter may or may not be associated with thickening of both adrenal glands. Multiple small nodules favor bilateral hyperplasia. Since a functional adenoma requires surgical resection, while bilateral hyperplasia is treated conservatively, differentiating between these entities is very important. When differentiation is impossible with ultrasound or CT, adrenal venography with venous blood sampling or adrenal scintigraphy may be necessary.

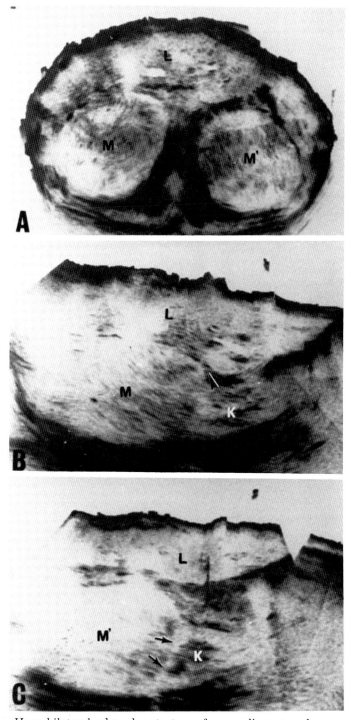

Figure 13.18.   Huge bilateral adrenal metastases from malignant melanoma causing adrenal insufficiency. *A*, Transverse scan 11 cm above umbilicus. The right adrenal mass (*M*) markedly indents the liver (*L*) simulating a liver mass. The left adrenal mass (*M*) occupies most of the space behind the left lobe of the liver. *B*, Longitudinal scan 6 cm to the right of the midline. The mass is similar to a large liver mass. A notch (*arrowhead*) between the liver and the mass inferiorly indicates that the mass is extrahepatic in origin. The right kidney (*K*) is displaced inferiorly. *C*, Longitudinal scan 6 cm to the left of the midline. The left adrenal mass (*M*) indents (*arrowheads*) and displaces the kidney inferiorly.

Adrenal carcinomas are usually discoverd when large because symptoms appear late even when they are functional; production of hormones by a functional carcinoma is usually not as profuse as by a functional adenoma. Therefore, carcinomas are easy to detect because of their large size. Small metastatic tumors of the adrenal gland, however, are frequently seen on general abdominal scanning as part of the workup for malignancies. Bilateral adrenal metastases (Figs. 13.17 and 13.18) are not uncommon, especially from lung cancer (21, 22). Complete replacement of both adrenal glands may cause adrenal insufficiency (23).

An adrenal adenoma or carcinoma may un-dergo necrosis or hemorrhage which may result in an echo-free mass similar to a cyst (20) (Fig. 13.16). It may have a thin smooth wall or a thick smooth or shaggy wall (20). The echo-free center may represent liquified or nonliquified necrosis. Some hemorrhage or necrosis with much fragmented tissue debris may, however, cause strong echoes. Neuroblastomas are usually highly echogenic (20) (Fig. 13.19) due to hemorrhage, necrosis, and calcification. The formation of rosettes, which consist of nerve fibrils surrounded by tumor cells, probably also causes echoes. A fibrofatty mass resulting from old inflammation may appear as an ill-defined echogenic mass (20). However, some other inflammatory

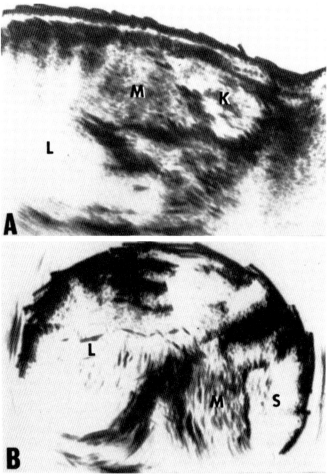

Figure 13.19. Neuroblastoma of the left adrenal gland. *A,* Posterior longitudinal scan shows a highly echogenic mass (*M*) anterosuperior to the kidney (*K*) representing neuroblastoma. The kidney is markedly indented. *L,* liver. *B,* Anterior transverse scan 12 cm above umbilicus. The adrenal mass (*M*) is medial to the spleen (*S*).

masses, e.g., tuberculoma, may be poorly echogenic (13).

Bilateral adrenal masses occur most frequently in metastatic malignant disease, especially lung cancer (21, 22). Pheochromocytoma may also be multiple (10% of patients) (Fig. 13.20). Such masses may be bilateral or unilateral. When unilateral, a dumbbell-shaped mass or a small mass arising from a larger one (budding appearance) may be seen (13). The two masses may appear as a single irregular mass. One of the bilateral adrenal masses may be much larger than the other. When a large mass is first discovered, a smaller mass may be easily overlooked. Since only complete excision of all of the masses will ensure eradication of the disease, one should carefully search the other adrenal area even after a mass is found in one gland. The examination should also include other parts of the abdomen, especially the para-aortic region, since extra-adrenal pheochromocytomas occur (10%).

Adrenal cysts are, like cysts elsewhere, echo-free lesions with smooth, round, thin walls. They are mostly of lymphangiomatous origin but may also result from old hematoma or necrosis in a tumor or an echinococeal cyst. Unlike renal cysts, calcification (Fig. 13.21) is frequently (about 15%) seen in benign adrenal cysts. The calcified wall appears as a thick, strongly echogenic ring which may cast an acoustic shadow if it is heavily calcified. A calcified normal-sized adrenal gland may result from an old hemorrhage (24). Strong echoes with acoustic shadows may be seen in a normal-sized gland.

Myelolipomas are also highly echogenic (25, 26) due to strong acoustic interfaces between fat and other cellular elements in the mass as well

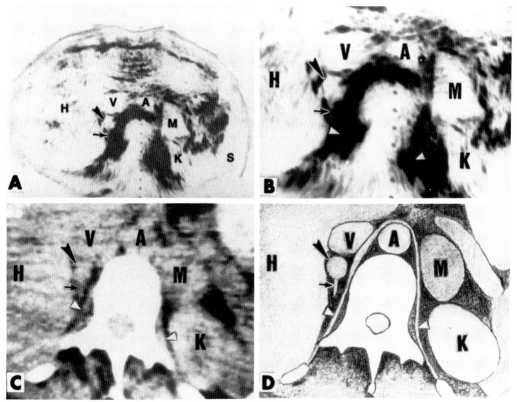

Figure 13.20. Bilateral pheochromocytomas in 49-year-old woman with multiple endocrine neoplasia, type II. *A*, Anterior transverse scan. *B*, Close-up of *A*. *C* and *D*, Corresponding CT scan close-up and drawing. A small mass (*large black arrowhead*) of 1.5 cm size is in the anteromedial ridge of the apex of the right gland. Normal medial wing (*arrow*) of the same gland can be seen. A larger mass (*M*) is located in the left gland. *H*, liver; *V*, inferior vena cava; *A*, aorta; *K*, kidney. (Reprinted with permission from Yeh (11).)

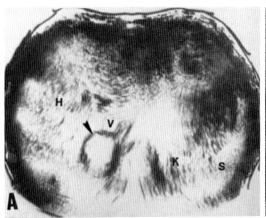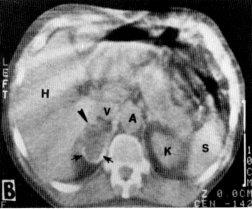

Figure 13.21. Adrenal cyst, calcified. *A*, Transverse sonographic scan 15 cm above the umbilicus. A cystic lesion (*arrowhead*) is seen behind the inferior vena cava (*V*). *H*, liver; *K*, kidney; *S*, spleen. *B*, Corresponding CT scan. The lesion (*arrowhead*) is of water density within a calcified rim (*arrows*). (Reprinted with permission from Yeh et al. (19).)

as calcification. The echoes may be as strong as the para-adrenal fat, so a relatively small-sized lesion may not be readily identifiable and the exact extent of a larger lesion may not be apparent.

The adrenal gland may become thickened in hyperplasia. However, this is more easily discerned on CT than on ultrasonography, especially in patients with Cushing's syndrome, due to the abundance of retroperitoneal fat which degrades the ultrasonic image but improves the visualization of the gland on CT. Furthermore, while the normal adrenal gland is quite variable in size, only about 50% of patients with bilateral hyperplasia have grossly enlarged adrenal glands. Although the convex contour of the gland seen on a radiograph (e.g., retroperitoneal pneumograph) (27) and on a longitudinal oblique sonogram (28) has been considered to indicate hyperplasia or tumor, in fact, a convex contour is frequently seen in the normal gland on insufflation and venographic studies in vitro (29) and on studies of anatomical specimens (Fig. 13.1). The convex contour is most frequently seen on the medial border of the right gland and superior medial border of the left gland (29). In general, unless the glands are markedly thickened or multiple hyperplastic nodules are seen, bilateral hyperplasia cannot be diagnosed with certainty by sonography and CT.

Differential Diagnosis of Adrenal Lesions

A mass in the upper pole of the kidney may simulate an adrenal mass. Differentiation between intra- and extra- (e.g., adrenal) renal masses may be difficult. However, when the main bulk of the mass is within the expected renal contour, the mass is most likely of renal origin. A well-defined demarcation may be seen between the mass and the adjacent renal parenchyma whether the mass is of renal or adrenal origin (20). Therefore, the presence of such a demarcation does not necessarily indicate an adrenal (or extrarenal) origin of the mass. Furthermore, a demarcation between a mass and the kidney may not be seen due to inadequate scanning technique (13) (Fig. 13.22) or technical limitations.

A large medial tubercle of the spleen may be mistaken for an adrenal mass, especially when only posterior longitudinal scans are done (13) (Fig. 13.23). On a careful anterior or posterior transverse scan, however, no demarcation is present between the tubercle and the rest of the spleen. The same sonographic texture will be seen in the tubercle and the spleen proper. The "pseudomass" on a posterior longitudinal scan is superior to the kidney rather than anterosuperior to the kidney as is an adrenal mass.

An accessory spleen located medial to the spleen may simulate an adrenal mass due to its suprarenal location on the posterior longitudinal scan. On anterior transverse scan, however, the "mass" can be clearly seen to be located lateral to the site of the adrenal gland.

The esophagogastric junction is located on the left anterior to the aorta and may simulate a small left adrenal mass on longitudinal oblique scan (18). It can be differentiated from an ad-

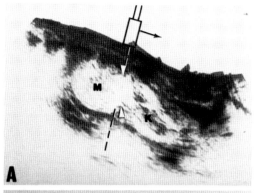

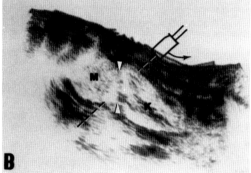

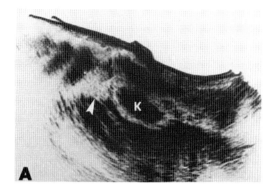

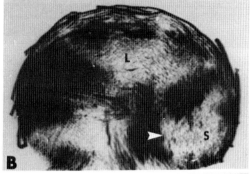

Figure 13.22. Scanning technique affecting the demarcation between adrenal mass (*M*) and kidney (*K*). *A*, The demarcation (*arrowheads*) between an adrenal mass, a pheochromocytoma, and the kidney is not seen because the interface is parallel to the ultrasound beam. *B*, By tilting the transducer and rescanning, the demarcation is now delineated. (Reprinted with permission from Mitty and Yeh (13).)

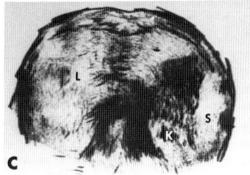

Figure 13.23. Spleen simulating an adrenal mass on posterior scanning. *A*, Left posterior longitudinal scan shows a mass-like structure (*arrowhead*) superior to the kidney (*K*) simulating an adrenal mass. *B*, Anterior transverse scan 16 cm above umbilicus. The mass-like structure actually represents the medial portion (*arrowhead*) of the spleen (*S*). *L*, liver. *C*, Anterior transverse scan 13 cm above umbilicus. The left kidney (*K*) is in the corresponding location to the medial portion of spleen as in *B*, i.e., the kidney is below the medial portion of the spleen.

renal mass on anterior transverse scan since it is located anterior to the adrenal site and echogenic mucosa may be seen within it (30). It indents the liver, forming an esophageal impression. A small adrenal mass is very unlikely to contain strong central echoes and to indent the liver. The second portion of the duodenum may also be mistaken for a right adrenal mass. It is usually located lateral to the inferior vena cava rather than posterior or posterolateral to the cava as is an adrenal mass. Real-time scanning may reveal peristaltic motion, and compressibility of the structure indicates a duodenal origin.

An enlarged para-aortic lymph node or retropancreatic node may simulate an adrenal mass. When the normal adrenal gland is clearly seen separate from the mass, an extra-adrenal mass or enlarged lymph node can be diagnosed. However, if the mass appears attached to the adrenal gland, it is difficult to determine whether the mass is intra- or extra-adrenal in origin. Angiography may be necessary to demonstrate feeding vessels so that the origin of the mass can be determined.

A segment of tortuous splenic artery in the

left adrenal area may be mistaken for a long (or wide) adrenal gland. However, this rarely occurs. An aneurysm of splenic artery, a segment of tortuous aorta, a dilated tortuous splenic vein, or a varicose vein may be mistaken for an adrenal lesion. Using the real-time scanner to observe pulsation or continuation to the vessel may be helpful in diagnosis.

A mass in the tail of the pancreas may simulate a left adrenal tumor. A pancreatic tumor is usually more anteriorly or laterally located than an adrenal mass. Continuity between the normal body of the pancreas and the tumor can be seen. A large left adrenal tumor will displace the pancreas and/or splenic vein anteriorly. On longitudinal oblique scan, a segment of normal pancreas may simulate an adrenal tumor (11). Anterior transverse scanning will clarify the anatomy.

DIAGNOSTIC ACCURACY AND CLINICAL APPLICATION OF ULTRASOUND

The accuracy of adrenal ultrasonography varies greatly depending on the technique used, the experience and skill of the operator, and the effort in scanning. Although an expensive system may be quite helpful, a standard machine even with a 2.25 MHz collimated transducer is usually sufficient to obtain high accuracy (11). With the longitudinal oblique scanning method, the normal right adrenal gland can be seen in 90% and the normal left adrenal gland in 80% of patients. However, this approach visualizes only a portion of the adrenal gland, and some small masses are difficult to discern within the contour of the gland since visualization of a small adrenal mass depends on a subtle focal alteration of echo pattern. On an anterior transverse scan, the normal right adrenal gland is seen in only 78% and the left gland in 44% of normal individuals. However, the thickness of the adrenal gland is visualized, and the entire adrenal area can be thoroughly examined. The accuracy for detecting a mass lesion is greater with this approach. Although the normal gland, which is only 0.3 to 0.6 cm in thickness, is not always clearly seen, a mass as small as 1.2 cm in size can be delineated and clearly distinguished from a normal gland. With longitudinal oblique scanning, a sensitivity of 89%, specificity of 97%, and overall accuracy of 95% were observed in 81 adrenal glands (28). With anterior transverse scanning, a sensitivity of 97%,

specificity of 96.5%, and an overall accuracy of 96.6% were achieved for detecting mass lesions in 148 glands; 10 of the masses detected were less than 3.6 cm in size, and five were less than 2.5 cm in size (11). Many of these patients were scanned with a 2.25-MHz collimated transducer. The masses not detected were usually small left adrenal masses in obese patients or in patients with excessive bowel gas. The accuracy of CT (19, 31–34) in detecting adrenal masses is similar to that of well-performed ultrasonography. The masses missed with CT are mainly in patients with scanty perirenal fat or in whom there are artifacts caused by biological motion obscuring the adrenal areas. Although the artifacts have decreased with new equipment, they still occur, especially when the patient is uncooperative or in the presence of multiple surgical clips. The latter have made the detection of recurrent tumor in patients with previous resection of pheochromocytoma difficult (31). Some tumors, such as aldosteronomas, may be difficult to discern because they have an acoustic density similar to the surrounding fat (Fig. 13.13). The low density of these tumors may be due to a high cholesterol or fat content (35).

Adrenal scintography with [131]I-19-iodocholesterol may detect functional adrenal tumors or hyperplasia (36–39). However, a delay of 4 to 15 days after the injection of isotope may be necessary before useful images can be obtained, and small masses (less than 3 cm in size) may not be seen. Nevertheless, detection of hyperfunction is possible before adrenal enlargement, and adenomas can be distinguished from nodular hyperplasia.

Adrenal venography is useful in detecting small aldosteronomas. By venous blood sampling and venography, masses can be localized or visualized (40). This is particularly helpful when the findings on CT or ultrasonography are negative or equivocal.

In clinical practice, ultrasound or CT will be the initial imaging procedure for the evaluation of the patient suspected of having adrenal disease. The choice between the two modalities will depend on the patient's age and body habitus, the availability of equipment, and the experience of the ultrasonographer. In children, thin adults, or pregnant women (Fig. 13.24), ultrasonography is the method of choice because of the lack of ionizing radiation. When examination of both ovaries is also required, such as in young women with hirsutism, ultrasonography is valuable since it will clearly delineate the ovaries, will

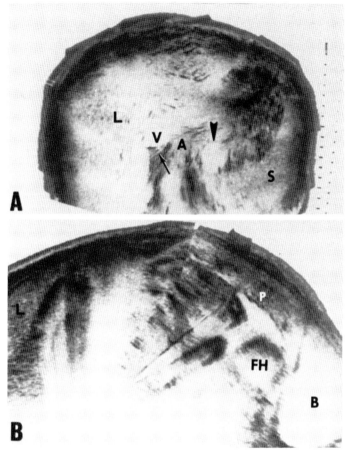

Figure 13.24. An adrenal adenoma causing Cushing's syndrome in a pregnant woman. *A,* Transverse scan 14 cm above umbilicus. A mass (*arrowhead*) is seen in the left adrenal region. The right adrenal gland (*arrow*) is normal. *L,* liver; *A,* aorta; *V,* inferior vena cava; *S,* spleen. *B,* Longitudinal scan at midline showing a fetus in the uterus. *FH,* fetal head; *P,* placenta; *B,* bladder.

show tiny ovarian cysts if present, and radiation to the gonads can be avoided. For very obese patients, however, CT is preferable. Scintigraphy may be performed in patients with functional abnormalities, especially when hyperplasia is suspected. However, since the appropriate isotopes are approved for use only at certain academic centers, this modality is not often available. Angiography is particularly useful in patients with hyperaldosteronism, especially when other modalities fail to locate the lesion.

References

1. Binholtz JC: Ultrasound imaging of adrenal mass lesions. *Radiology* 109:163–166, 1973.
2. Davidson JK, Morley P, Hurley GD, Holford NGH: Adrenal venography and ultrasound in the investigation of the adrenal gland: an analysis of 53 cases. *Br J Radiol* 48:435–450, 1975.
3. Ghorashi B, Holmes JH: Gray scale sonographic appearance of an adrenal mass: a case report. *J Clin Ultrasound* 4:121–123, 1976.
4. Holm HH, Kristensen JK, Rasmussen SN, Pedersen JF: Ultrasonic diagnosis of juxtarenal masses. *Scand J Urol Nephrol* 6 (Suppl 15):83–88, 1972.
5. Holm HH: Ultrasonic scanning in the diagnosis of space-occupying lesions of the upper abdomen. *Br J Radiol* 44:24–36, 1971.
6. Lyons EA, Murphy AV, Arneil GC: Sonar and its use in kidney disease in children. *Arch Dis Child* 47:777–786, 1972.
7. Pitts WR Jr, Kazam E, Gershowitz M, Muecke EC: A review of 100 renal and perinephric sonograms with anatomic diagnosis. *J Urol* 114:21, 1972.
8. Brascho DJ: Clinical applications of diagnostic ultrasound in abdominal malignancy. *South Med J* 65:1331, 1972.
9. Holm HH, Rasmussen SN, Kristensen JK: Errors and pitfalls in ultrasonic scanning of the abdomen. *Br J Radiol* 45:835, 1972.
10. Pond GD, Haber K: Echography: a new approach

to the diagnosis of adrenal hemorrhage of the newborn. *J Can Assoc Radiol* 27:40–44, 1976.

11. Yeh HC: Sonography of the adrenal glands: normal glands and small masses. *AJR* 135:1167–1777, 1980.

12. Sample WF: A new technique for the evaluation of the adrenal gland with gray scale ultrasonography. *Radiology* 124:463–469, 1977.

13. Mitty HA, Yeh HC: *Radiology of the Adrenals with Sonography and CT.* Philadelphia, WB Saunders, 1982.

14. Brownlie K, Kreel L: Computer assisted tomography of normal suprarenal glands. *J Comput Asst Tomogr* 2:1–10, 1978.

15. Karstaedt H, Segel SS, Stanley RJ, Melson GL, Levitt RG: Computed tomography of adrenal gland. *Radiology* 129:723–730, 1978.

16. Davies DV: *Gray's Anatomy*, ed 34. London, Longmans, Green, 1967, pp 1601–1605.

17. Netter FH: *Endocrine System and Selected Metabolic Diseases* (The CIBA Collection of Medical Illustrations, Vol 4). Summit, NJ, CIBA Pharmaceutical Company, 1965, pp 78–79.

18. Sample WF, Sarti DA: Computed tomography and gray scale ultrasonography of the adrenal gland: a comparative study. *Radiology* 128:377, 1978.

19. Yeh HC, Mitty HA, Rose J, Wolf BS, Gabrilove JL: Ultrasonography of adrenal masses: usual features. *Radiology* 127:467–474, 1978.

20. Yeh HC, Mitty HA, Rose J, Wolf BS, Gabrilove JL: Ultrasonography of adrenal masses: unusual manifestations. *Radiology* 127:475–483, 1978.

21. Forsythe JR, Gosink BB, Leopold GR: Ultrasound in the evaluation of adrenal metastases. *J Clin Ultrasound* 5:31–34, 1977.

22. Robbins SL: *Pathology*, ed 3. Philadelphia, WB Saunders, 1967, pp 1219–1240.

23. Weber CL, Murphy ML: Adrenal hypofunction secondary to adenocortical destruction by metastatic carcinoma of the lung. *J Ark Med Soc* 68:181, 1971.

24. Pery M, Kaftori JK, Bar-Maor JA: Sonography for diagnosis and follow-up of neonatal adrenal hemorrhage. *J Clin Ultrasound* 9:397–401, 1981.

25. Behan M, Martin EC, Meucke EC, Kazam E: Myelolipoma of the adrenal: two cases with ultrasound and CT findings. *AJR* 129:993–996, 1977.

26. Scheible W, Ellenbogen PH, Leopold GR, Siao NJ: Lipomatous tumors of the kidney and adrenal: apparent echographic specificity. *Radiology* 129:153–156, 1978.

27. McLelland R, Landes RR, Ransom CL: Retroperitoneal pneumography: a safe method using carbon dioxide. *Radiol Clin North Am* 3:113–128, 1965.

28. Sample WF: Adrenal ultrasonography. *Radiology* 127:461, 1978.

29. McLachlan MSF, Robert EE: Demonstration of normal adrenal gland by venography and gas insufflation. *Br J Radiol* 44:664–671, 1971.

30. Yeh HC, Rabinowitz JG: Ultrasonography of normal or the dilated stomach, correlation with computed tomography. *Appl Radiol* 11:121–127, 1982.

31. Dunnick NR, Doppman JL, Gill JR, Strott CA, Keiser HR, Brennan MF: Localization of functional adrenal tumors by computed tomography and venous sampling. *Radiology* 142:429–433, 1982.

32. Abrams HL, Siegelman SS, Admas DF, Sanders R, Finberg HJ, Hessel SJ, McNeil BJ: Computed tomography versus ultrasound of adrenal gland: a prospective study. *Radiology* 143:121–128, 1982.

33. Laursen K, Damgaard-Pederson K: CT for pheochrocytoma diagnosis. *AJR* 134:277–280, 1980.

34. Dunnick NR, Schaner EG, Doppman JL, Strott CA, Gill JR, Javadpour N: Computed tomography in adrenal tumors. *AJR* 132:43–46, 1979.

35. Schaner EG, Dunnick NR, Doppman JL, Strott CA, Gill JR Jr, Javadpour N: Adrenal cortical tumors with low attenuation coefficient: a pitfall in computed tomography diagnosis. *J Comput Asst Tomogr* 2:11, 1978.

36. Beierwaltes WH, Lieberman LM, Ansari AN, Nishiyama H: Visualization of human adrenal glands in vivo by scintillation scanning. *JAMA* 216:275, 1971.

37. Troncone L, Galli G, Salvo D, Barbarino A, Bonomo L: Radioisotopic study of the adrenal glands using I^{131}-19-iodocholesterol. *Br J Radiol* 50:340, 1977.

38. Thrall JH, Freitas JE, Beierwaltes WH: Adrenal scintigraphy. *Semin Nucl Med* 8:23, 1978.

39. Gross MD, Valk TW, Swanson DP, Thrall JH, Grekin RJ, Beierwaltes WH: The role of pharmacologic manipulation in adrenal cortical scintigraphy. *Semin Nucl Med* 11:128–148, 1981.

40. Mitty HA, Nicolis GL, Gabrilove JL: Adrenal venography: clinical radiographic correlation in 80 patients. *AJR* 119:564–575, 1973.

CHAPTER 14

The Role of Ultrasound in Pediatric Uroradiology*

DIANE S. BABCOCK, M.D.
JOHN R. BABCOCK, M.D.

The use of ultrasound in evaluation of the pediatric patient initially lagged behind its use in the adult patient, but its value is now recognized. The small size and relative lack of body fat make the child an ideal patient for ultrasound. Higher frequency transducers with their increased resolution can be employed. In the pediatric patient ultrasound was initially used to evaluate renal masses and to diagnose hydronephrosis (1, 2). The diagnostic capabilities and clinical usefulness of ultrasonography have expanded to include many clinical problems and disease processes of the pediatric urological patient (3–5). Improved resolution of scanners and the development of gray-scale ultrasonography have resulted in expanded diagnostic use in evaluating changes in the parenchymal echo pattern produced by various renal diseases from those of the normal renal parenchyma (6). Ultrasound is also useful for repetitive examinations in the follow-up and management of pediatric urological problems, and it avoids the irradiation of conventional methods.

TECHNICAL CONSIDERATIONS

For examining the kidneys, the traditional longitudinal and transverse scans are performed with the patient in the prone position. Scans in the supine and decubitus positions should also be obtained since the parenchymal anatomy of the right kidney is best shown when the liver is used as an acoustical window. Scans of the left kidney and spleen can be obtained by coronal sector scans in the decubitus position. To demonstrate parenchymal detail, single-sector scans of the kidney should be obtained, thus scanning each area of tissue only once and avoiding compound images.

The bladder is routinely examined in longitudinal and transverse planes with the bladder distended. Re-examination is performed after bladder emptying to evaluate bladder residual in patients with neurogenic bladders and urinary tract infections.

In the ultrasonographic examination of the pediatric patient, special consideration must be given to immobilization and to maintenance of normal body temperature. In our scanning rooms an overhead servo-control heater (Solaroid Electric Infrared Heater, Aitken Products, Geneva, OH, and Proportional Temperature Controller, Yellow Springs Instrument, Yellow Springs, OH) is suspended over the baby. The couplant, either gel or mineral oil, is warmed. Sedation frequently aids in immobilization, and chloral hydrate in an oral dose of 50 mg/kg is routinely used with nursing service monitoring the patient. The transducer having the highest possible frequency should be used to optimize the resolution of small structures. In newborns and young infants, a 5.0 or 7.5 MHz, 6-mm face, short internal focused transducer is routinely used; a 5.0 or 3.5 MHz, 13-mm face, medium-focused transducer is used for larger infants and older children.

NORMAL RENAL ANATOMY OF THE INFANT

The normal intrarenal anatomy of the adult patient has been described in detail (7, 8). The kidney of the normal infant has several features which differ from those in the kidney of the normal adult patient (Fig. 14.1). The central echo complex is much less dense relative to the renal parenchyma. It has been postulated that this is due to less peripelvic fat in the infant than in the adult (9). We have noted that the

* We thank Marsha Ellington, Theresa Adams, and Debora Root for technical assistance; and Marlena Tyre for assistance in manuscript preparation.

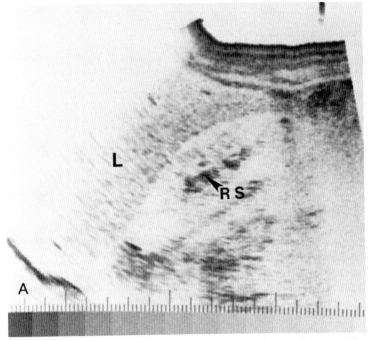

Figure 14.1. Normal kidney. Longitudinal supine view of right kidney. *A*, Normal kidney in adult or older child elliptical in shape with densely echogenic renal sinus (*RS*). Renal cortex less echogenic than adjacent liver (*L*)

echogenicity of the renal cortex in the normal infant differs from that of the adult in that it is the same as the echogenicity of the adjacent normal liver, rather than being less, as in the adult patient (10). The medullary pyramids in the infant are larger relative to the rest of the kidney and tend to appear more prominent. The corticomedullary differentiation is generally greater in the infant kidney than in the adult (Fig. 14.1), possibly because of increased resolution from higher frequency transducers and less overlying body tissue. These findings indicate that the pyramids in the infant kidney can easily be confused with multiple cysts by those not familiar with the differences; normal pyramids line up around the central echo complex in a characteristic pattern and can, therefore, be differentiated from cysts. Also, the position of the arcuate artery can help to identify a structure as a pyramid.

Urinary Bladder

The normal bladder is a fluid-filled structure in the lower pelvis which has a thin wall when it is distended. A crude measurement of bladder volume can be obtained by measuring antero-posterior, transverse, and longitudinal dimensions and using the volume for a cube. In the normal patient the urinary bladder empties completely with voiding. Bladder residual can be estimated by measuring the residual volume after voiding.

CONGENITAL ANOMALIES OF THE URINARY TRACT

Anomalies of the urinary tract are the most common congenital malformations found in children, with a reported incidence of about 10% (3); however, many of these anomalies are of minor or no importance. In most cases, all but the most minor anomalies of the urinary tract can be diagnosed easily by ultrasonography without subjecting patients to the hazards of ionizing radiation and contrast material. Ultrasound is recommended as a screening procedure in those suspected of having congenital anomalies, i.e., patients with syndromes which often include urinary tract anomalies, in patients with recurrent urinary tract infections, or failure to thrive.

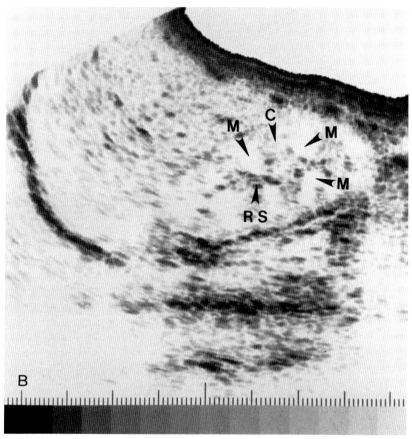

Figure 14.1. *B*, Normal infant kidney; renal sinus (*RS*) less echogenic than in adult patient. Renal cortex (*C*) equal in echogenicity to adjacent liver. Renal medullary pyramids (*M*) in infant are larger relative to rest of kidney and appear prominent. (Reprinted with permission from Babcock (6).)

Anomalies of the kidney include supernumerary kidneys and renal agenesis. Bilateral renal agenesis is rare and is incompatible with life. The associated oligohydramnios results in Potter's syndrome and pulmonary hypoplasia, causing death. The absence of kidneys is readily detectable with portable real-time ultrasound equipment in the newborn nursery for these critically ill infants.

Unilateral renal agenesis is caused by failure of development of the nephrogenic blastema and the ureteric bud from the Wolffian ducts. The ureterovesical orifice and adjacent portion of the trigone are also absent in the majority of cases. Genital anomalies are frequently associated and, in females, may range from an ipsilateral absence of the oviduct to a unicornuate uterus with an absent ovary and atretic vagina (Fig. 14.2). In males the ipsilateral vas deferens, seminal vesicle, or ipsilateral testicular appendages may be absent. Compensatory hypertrophy of the contralateral kidney is usually present. Ultrasonography easily demonstrates the solitary hypertrophied kidney and the absence of the opposite kidney, although at times it may be difficult to completely exclude a small hypoplastic or damaged kidney. When the kidney is absent, the bowel—either the hepatic or splenic flexure—fills in the renal fossa and can be mistaken for an abnormal kidney if a careful examination is not performed. When unilateral renal agenesis is found, the associated anomalies of the genital tract should be sought (11).

Anomalies of kidney position—such as malrotation, ectopia, and ptosis—can be recognized by ultrasonography when abnormal position or orientation of the renal axis is seen. When the kidney is not seen in normal position in the

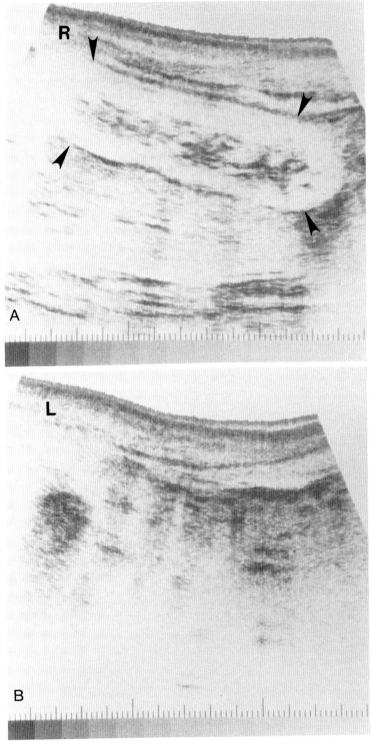

Figure 14.2.   Unilateral renal agenesis with bicornuate uterus. Longitudinal prone scans of right flank (*A*), left flank (*B*), and transverse prone scan (*C*) demonstrate solitary right kidney (*arrows*) with bowel gas occupying left renal fossa. *D,* Transverse scan of uterus demonstrates two cornu (*C*).

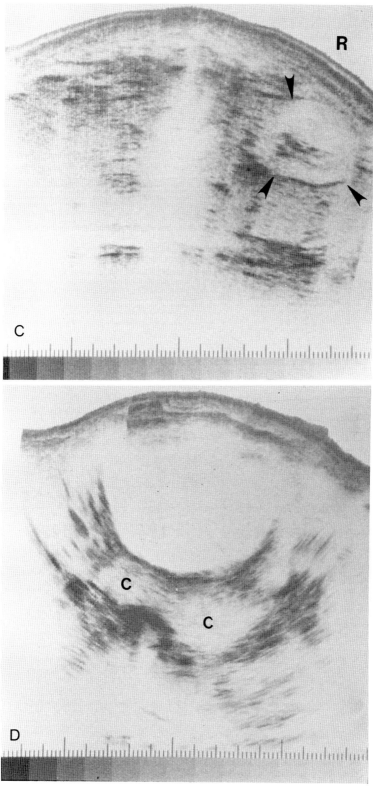

Figure 14.2, *C* and *D*.

renal fossa, then a careful search of the pelvis and lower abdomen should be performed to look for an ectopic kidney. The horseshoe kidney is the most common type of fusion anomaly with fusion of the lower poles by a band of functioning renal parenchyma or fibrous tissue. The band of renal parenchyma can be identified anterior to the spine on abdominal ultrasonography, and the abnormal axis of the kidneys, with the lower poles positioned more medially than the upper poles, can be recognized.

Duplication of the renal pelvis and ureter is a frequent anomaly of the urinary tract, estimated to occur in 0.7% of the general population, and may be partial or complete and unilateral or bilateral. Associated anomalies, such as ectopic insertion of the ureter, ureteroceles, or structural renal anomalies, are common (12). The normal renal sinus forms a continuous echogenic area within the center of the kidney (Fig. 14.1A). With a duplication the renal sinus will be divided into two portions by a band of hypoechoic renal parenchyma representing a column of Bertin. One portion of the duplicated collecting system may be hydronephrotic (Fig. 14.3); in such cases, a source of obstruction should be searched for in the ureter and bladder. The upper pole collecting system, which may be small and nonfunctioning, may insert abnormally low in the urinary bladder or urethra, or it may be obstructed distally by a ureterocele (Fig. 14.4). Ultrasound is useful in detecting small duplications not visible on radiography.

Ultrasonography can be helpful in the evaluation of intersex problems to gain knowledge of the internal genital anatomy. The vagina and uterus are easily demonstrated in infants and children of all ages. Their size and configuration can be evaluated. Ovaries are more difficult to identify, particularly in infants, but can frequently be demonstrated in the older child (13). The appearance of the external and internal genital anatomy as well as the sex chromosome pattern are necessary for prompt assignment of sex in the neonatal period.

HYDRONEPHROSIS

A number of studies have documented the ability of ultrasound to demonstrate hydronephrosis even in its mild form (14). Ultrasonography demonstrates fluid-containing areas within the renal sinus that conform anatomically to the renal collecting system. With the resolution possible with the latest equipment, the normal renal calyx and infundibulum can sometimes be identified. The minimal dilatation that occurs with hydration after intravenous urography or partial obstruction of the distal ureter by a distended urinary bladder is a possible source of false positives. Documentation of the degree of hydration of the patient and rescanning the kidneys with the bladder empty will resolve this problem in most cases.

Sonography is recommended as a screening procedure to look for hydronephrosis for the initial diagnosis, for follow-up examinations to evaluate changes in the degree of hydronephrosis, and to determine the thickness of the renal cortical mantle. The salvagability of the kidneys is best determined by nuclear isotope studies that more properly assess renal function.

Ureteropelvic Junction Obstruction

Ureteropelvic junction obstruction is the most common congenital obstruction of the urinary tract but can occur at any age and may be unilateral or bilateral (15). It can occur in utero and may be the etiology of a multicystic kidney (16). It most commonly presents as a palpable abdominal mass; however, abdominal pain due to intermittent obstruction and hematuria may also occur. Its etiology may be congenital bands, aberrant blood vessels, or intrinsic abnormalities of the muscle fibers in the pelvis, although no single cause has been established.

Ultrasonography demonstrates dilatation of the renal pelvis and renal calices with a normal caliber ureter (Fig. 14.5). Sonography can also be used to assess the renal cortical thickness and to provide an estimation of prognosis. If the obstruction is severe enough to cause significant renal damage, function may be too poor to demonstrate the anatomy on excretory urography, whereas sonography, which does not rely on renal function, provides an immediate diagnosis. If the child is too sick for immediate surgery, percutaneous nephrostomy can be performed under ultrasound guidance as a temporizing procedure (17). Postoperatively, ultrasonography can be used to evaluate the residual degree of pelvicalyceal dilatation and the thickness of the renal parenchyma, obviating the need for frequent urography.

Ultrasonography and excretory urography demonstrate the degree of dilatation and the apparent site of obstruction, but the functional

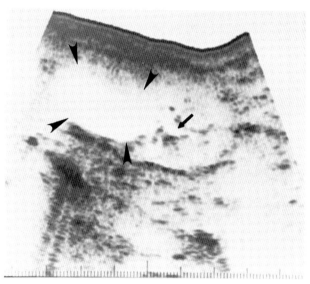

Figure 14.3. Duplication of the renal sinus. Longitudinal prone scan shows hydronephrotic upper pole (*arrowheads*) and normal lower pole (*arrow*) collecting system in patient with duplication and obstruction of upper system.

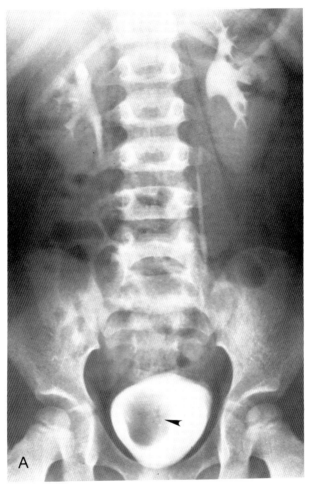

Figure 14.4. Duplicated collecting system with ureterocele. *A,* Excretory urogram shows somewhat small right kidney with fewer calices compared to left and filling defect in bladder.

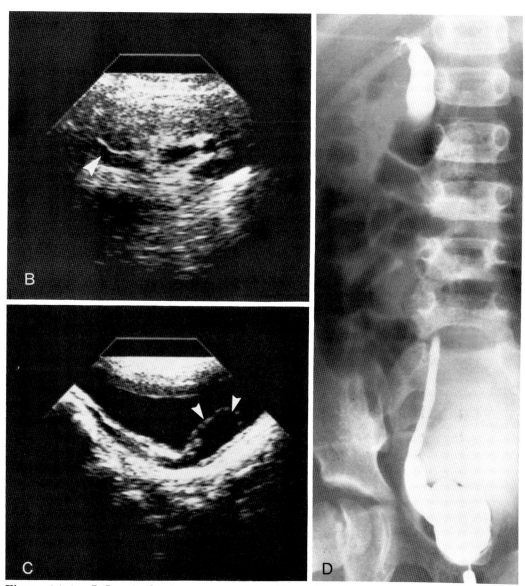

Figure 14.4. *B,* Longitudinal prone scan, right kidney, dilated upper pole ureter demonstrated medial to upper pole right kidney (*arrow*). *C,* Longitudinal scan of urinary bladder shows dilated lower right ureter with ureterocele (*arrows*) bulging into bladder. *D,* Retrograde injection of ureterocele shows contrast material filling small upper pole and its dilated ureter.

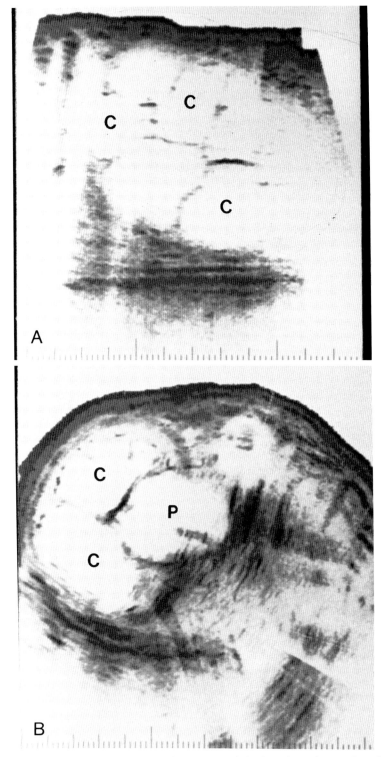

A

B

Figure 14.5. Marked hydronephrosis with ureteropelvic junction obstruction. Longitudinal prone (*A*) and transverse prone (*B*) scans demonstrate enlarged kidney with markedly dilated calices (*C*) and renal pelvis (*P*). Renal parenchyma diffusely thinned. Ureter was not dilated.

degree of obstruction is better evaluated by the Whitaker test or a Lasix renogram.

Ureterovesical Junction Obstruction

Obstruction at the ureterovesical junction can occur due to stricture, following ureteral reimplantation, from edema, or with a congenital ectopic ureter and ureterocele. Ultrasonography demonstrates dilatation of the ureter down to its insertion into the bladder (18). With a ureterocele, the distal ureter is dilated, bulbous in shape, and bulges into the bladder (Fig. 14.4). A ureterocele is a dynamic structure, and observation with real-time ultrasound usually demonstrates the ureterocele changing in size as the urine flows through it and is intermittently emptied into the bladder.

Urethral Obstruction

The most common cause of severe urinary tract obstruction in the male infant is posterior urethral valves. Infants usually present with a palpable abdominal mass or masses due to the distended bladder and kidneys and a poor voiding stream. The majority are discovered during the first year of life, but occasionally older children and adults are discovered to have hydronephrosis secondary to posterior urethral valves (19). Ultrasonography in these patients will demonstrate bilateral hydroureteronephrosis and an abnormally thickened bladder wall due to muscular hypertophy (Fig. 14.6). Angled views of the lower bladder in coronal and sagittal plane may demonstrate the dilated posterior urethra proximal to the valves. Although the diagnosis can frequently be made by careful ultrasound examination of the entire urinary tract, a voiding cystourethrogram is performed to confirm the diagnosis.

Nonobstructive Causes of Urinary Tract Dilatation

Infection, bladder distention, and vesicoureteral reflux can all cause dilatation without obstruction which is difficult to distinguish from obstructive hydronephrosis. Vesicoureteral reflux can cause urinary tract dilatation and may be associated with renal scarring, which can frequently be identified by ultrasound. There has been recent interest in the ultrasound diagnosis of vesicoureteral reflux, and a recent paper reported accurate diagnosis of grades 2B, 3, and 4 reflux when compared to static cystograms (20). Similarly, ultrasonic examinations can be used to monitor the continued presence or absence of reflux in patients following operative and nonoperative treatment.

Patients with neurogenic bladders may develop urinary tract dilatation secondary to incomplete emptying, urinary tract infections, and reflux. Serial ultrasonography has proven useful to evaluate the degree of dilatation and renal scarring and can be substituted for radiographic procedures in the follow-up management of these patients, thereby lessening the cumulative radiation dose that these children receive.

In the Eagle-Barrett ("prune belly") syndrome dilatation of the ureters and bladder is seen and is due to an insufficient amount of muscle or structurally abnormal muscle in the ureter and bladder wall. Absent abdominal musculature and cryptorchidism are also present in these patients (21). Ultrasonography can be of diagnostic and prognostic value in evaluating the degree of dilatation and thickness of the renal parenchyma. Often a cystourachal remnant can be seen in the dome of the bladder.

EVALUATION OF ABDOMINAL MASSES

With the advent of the newer imaging modalities in diagnostic radiology, such as ultrasound and computed tomography, it has become necessary to develop new combined imaging approaches to specific clinical problems. Since approximately 85% of abdominal masses in children, particularly neonates, involve the kidneys or retroperitoneal structures, visualization of these structures is of paramount importance. In the past, the excretory urogram has been performed as the first procedure since it provides both physiological and anatomical information regarding the kidneys and the retroperitoneal structures. However, in children with renal function too poor to allow satisfactory visualization of the urinary tract, or in newborn infants, ultrasound often provides more information. In addition, a poorly functioning kidney on excretory urography is better evaluated by ultrasound. Currently, the initial work-up of the abdominal mass in a child includes ultrasonography and usually a plain film of the abdomen to look for calcifications within the mass and displacement or obstruction of the bowel gas. The site of origin of the mass is determined by ultrasound—whether originating from the kidney or

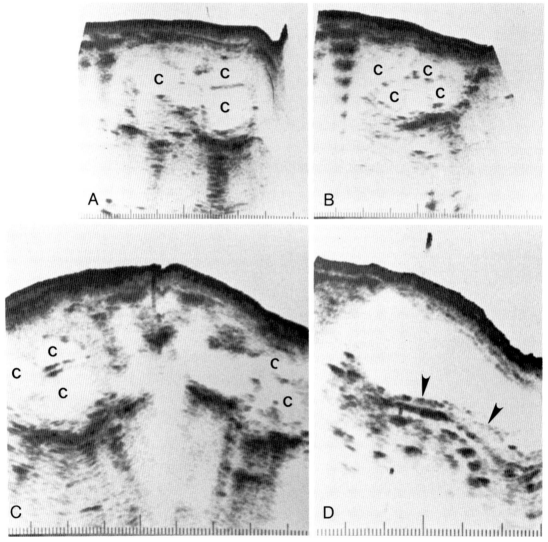

Figure 14.6. Hydronephrosis and posterior urethral valves. Longitudinal prone scans of left kidney (*A*), right kidney (*B*), and transverse prone scan (*C*) demonstrate bilateral marked hydronephrosis. *C*, Dilated calices. *D*, Longitudinal scan of urinary bladder shows dilatation with thickening and irregularity of wall due to muscular hypertrophy (*arrowheads*).

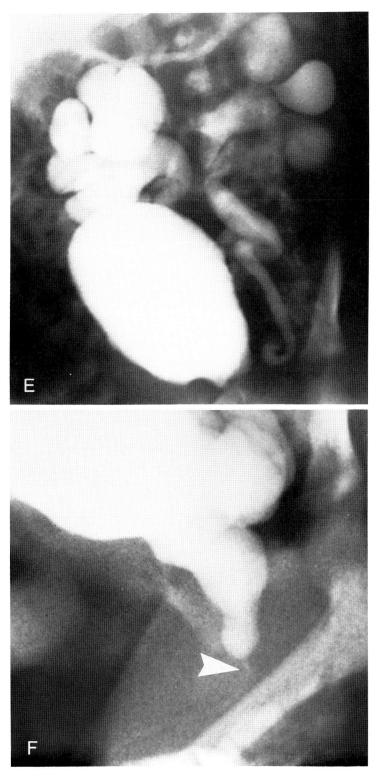

Figure 14.6. *E* and *F,* Cystourethrogram shows reflux with hydronephrosis, trabeculated bladder, and dilated posterior urethra proximal to valves (*arrowhead*).

other organ, such as the adrenal gland or liver. Ultrasound has an advantage over the excretory urogram in that if a mass arises from an organ other than the urinary tract it can still be evaluated. Information about the mass, including whether it is cystic or solid and, if solid, the echo texture, can be used to aid in the differential diagnosis of the mass. Evidence of metastasis in the draining lymph nodes and the liver can also be searched for with ultrasound.

Cystic Renal Masses

The most common renal masses in children are benign and are cystic. In our experience they are almost equally divided between hydronephrosis and multicystic dysplasia of the kidney. Multicystic dysplasia of the kidney is usually a unilateral disease with multiple cysts of varying size and dysplastic renal parenchyma, including areas of proliferation of connective tissue, cartilage, and other components. The ureter is usually small in caliber, atretic, or both. The renal artery is also often small or is absent.

The characteristic ultrasonographic pattern of a multicystic dysplastic kidney (Fig. 14.7) is a multiloculated cystic mass, having curvilinear septa within it that divide it into cysts of varying size (22, 23). Varying amounts of solid dysplastic renal parenchyma can also be identified within the cystic mass. The outline of the dysplastic kidney is lobulated and the cysts have no organization, whereas the severely hydronephrotic kidney usually maintains its reniform shape and dilated calices are arranged around a larger, more medial pelvis.

The differential diagnosis can usually be confidently made by ultrasound between the hydronephrotic kidney and the multicystic dysplastic kidney; however, in some cases the ultrasound is not diagnostic, and nuclear scan or excretory urography may be helpful since little excretion is seen with the multicystic dysplastic kidney owing to the absence of functioning parenchyma. Severely hydronephrotic kidneys, however, can also sometimes have little excretion. Unilateral multicystic dysplasia of the kidney is a benign disorder. If the diagnosis can be confidently made by ultrasonography and other imaging modalities, then surgery can be delayed until the neonate is older or can even be avoided in some cases (22).

Simple renal cortical cysts are an acquired lesion with increasing incidence with age. Although they are primarily lesions of adults, they can occasionally occur in childhood or even in neonates. Ultrasonography will show a round, sonolucent mass without internal echoes, a sharply defined, smooth border, and an increased through transmission. Since the possibility of a hypovascular cystic Wilms' tumor always exists and true simple cysts are rare in children, a cyst puncture under sonographic or fluoroscopic guidance is usually performed for laboratory analysis of the fluid.

Solid Renal Masses

The most common intra-abdominal malignant tumor in childhood is the Wilms' tumor or nephroblastoma (24, 25). The peak incidence of occurrence is between the ages of 2 and 5 years, with an incidence of bilateral tumors of about 5%. The patient usually presents with an asymptomatic abdominal mass which is often quite bulky. Other symptoms such as fever or microscopic hematuria are only rarely present. Wilms' tumor has been associated with other congenital anomalies, including aniridia, hemihypertrophy, Beckwith-Wiedemann's syndrome (organomegaly involving the kidney, adrenal cortex, and liver), trisomies 8 and 18, and genitourinary tract anomalies (cryptorchidism, hypospadias, duplication of the urinary tract, and horseshoe kidney). Patients with these other anomalies can be regularly screened with ultrasonography of the kidneys rather than repeated radiographic procedures.

Ultrasonography of a Wilms' tumor typically demonstrates a bulky mass expanding within the renal parenchyma resulting in distortion and displacement of the pelvicalyceal system (Fig. 14.8). The mass is primarily echogenic and solid but may have sonolucent areas of necrosis, hemorrhage, and liquifaction within it (24). The tumor may spread into the renal vein and inferior vena cava, and these structures should be imaged by ultrasonography looking for tumor thromboses. If the vena cava is normal by ultrasound, a contrast inferior venacavogram is not necessary. However, if there is any abnormality in the visualization of the entire cava or if tumor thrombosis is definitely seen, an inferior venacavogram is then necessary.

Since about 5% of Wilms' tumors are bilateral, the opposite kidney should be carefully scanned for a second primary. Ultrasonography of liver metastasis shows alteration from the

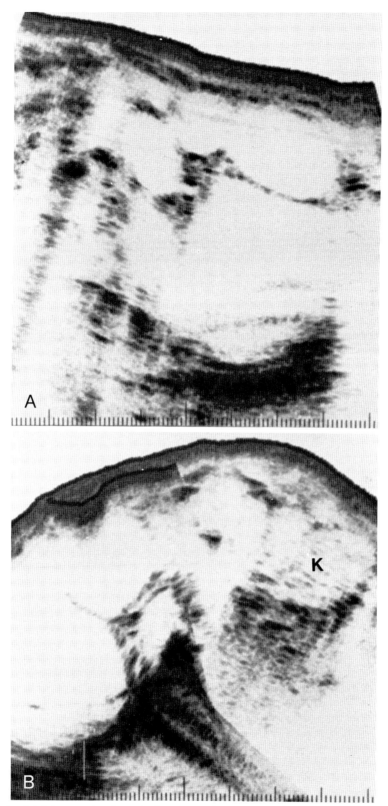

Figure 14.7. Multicystic dysplastic kidney in newborn with abdominal mass. Longitudinal prone (*A*) and transverse prone (*B*) views demonstrate multiloculated cystic mass in position of left kidney. Excretory urography showed no function of left kidney. *K*, normal right kidney. (Reprinted with permission from Babcock (6).)

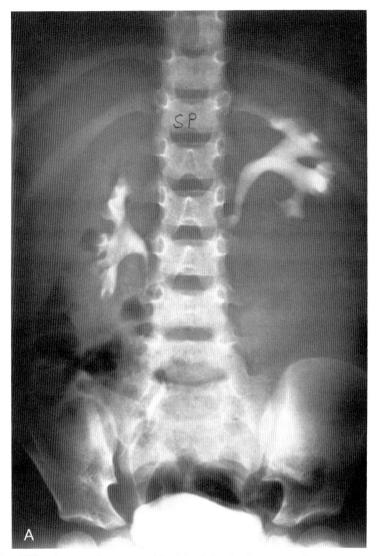

Figure 14.8. Wilms' tumor in 3-year-old with abdominal mass. *A,* Excretory urography shows large mass distorting and displacing left kidney.

normal homogeneous parenchymal echo pattern of the liver with areas that are decreased or increased in echogenicity.

Other primary renal tumors occur less commonly in children. The congenital Wilms' tumor or mesoblastic nephroma is a benign hamartoma seen in newborns. Its ultrasound pattern is similar to Wilms' tumor, but the younger age of presentation aids in diagnosis (26). Renal cell carcinoma can occur in older children and has an appearance similar to Wilms' tumor.

Other rare renal tumors seen in children include angiomyolipomas, rhabdomyosarcomas, leiomyosarcomas, hemangiomas, hemangioperi-cytomas, cystadenomas (multilocular cysts), and mucosal epithelial tumors. The angiomyolipoma is a hamartoma containing vascular, fatty, and muscular tissue seen particularly in patients with tuberous sclerosis. The diagnosis can be made if fat can be identified within the tumor either on ultrasound or CT (27). Other tumors require histological material for accurate diagnosis.

The Enlarged Kidney

Polycystic disease of the kidney frequently presents as bilateral abdominal masses which

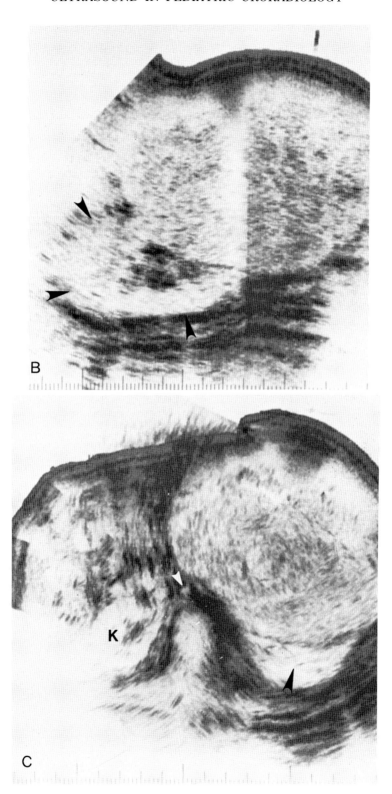

Figure 14.8.   Longitudinal (*B*) and transverse supine (*C*) scans demonstrate echogenic solid mass arising from lower pole of left kidney (*black arrowheads*). Mass crosses midline anterior to aorta (*white arrowhead*). *K*, Normal right kidney.

are actually enlarged kidneys. Two types of polycystic kidney disease were described by Osathanondh and Potter (28); both can have a spectrum of severity. The infantile type (Potter type I) has an autosomal recessive inheritance. Classically, the kidneys in this condition are bilaterally large and sponge-like with impaired function. The thousands of so-called cysts are actually dilated collecting tubules. Periportal fibrosis in the liver is a part of the disease. Blyth and Ockenden (29) have divided this recessive type of polycystic kidney disease into four groups: perinatal, neonatal, infantile, and juvenile, according to the percentage of tubules affected and the clinical and pathological presentation and course.

The classical infantile type of polycystic kidney disease (perinatal type) presents with bilat-

erally enlarged kidneys having poor function on excretory urography (Fig. 14.9). Delayed films demonstrate linear radial streaking of the contrast material in the dilated tubules. Ultrasonography in these patients shows bilaterally massively enlarged kidneys with poorly defined borders, increased dense echoes throughout the renal parenchyma, and good sound transmission (30–32). The central echo complex is obliterated by the dense parenchymal echoes. This increased echogenicity is caused by the sound beam being reflected by the walls of the multiple, dilated tubules. Increased echogenicity in the liver, owing to hepatic fibrosis, can sometimes be demonstrated in these patients.

The adult type of polycystic renal disease (Potter type III) is transmitted by autosomal dominant inheritance. Cystic dilatations in this

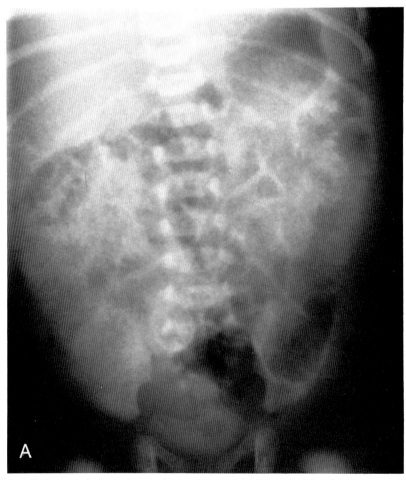

Figure 14.9. Polycystic kidney disease in newborn with bilateral abdominal masses. *A*, Excretory urogram (delayed film) demonstrates linear radial streaking of contrast material in dilated tubules.

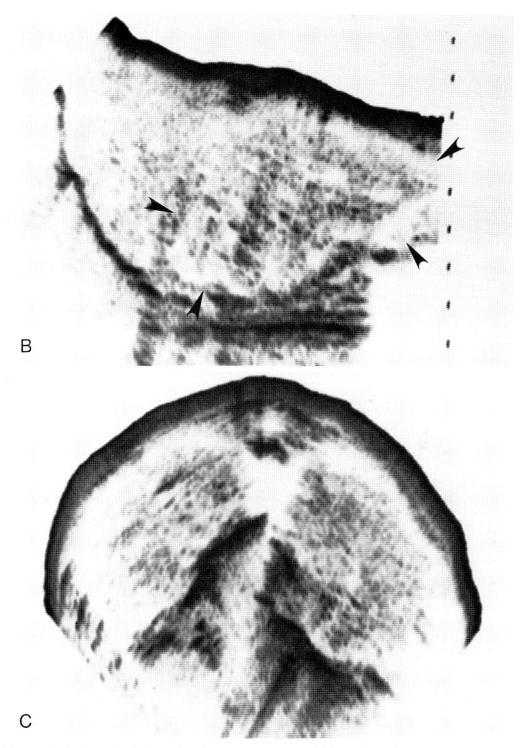

Figure 14.9.   Longitudinal supine ultrasound scan, right kidney (B) and transverse prone scan of both kidneys (C) show enlarged kidneys with increased dense echoes throughout renal parenchyma and obliteration of renal sinus. (Reprinted with permission from Babcock (6).)

condition involve the proximal convoluted tubules and Bowman's capsule, as well as the collecting tubules. In the classic form, the cysts enlarge with age and the disease is usually not diagnosed clinically until middle age, when renal function is diminished. The condition can become manifest in childhood with subtle findings of increased echogenicity of the kidneys; small cysts can sometimes be identified before the excretory urogram demonstrates any abnormalities (33). Ultrasound examination has been proposed as a screening test for families with this disease (34). Several cases have been reported in which the radiographic and sonographic findings resemble those in the recessively inherited type I polycystic kidney disease (35); the ultrasound findings in these patients may differ from those in the type I disease in that the cysts are large enough to be resolved on the ultrasound scan (Fig. 14.10).

Renal vein thrombosis can be seen in the neonate as a complication of dehydration, sepsis, or both; it can occur in older children secondary to such processes as glomerulonephritis, tumor, or renal transplantation. In renal vein thrombosis the entire kidney becomes enlarged and edematous; ultrasound examination (Fig. 14.11) reveals nephromegaly and distortion of the normal architecture, with increased echogenicity of the renal cortex diffusely or in multiple localized areas throughout the kidney (36). The findings are usually unilateral, although they are occasionally bilateral and are similar to those in lymphoma. On follow-up examinations the kidney may return to normal or become small and atrophic.

URINARY TRACT INFECTION

With acute pyelonephritis both ultrasonography and excretory urography frequently demonstrate no abnormality (37). Ultrasound findings, when present, include swelling of the affected kidney and decreased echogenicity of the renal parenchyma due to edema. Occasionally,

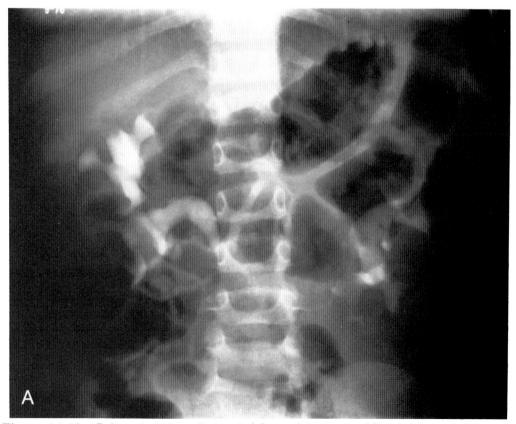

Figure 14.10. Polycystic kidney disease (adult type) in 3-year-old with bilateral abdominal masses and mildly elevated blood urea nitrogen since birth. *A,* Excretory urogram shows enlarged kidneys with distortion and splaying of renal calices about multiple intrarenal cysts.

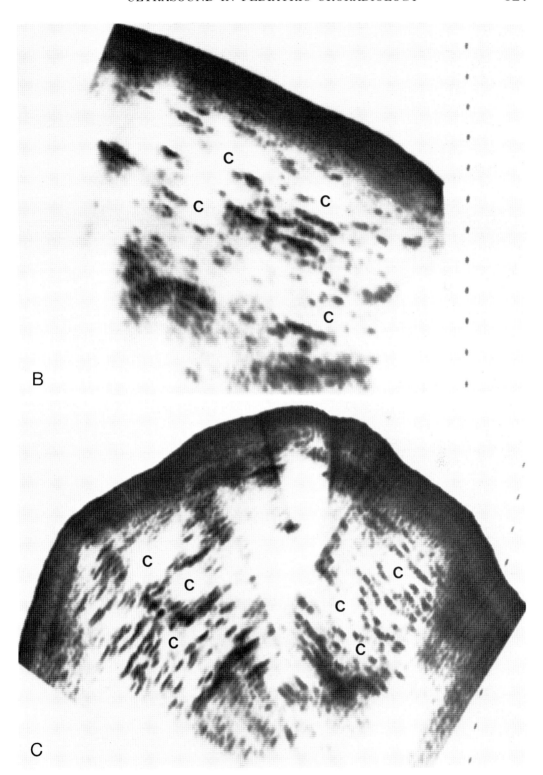

Figure 14.10.   Longitudinal prone (*B*) and transverse prone (*C*) ultrasound scans demonstrate bilateral renal enlargement with multiple cysts (*C*) of varying sizes throughout both kidneys. (Reprinted with permission from Babcock (6).)

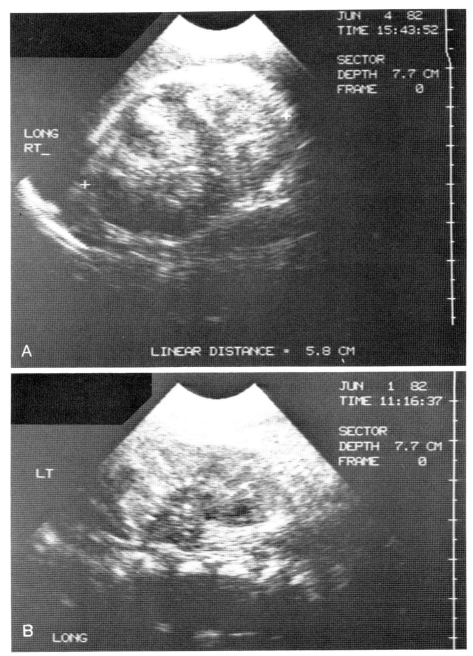

Figure 14.11. Renal vein thrombosis in newborn infant. Longitudinal supine scans of right (*A*) and left (*B*) kidneys demonstrate enlarged right kidney with abnormal patchy areas of increased and decreased echogenicity obscuring normal landmarks. Normal left kidney for comparison.

acute pyelonephritis or infectious interstitial nephritis will be focal, involving only one portion of the kidney (acute lobar nephronia). Ultrasound and excretory urography will reveal a localized renal mass (Fig. 14.12); this will be relatively anechoic on ultrasound and will disrupt the corticomedullary definition, producing

some low level echoes (38). Lobar nephronia may mimic a renal tumor or abscess; however, tumors are rarely as sonolucent as acute lobar nephronia. Sequential examinations demonstrate rapid change, with resolution of the mass in response to antibiotic therapy.

Sonography is useful when a complication of

the infection, such as an abscess or infected cyst, is suspected. Sonography will demonstrate a mass which may be partially fluid filled but is irregular in outline and does not have the characteristics of a simple cyst (39). The perinephric space is also well visualized by ultrasonography, and perinephric abscesses which may be difficult to identify on excretory urography can be visualized with ultrasonography. Ultrasound can also be used for percutaneous aspiration of the abscess for culture and for placement of a percutaneous drainage tube (40).

Chronic pyelonephritis may result in the small kidneys indicative of end-stage renal disease (Fig. 14.13). The kidneys usually have increased echogenicity and irregular outline owing to scars. There is a reversal of the normal relationship between the liver and the kidney, the renal cortex being more echogenic than the liver parenchyma. These findings are not specific,

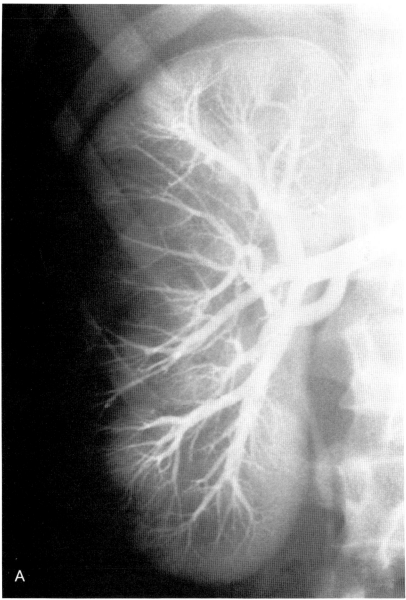

Figure 14.12. Acute focal bacterial nephritis (acute lobar nephronia) in 13-year-old boy with right-sided abdominal pain and normal urinalysis. *A*, Angiography demonstrates avascular mass in mid-right kidney.

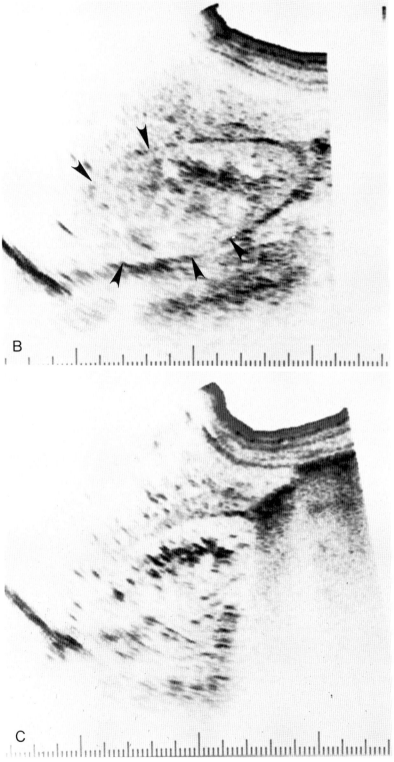

Figure 14.12. *B,* Longitudinal decubitus ultrasound scan shows swelling of upper half of right kidney (*arrowheads*) with distortion of renal sinus echoes which do not appear to be in center of kidney. Radioisotope scan showed cold mass in area. *C,* Two weeks after treatment with antibiotics, mass and swelling have resolved. (Reprinted with permission from Babcock (6).)

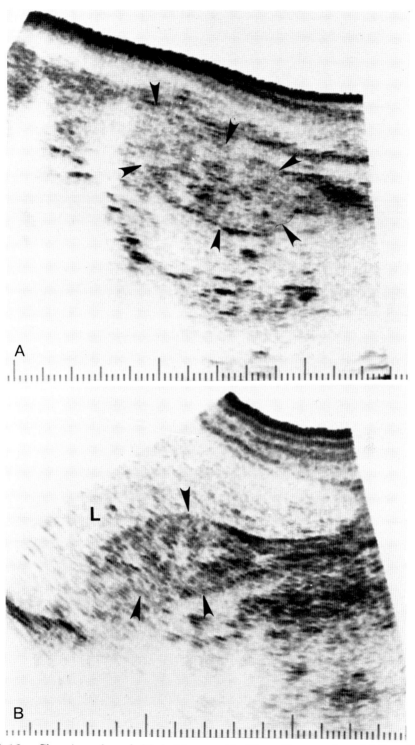

Figure 14.13. Chronic pyelonephritis in 11-year-old with rapid onset of renal failure. Nonfunctioning kidneys on excretory urography. Longitudinal prone (*A*) and longitudinal supine (*B*) views show bilaterally small kidneys (*arrowheads*), smooth in outline, with diffuse increased echogenicity relative to adjacent liver (*L*)—reverse of normal relationship, with renal parenchyma more echogenic than liver parenchyma. (Reprinted with permission from Babcock (6).)

however, and can also been seen in chronic glomerulonephritis and hypertensive or ischemic disease.

RENAL FAILURE

An important use of ultrasonography is for the evaluation of patients with renal failure where poor function precludes excretory urography. By evaluating the renal size, contour, and laterality of involvement, a systematic approach to the diagnosis of renal disease in renal failure can be performed. Ultrasound can determine whether kidneys are present in a newborn with suspected absent or hypoplastic kidneys. It can differentiate renal failure due to obstruction and medical renal diseases.

References

1. Teele RL: Ultrasonography of the genitourinary tract in children. *Radiol Clin North Am* 15:109–128, 1977.
2. Shkolnik A: B-mode ultrasound in the nonvisualizing kidney in pediatrics. *AJR* 128:121–125, 1977.
3. Kangarloo H, Sample WF: *Ultrasound of the Pediatric Abdomen and Pelvis: A Correlative Imaging Approach.* Chicago, Year Book Medical Publishers, 1980, pp 20–115.
4. Frank JL, Potter BM, Shkolnik A: Neonatal ultrasonography. *Clin Diagn Ultrasound* 2:159–174, 1979.
5. Markle BM, Potter BM: Surgical diseases of the urinary tract. *Clin Diagn Ultrasound* 8:135–164, 1981.
6. Babcock DS: Medical diseases of the urinary tract and adrenal glands. *Clin Diagn Ultrasound* 8:113–134, 1981.
7. Cook JH III, Rosenfield AT, Taylor KJW: Ultrasonic demonstration of intrarenal anatomy. *AJR* 129:831–835, 1977.
8. Rosenfield AT, Taylor KJW, Crade M, DeGraaf CS: Anatomy and pathology of the kidney by gray scale ultrasound. *Radiology* 128:737–744, 1978.
9. Behan M, Kazam E: The echogenic characteristics of fatty tissues and tumors. *Radiology* 129:143, 1978.
10. Haller JO, Berdon WE, Friedman AP: Increased renal cortical echogenicity: a normal finding in neonates and infants. *Radiology* 142:173–174, 1982.
11. Fried AM, Oliff M, Wilson EA, Whisnant J: Uterine anomalies associated with renal agenesis: role of gray scale ultrasonography. *AJR* 131:973, 1978.
12. Kelalis PP: Renal pelvis and ureter. In Kelalis PP, King LR, Bellman AB: *Clinical Pediatric Urology.* Philadelphia, WB Saunders, 1976, pp 503–558.
13. Babcock DS, Han BK: Ultrasonography of the pediatric pelvis. *Clin Diagn Ultrasound*, in press.
14. Ellenbogen PH, Scheible FW, Talner LB, Leopold GR: Sensitivity of gray scale ultrasound in detecting urinary tract obstruction. *AJR* 130:731–733, 1978.
15. Griscom NT: The roentgenology of neonatal abdominal masses. *AJR* 93:447–463, 1965.
16. Felson B, Cussen LJ: The hydronephrotic type of unilateral congenital multicystic disease of the kidney. *Semin Roentgenol* 10:113–124, 1975.
17. Babcock JR, Shkolnik A, Cook WA: Ultrasound-guided percutaneous nephrostomy in the pediatric patient. *J Urol* 121:327–329, 1979.
18. Chopra A, Teele RL: Hydronephrosis in children: narrowing the differential diagnosis with ultrasound. *J Clin Ultrasound* 8:473–478, 1980.
19. Kelalis PP: Anterior urethra. In Kelalis PP, King LR, Bellman AB: *Clinical Pediatric Urology.* Philadelphia, WB Saunders, 1976, pp 334–336.
20. Kessler RM, Altman DH: Real-time sonographic detection of vesicoureteral reflux in children. *AJR* 138:1033, 1982.
21. Duckett JW Jr: The prune-belly syndrome. In Kelalis PP, King LR, Bellman AB: *Clinical Pediatric Urology.* Philadelphia, WB Saunders, 1976, pp 615–635.
22. Bearman SB, Hine PL, Sanders RC: Multicystic kidney: a sonographic pattern. *Radiology* 118:685–688, 1976.
23. Sumner TE: Preoperative diagnosis of unilateral multicystic kidney with hydronephrosis. *Urology* 11:519, 1978.
24. Jaffe MH, White SJ, Silver TM, Heidelberger KP: Wilms' tumor: ultrasonic features, pathologic correlation, and diagnostic pitfalls. *Radiology* 140:147–152, 1981.
25. Caffe J: *Pediatric X-ray Diagnosis,* ed 7. Chicago, Year Book Medical Publishers, 1978, p 934.
26. Hartman DS, Lesar MSL, Madewell JE, Lichtenstein JE, Davis CJ Jr: Mesoblastic nephroma: radiologic-pathologic correlation of 20 cases. *AJR* 136:69–74, 1981.
27. Scheible W, Ellenbogen PH, Leopold GR, Siao NT: Lipomatous tumors of the kidney and adrenal: apparent echographic specificity. *Radiology* 129:153–156, 1978.
28. Osathanondh V, Potter EL: Pathogenesis of polycystic kidneys: historical survey. *Arch Pathol* 77:459–512, 1964.
29. Blyth H, Ockenden BG: Polycystic disease of the kidneys and liver presenting in childhood. *J Med Genet* 8:257, 1971.
30. Thomas JS, Sumner TE, Crowe JE: Neonatal detection and evaluation of infantile polycystic disease by gray scale echography. *J Clin Ultrasound* 6:343–344, 1978.
31. Metreweli C, Garel L: The echographic diagnosis of infantile renal polycystic disease. *Ann Radiol* 23:103–107, 1980.
32. Boal DK, Teele RL: The sonography of infantile polycystic kidney disease. *AJR* 135:575, 1980.
33. Wolf B, Rosenfield AT, Taylor KJW, Rosenfield N, Gottlieb S, Hsia YE: Presymptomatic diagnosis of adult onset polycystic kidney disease by ultrasonography. *J Genet* 14:1, 1978.
34. Rosenfield AT, Lipson MH, Wolf B, Taylor KJW, Rosenfield NS, Hendler E: Ultrasonography and nephrotomography in the presymptomatic diagnosis of dominantly inherited (adult-onset) polycystic kidney disease. *Radiology* 135:423–427, 1980.

35. Haller JO, Schneider M: *Pediatric Ultrasound.* Chicago, Year Book Medical Publishers, 1980.
36. Rosenberg ER, Trought WS, Kirks DR, Sumner TE, Grossman H: Ultrasonic diagnosis of renal vein thrombosis in neonates. *AJR* 134:35–38, 1980.
37. Silver TM, Kass EJ, Thornburg JR, Konnak JW, Wolfman MJ: The radiologic spectrum of acute pyelonephritis in adults and adolescents. *Radiology* 118:65, 1976.
38. Rosenfield AT, Glickman MG, Taylor KJW, Crade M, Hatson J: Acute focal bacterial nephritis (acute lobar nephroma). *Radiology* 132:553–561, 1979.
39. Carroll B, Silverman PM, Goodwin DA, McDougal IR: Ultrasonography and indium 111 white blood cell scanning for the detection of intra-abdominal abscesses. *Radiology* 140:155–160, 1981.
40. van Sonnenberg E, Ferrucci JT Jr, Mueller PR, Wittenberg J, Simeone FJ: Percutaneous drainage of abscesses and fluid collections: technique, results, and applications. *Radiology* 142:1–10, 1982.

CHAPTER 15

Ultrasonography of the Renal Transplant

DARYL H. CHINN, M.D.
HEDVIG HRICAK, M.D.

Since 1956 when the first successful human renal transplant was performed, over 50,000 renal transplant operations have been done for the treatment of chronic renal failure (1). Significant improvements in our understanding of transplant immunology have allowed favorable selection of donor-recipient combinations. Additionally, advances in immunosuppressive therapy have permitted increased allograft survival while simultaneously decreasing the occurrence of life-threatening infections secondary to immunosuppression. These improvements have led to prolonged allograft survival (60 to 80% two-year survival for cadavaric grafts depending on tissue matching) (2).

With the significant technological improvements which have occurred in ultrasound over the past decade, the ability of ultrasound to evaluate the transplant allograft has been gradually appreciated. We shall focus on the application of sonography to two commonly encountered clinical problems. These are the problems of acute renal failure in the early post-transplant setting and the problem of peritransplant fluid collections. Prior to the discussion of these pathological states, the techniques of scanning the allograft and the sonographic appearance of the normal transplant allograft will be described.

SCANNING TECHNIQUE

The sonographic imaging of the renal allograft can be performed easily throughout the postoperative course of the renal transplant. Even in the immediate postoperative period, sonography is safe and easily performed. By observing certain precautions, the theoretical risk of a wound infection introduced by the ultrasound transducer can be virtually eliminated.

By scanning alongside the wound and angling the transducer toward the allograft, adequate images of the allograft can often be obtained without necessitating removal of the wound bandages. Furthermore, these images are usually superior to those obtained directly over the wound, since sutures and wound fibrosis, which may degrade the ultrasound image, are avoided.

If scanning over the wound is necessary, sterile coupling gel and a sterile covering of the transducer should be used to limit the theoretical risk of introducing a wound infection.

Both static B-arm and real-time scanners should be employed in the routine evaluation of the renal allograft. Due to wider field of view, static B-scanners offer a superior evaluation of the entire allograft bed. Furthermore, the allograft length and, therefore, renal volume are more accurately evaluated. Rarely can the entire length of the kidney be measured with current linear array transducers. Mechanical sector real-time devices are inaccurate in measuring allograft length.

Optimal scanning of the allograft is along its anatomical coronal plane. This axis permits optimal assessment of renal length, renal parenchyma, corticomedullary junction, renal collecting system, and renal sinus. Even with angling the transducer at the skin and obliquing the patient, this optimal coronal scanning plane is occasionally unobtainable as it may be obscured by the iliac wing.

To obtain the optimal coronal plane with static B-scanners, it is necessary to mark the upper and lower poles of the kidney on the patient's skin. Then longitudinal scans through the upper and lower poles at various degrees of medial angulation should yield the optimal scanning plane. Occasionally a real-time transducer is used to "line up" the coronal section for static B-scanning. A scan plane perpendicular to this coronal plane through the mid-portion of the allograft will be most accurate in defining anterior-posterior dimension and width of the allograft, which are necessary to calculate allograft volume.

Real-time ultrasound is particularly useful in instances of pelvicaliectasis. It can effectively trace the ureters, and in the case of obstruction it can often define the level of obstruction.

The small transducer surface area of current mechanical sector scanners permits greater angulation than with static scanners and is occasionally more useful in allografts of unusual orientation. Finally, the ability of real-time to detect motion is indispensable in identifying bowel peristalsis, arterial pulsation, or ureteral peristalsis.

SONOGRAPHIC APPEARANCE OF THE NORMAL RENAL ALLOGRAFT

The sonographic appearance of the allograft is dependent upon its anatomical relationship in the iliac fossa. Generally, a donor kidney is transplanted into the contralateral iliac fossa of the recipient. Thus, the dorsal aspect of the transplant is oriented to the ventral aspect of the recipient. The renal hilum is medial to the allograft parenchyma. The transplant renal artery is anastomosed end-to-end to the internal iliac artery. The transplant renal vein is anastomosed end-to-side to the external iliac vein. The allograft ureter is anastomosed to the bladder via a ureteroneocystostomy. Therefore, the most anterior structure is the renal pelvis followed by the renal artery and vein. The knowledge of this relationship is mandatory for interventional procedures. This idealized anatomical arrangement may be altered depending on the specific surgical setting.

The allograft is easily scanned sonographically due to its superficial location. The visualization of the allograft is rarely obscured by bowel gas. With ultrasound, the graft is readily demonstrated in the iliac fossa overlying the iliac vessels and psoas muscle. The renal hilum is identified medial to the renal parenchyma. Usually, specific identification of the allograft pelvis and ureter can be made. When pelvicaliectasis is present, intercommunications with the intrarenal collecting system makes the identification of the pelvis and ureter easier. Additionally, the pelvis and ureter can be identified anatomically since they lie anterior to the allograft artery and vein. If pulsations originating

in a vessel are seen, then the artery is clearly identified.

Using current high resolution, focused ultrasound equipment, the internal architecture of the allograft is well displayed. The renal parenchyma can be divided into the poorly echogenic cortex and the triangular hypoechoic centrally located medulla. The corticomedullary junction is distinct. Intense, focal echoes at the corticomedullary junction represent the arcuate vessels. Central to the medulla is the strongly echogenic renal sinus, which is comprised of hilar adipose tissue, blood vessels, and renal collecting system (Fig. 15.1).

When the allograft is carefully scanned, the site and shape of the graft may be assessed. The normal graft is elliptical in shape. Reported ratio of anterior-posterior diameter divided by allograft length is 0.36 to 0.54 (3).

Following transplantation, the allograft, which provided approximately one-half the renal clearance of the donor, must solely provide all the renal clearance function of the recipient. Therefore, compensatory hypertrophy of the allograft occurs. Although quite remarkable degrees of compensatory hypertrophy have been described, the usual degree of hypertrophy is modest. Using the modified formula for the volume of prolate ellipse ($V = L \times W \times AP \times 0.49$), normal allograft hypertrophy compared to a baseline study was approximately 16% (range 7 to 25%) at 2 weeks and approximately 22% (range 14 to 32%) at 3 weeks (4). Despite hypertrophy, the normal elliptical shape of the allograft is preserved (3). In one case a 16-year-old patient received a kidney from a 16-month-old donor; the calculated filtration rate increased six times in 4 weeks, and the allograft length increased from 7 to 11.5 cm in 8 weeks (5).

Mild dilatation of the intrarenal collecting system in the immediate post-transplant period is seen frequently and is considered a normal finding (Figs. 15.1 and 15.5A). The exact etiology of the dilatation is not known with certainty, but transient edema at the site of ureteroneocystostomy leading to temporary partial obstruction of the distal ureter is a likely cause (6). Other proposed etiologies of the "normal" dilatation are prolonged ischemia of the ureter during allograft acquisition and disturbed ureteral innervation (7). Regardless of the cause, temporary mild dilatation of the collecting system normally occurs during the immediate postsurgical period.

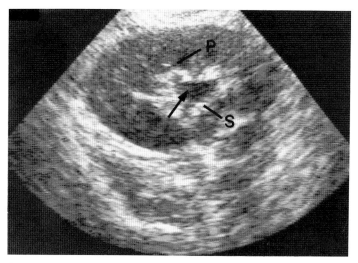

Figure 15.1. Longitudinal scans of a normal allograft. The normal renal sinus (*s*) is very echogenic. Mild dilatation of the intrarenal collecting system (*arrow*) is a normal finding in the immediate postsurgical period. *P*, medullary pyramids.

ACUTE POST-TRANSPLANT RENAL FAILURE

Renal failure in the immediate post-transplant period is an extremely difficult problem faced by the transplant team. The incidence of this problem varies widely depending upon the specifics of the transplant procedure (i.e., living related versus cadavar kidney; modality and duration of allograft preservation; operative technique; immunological compatibility of donor and recipient; type of prophylactic immunosuppression). The differential diagnosis encompasses a wide range of pathophysiological processes including arterial obstruction, arterial stenosis, renal vein thrombosis, pyelonephritis, ureteral obstruction, cytomegalovirus infection, acute rejection, and acute tubular necrosis. Although insufficient data are available to permit generalizations concerning the sonographic appearance of the less common entities, current data strongly suggest that the three most common causes of early allograft failure (acute tubular necrosis, acute rejection, and ureteral obstruction) can be distinguished sonographically.

Acute Rejection

The occurrence of allograft rejection is a theoretical possibility in all renal transplants, except in the rare instance when the donor and recipient are immunologically identical. Not surprisingly, the incidence of rejection episodes is high (up to 93% in cadavar kidneys) (8). To better appreciate the sonographic features of acute rejection, the pathology will be briefly reviewed.

Traditionally, the rejection process has been simplistically categorized into hyperacute, accelerated acute, acute, and chronic. The hyperacute rejection is a separate pathogenetic phenomenon and will not be discussed. The latter three categories are of similar pathogenesis; the distinction between them is vague, and significant overlap in the histological appearance exists. For the purposes of this discussion, the pathological and sonographic appearance of acute and accelerated acute rejection will be considered a distinct entity.

Acute rejection typically occurs during the first weeks following transplantation. However, due to the current routine use of prophylactic immunosuppresion which may delay the rejection process, the exact chronological onset of the process is highly variable (9). Acute rejection has been reported as early as 5 days or as late as 5 years following transplantation (10).

The histological features of acute rejection are very complex. Acute rejection may histologically be described as primarily vascular or cellular (Figs. 15.2 and 15.3). In reality, most cases demonstrate elements of both. In cellular rejection, mononuclear cells and edema infiltrate the renal interstitium. Vascular rejection is manifested by the intimal thickening of arteries and arterioles,

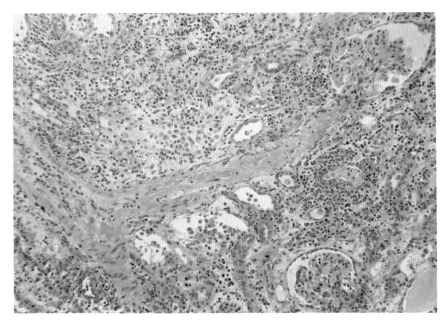

Figure 15.2.   Acute rejection, predominantly vascular type. Photomicrograph shows feature of both vascular and cellular acute rejection. Vascular rejection is predominant, demonstrating prominent intimal proliferation of intermediate-sized arteries. There is thrombosis of an artery as well. Diffuse interstitial mononuclear cell infiltration is present. Figure 15.6 is the ultrasound of this allograft.

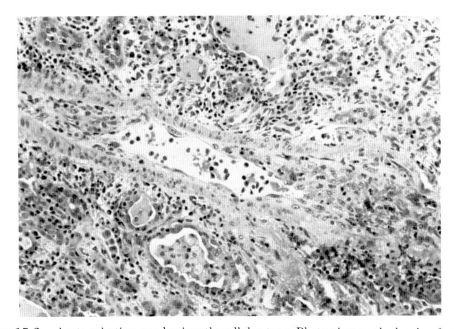

Figure 15.3.   Acute rejection, predominantly cellular type. Photomicrograph showing features predominantly of interstitial acute rejection. There is diffuse interstitial mononuclear cell infiltrate. Vascular changes are less pronounced, showing some intimal proliferation. Figure 15.10 is the ultrasound of this allograft.

with associated thrombosis. These vascular changes lead to infarction and interstitial hemorrhage (9). Histologically, changes of rejection are present in all renal compartments, including the cortex, medullary pyramids, and adipose tissue.

The sonographic features of acute rejection are complex and variable. Following recent technological improvements in ultrasound image quality, numerous studies have described renal parenchymal abnormalities associated with rejection (4, 11–20). The renal allograft becomes greatly enlarged and round in configuration (15, 19). The parenchymal abnormalities associated with acute rejection include hypoechoic enlarged medullary pyramids, indistinct corticomedullary junction, focal parenchymal sonolucent regions, increased cortical echogenicity, decreased cortical echogenicity, and decreased hilar echogenicity. Mild dilatation of the collecting system during acute rejection has been observed as well (21). In the following discussion, the relative merits of these ultrasonographic findings in the diagnosis of allograft rejection will be described.

The acutely rejecting allograft increses in size at a rate greater than that attributable to normal compensatory hypertrophy. Pathologically, the alteration in allograft size and shape is related to the extensive interstitial edema and cellular infiltration occurring during acute rejection. As early as 1970, the sonographic assessment of

allograft size and shape was promoted as a means of detecting allograft rejection (22). Recently, allograft size and shape have been quantified in a number of ways (4, 19). The anteroposterior diameter/longitudinal length ratio (AP/L) has been assessed. The results showed that in acute rejection the allograft assumed a globular shape with AP/L ratio greater than 0.55 (normal 0.36 to 0.54) (19). Also, there was a significant increase in allograft thickness with an anteroposterior diameter being greater than 5.5 cm (19). Allograft volumetric enlargement greater than the normal allowances for compensatory hypertrophy permitted detection of rejection in 84% (16 of 19) (4). Although there are reports suggesting that geometric criteria are insensitive in the detection of acute rejection (13), our enthusiasm for these criteria remains high. However, an isolated finding of increased allograft size is not specific for allograft rejection, since renal vein thrombosis (23), bacterial pyelonephritis, and CMV infection may also cause abnormal graft enlargement.

Many investigators have described swelling and decreased echogenicity of the medullary pyramids as an early sign of acute allograft rejection (4, 11–14, 16–18) (Figs. 15.4 to 15.6). Pathologically, this finding corresponds to the extensive interstitial peritubular edema which involves the medulla in acute rejection (9). Some observers claim that the apparent increase in

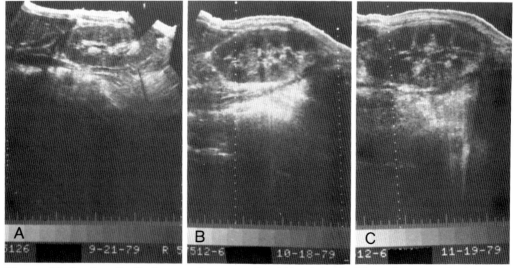

Figure 15.4. Longitudinal scans demonstrating (*A*) minimal, (*B*) moderate, and (*C*) severe acute rejection. Note the progressive globular appearance of the allograft. The medullary pyramids become larger, the corticomedullary junction becomes less distinct, and the renal sinus fat becomes less apparent with increasing severity of acute rejection.

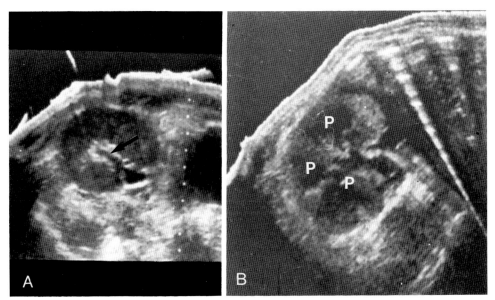

Figure 15.5. Transverse images immediately post-transplantation (*A*) and during acute rejection (*B*). The medullary pyramids (*P*) have increased in size and decreased in echogenicity. The corticomedullary junction has become indistinct. The mild dilatation of the intrarenal collecting system (*arrow*) is normal immediately post-transplantation (*A*).

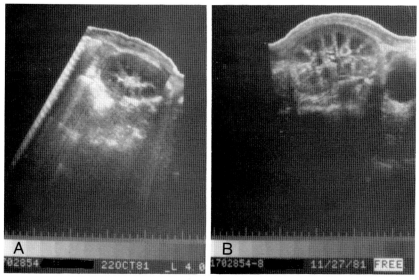

Figure 15.6. Longitudinal scans immediately post-transplantation (*A*) and during acute rejection (*B*). Pyramids have markedly enlarged and become hypoechogenic. Sinus fat has decreased in echogenicity. The entire allograft is globular.

pyramid size on sonography is actually a reflection of parenchymal edema in the adjacent cortex (6, 11), but others maintain that on pathological examination the medullary pyramids actually increase in size due to congestion, edema, and hemorrhage (12). Frick et al. (16) demonstrated increased size and hypoechogenicity of the medullary pyramids in 88% (44 of 50) of patients with acute rejection. Similarly, Hricak et al. (4) noted enlarged pyramids in 79% (15 of

19) of cases, and Heckemann et al. (19) demonstrated this feature in all (11 of 11) cases of acute rejection. Despite this demonstrated high sensitivity, one must be cautious in using this feature alone in diagnosing acute allograft rejection. The finding of enlarged, hypoechogenic medullary pyramids has been noted in normal kidneys (16, 18), especially following diuretic therapy (4), and occasionally in allografts experiencing acute tubular necrosis (16).

A closely related alteration in the appearance of the medullary pyramids in acute rejection is the sonographic indistinctness of the corticomedullary junction (4, 13, 14) (Fig. 15.5). Hricak et al. (4) described this feature in 58% (11 of 19) of patients with acute rejection. Histologically, the corticomedullary junction is one of the earliest sites within the allograft to be affected by edema and mononuclear cellular infiltration (9).

Recently, decreased echogenicity and decreased size of the renal hilum echoes have been correlated with acute rejection (Figs. 15.4 to 15.8). Pathological correlation has shown that during acute rejection, the interlobular and intralobular fibrous septa within the renal hilum enlarge in size due to edema and infiltrating mononuclear cells. Subsequently, the number and size of the hilar fat cells decrease. The observed decreased hilar echogenicity is a reflec-

tion of a decreased quantity of fat combined with a replacement of fat by edematous infiltrated fibrous septa (20) (Fig. 15.9, *A–C*). In two studies, Hricak et al. (4, 20) reported this sonographic finding in 25 of 33 (76%) cases with acute rejection. Heckemann et al. (19) noted this appearance in all (11 of 11) patients with acute rejection, and in no (0 of 21) normal renal transplants. Although this finding may be seen in cases of chronic rejection (12), in the setting of renal failure in the immediate post-transplant period, this appearance of the renal sinus is sensitive and specific in the diagnosis of allograft rejection. We have observed one case of chronic allograft infection demonstrating decreased central sinus echoes in the absence of rejection.

Multiple focal sonolucencies scattered throughout the allograft parenchyma have been described by numerous observers in acute allograft rejection (4, 11, 12, 15, 16). Pathologically, these focal regions of anechogenicity correspond to areas of parenchymal edema, hemorrhage, infarction, and necrosis (11, 12, 15). Singh and Cohen (15) described this feature in 70% (38 of 58) of cases. In a smaller series, focal sonolucencies were present in 36% (18 of 50) and 21% (4 of 19) of patients with acute rejection (4, 16). Multiple focal sonolucencies are fairly specific

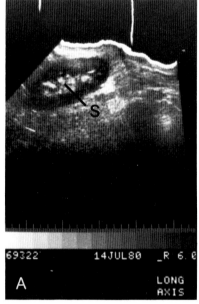
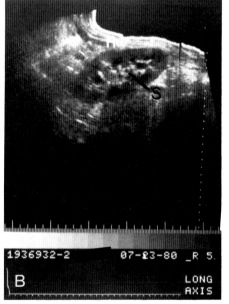

Figure 15.7. Longitudinal scans immediately post-transplantation (*A*) and during acute rejection (*B*) showing the marked interval decrease in the echogenicity of the renal sinus fat (*s*) with acute rejection.

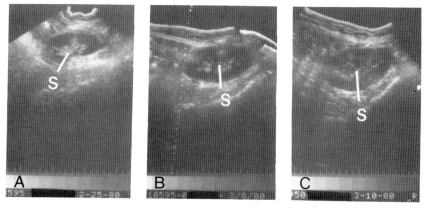

Figure 15.8. Longitudinal series of sonograms showing (*A*) baseline study, (*B*) moderate, and (*C*) severe changes of acute rejection. Note the progressive decrease in intensity of central sinus fat (*S*). The allograft has become globular.

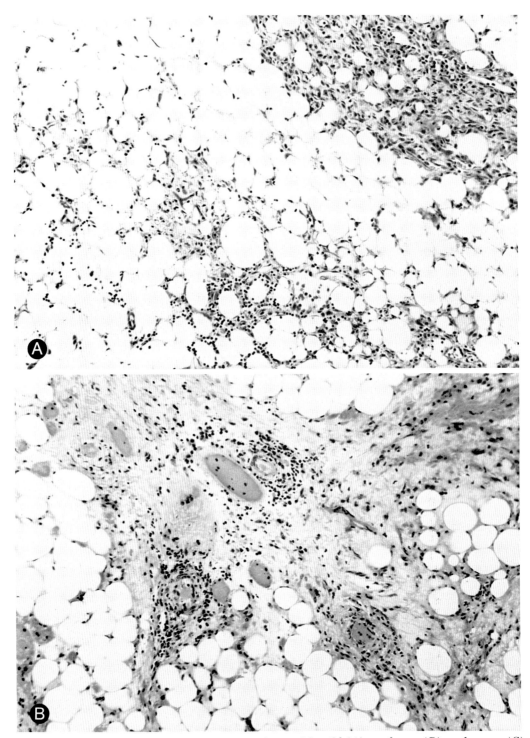

Figure 15.9. Histological specimens from patients with mild (*A*), moderate (*B*), and severe (*C*) acute rejection. The decreasing number of fat cells and the degree of infiltration of fibrous septa with mononuclear cells and collagen correlate with the severity of acute rejection.

for acute rejection. Rarely, multiple allograft abscesses (18) or multiple embolic infarctions might appear similarly.

In acute rejection, the cortical echogenicity has been described as both incresed (4, 12–14, 16, 17) (Fig. 15.10) or decreased (4, 13, 14, 19). These seemingly inconsistent findings undoubtedly both occur. Likely, they relate to the relative amount of interstitial edema versus cellular infiltration which would lead to hypoechogenicity or hyperechogenicity, respectively. How-

ever, the utility of this sign is limited, since the determination of normal cortical echogenicity is extremely difficult in the absence of an adjacent reference organ. Additionally, to suggest acute rejection solely whenever an alteration in cortical echogenicity occurs would likely lead to numerous false positive diagnoses.

In this review, the effectiveness of sonography in detecting acute allograft rejection has been unequivocally demonstrated. Although a small study comparing nuclear medicine with ultra-

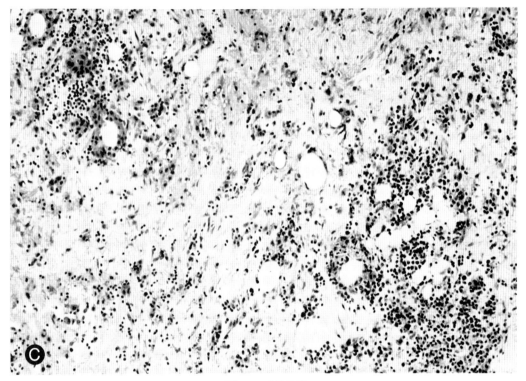

Figure 15.9C.

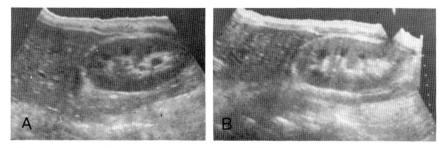

Figure 15.10.   Longitudinal scan; (A) normal and (B) during acute rejection. Note the increased cortical echogenicity as the primary evidence of acute rejection. Renal sinus fat and pyramids are basically unchanged. The histology of this renal biopsy was primarily cellular infiltration of the cortex.

sound has been performed (15), a large prospective study is necessary before the relative merits of each modality are defined.

In summary, acute allograft rejection can be detected sonographically. The signs of acute rejection reflect specific pathological alterations in the rejecting allograft. The major sonographic signs of acute allograft rejection in decreasing order of sensitivity are: an enlarged, globular allograft; swollen, hypoechogenic medullary pyramids; indistinct corticomedullary junction; decreased renal sinus echoes; and multiple focal parenchymal sonolucencies.

Acute Tubular Necrosis

Acute tubular necrosis (ATN) is a significant cause of renal failure in the immediate post-transplant period. (ATN is actually a misnomer for the renal failure resulting from tubular damage without the necessary presence of frank tubular necrosis.) Histological evidence of tubular damage may be identified in all renal allografts, but clinically significant episodes of ATN occur in up to 50% of cadaver renal transplants (24). Due to premortem events in the cadaver donor, such as hypotension, cardiac arrest, and disseminated intravascular coagulation, cadaver kidneys are more likely to suffer ATN than are living related kidneys. Additionally, preservation and storage of cadaver kidneys also increase the likelihood of ATN in cadaver renal allografts (1). Therefore, allograft renal failure immediately following surgery raises the possibility of ATN, especially in the cadaver renal transplant.

In contrast to acute rejection, ATN has a paucity of sonographic findings. Although rare cases of ATN may demonstrate medullary hypoechogenicity (16) and mild swelling, most clinical (4, 12) and experimental (25) series demonstrate that ATN is characterized by a lack of sonographic findings.

Obstructive Uropathy

Allograft urinary obstruction also may lead to allograft failure. Ureteral obstruction requiring repeat surgery occurs in 1 to 10% of renal transplants (26). The causes of obstruction are multiple, including intrinsic blockage (i.e., blood clots, calculi, tumors), ureteropelvic, ureteric, or ureterovesical stricture, and extrinsic compression (i.e., hematoma, lymphocele, or any pelvic mass) (Fig. 15.11).

Sonography easily detects dilatation of the renal pelvis and intrarenal collecting system. However, evaluation of the entire ureter is often difficult due to absence of an adequate acoustic window (Fig. 15.12). When the entire ureter is dilated, often its proximal and distal aspect can be identified if the allograft and bladder are used as acoustic windows. The mid-portion of the ureter often remains obscured.

Ultrasound accurately assesses the dilatation of the intra- and extrarenal collecting system, but the degree of dilatation does not reflect the presence or the severity of ureteral obstruction. The dilatation of the collecting system is a complex product of the amount of urine produced, compliance of the collecting system, and degree of ureteral outflow obstruction. In the renal allograft, urine production may be reduced by renal failure, and ureteral compliance may be decreased by cellular infiltration and edema which accompanies acute rejection (6, 21). Therefore, when urinary obstruction is clinically suspected, even a minimal dilatation of the pelvicalyceal system should not disuade one from performing additional diagnostic procedures, such as antegrade or retrograde pyelogram.

Similarly, one cannot presume that mild degrees of pelvicalyceal dilatation in the renal allograft represent obstruction. As noted previously, in the immediate post-transplant period transient edema at the ureteroneocystostomy may cause mild dilatation (6). A distended urinary bladder may cause dilatation of the ureter and intrarenal collecting system (27). The ureter may also be dilated during acute (6, 24) and chronic (6, 21) allograft rejection, in the absence of frank anatomical obstruction. Like the allograft parenchyma, the musculature of the ureter is infiltrated by edema and mononuclear cells during acute rejection (13). This leads to decreased ureteral peristalsis and subsequent ureteral dilatation, both of which may be detected sonographically (21) (Fig. 15.13). If unresponsive to therapy or inadequately treated, ureteral rejection may lead to ureteral fibrosis and ultimately frank obstruction requiring corrective surgery (28).

When dilatation of the collecting system is associated with an extrinsic mass, such as a lymphocele (Fig. 15.14), then one may be more certain that the dilatation is secondary to mechanical obstruction. Usually, however, the diagnosis of urinary tract obstruction and determination of the site of obstruction may only be

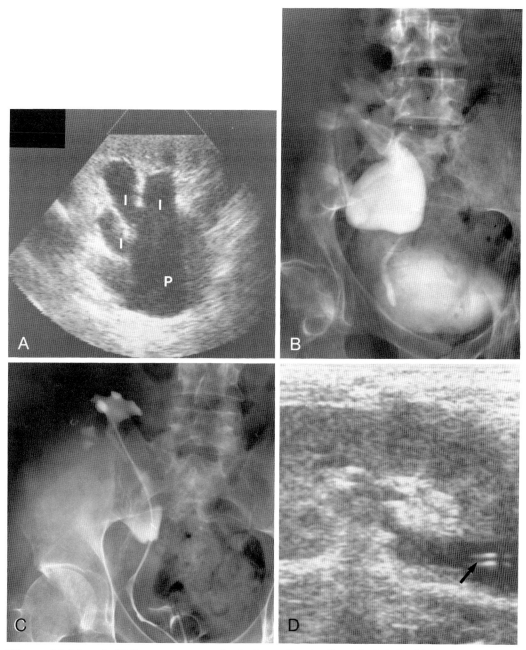

Figure 15.11.   *A*, Oblique sonogram of a hydronephrotic allograft. *I*, infundibular; *P*, pelvis. *B*, Delayed excretory urogram demonstrates high grade ureteropelvic junction obstruction. *C*, Retrograde decompression was performed. *D*, Longitudinal ultrasonogram shows interval resolution of hydronephrosis. *Arrow*, Stent.

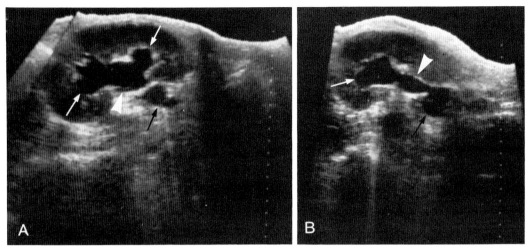

Figure 15.12. Longitudinal (*A*) nd oblique (*B*) images of a hydronephrotic allograft. Dilatation of the intrarenal collecting system and proximal ureter is present. The exact site of ureteral obstruction is obscured by overlying bowel gas. *Black arrow*, proximal ureter; *white arrow*, intrarenal collecting system; *white arrowhead*, pelvis.

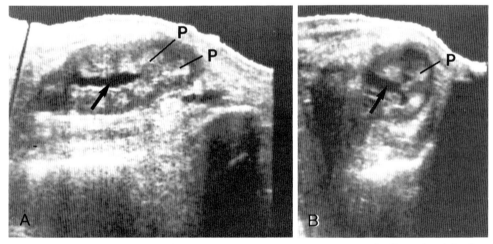

Figure 15.13. Longitudinal (*A*) and transverse (*B*) images of renal allograft with chronic rejection. The dilated intrarenal collecting system (*arrow*) was a result of multiple previous episodes of acute rejection. The echogenic medullary pyramids (*P*) represent nephrocalcinosis.

suggested by ultrasound, and requires confirmation with excretory urography, antegrade or retrograde pyelography, or nuclear scintigraphy.

PERITRANSPLANT FLUID COLLECTIONS

Another major application of ultrasound is the evaluation of peritransplant fluid collections. Lymphoceles, urinomas, hematomas, abscesses, and seromas may involve the transplant bed. The sonographic appearances of each are largely nonspecific, and ultimate diagnosis requires clinical correlation, needle aspiration, or surgical exploration. Lymphoceles, urinomas, and hematomas will briefly be discussed in order to describe their sonographic features which are unique to renal transplantation. The sonographic appearance of seromas and abscesses associated with renal transplantation is essentially the same as their appearance associated with other intra-abdominal surgical procedures. These two entities will not be discussed.

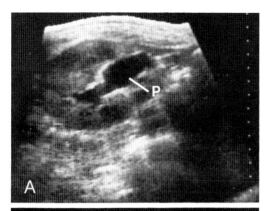

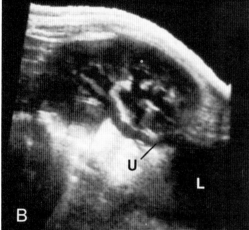

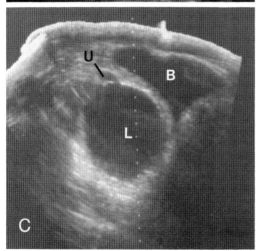

Figure 15.14. Transverse (*A*) and longitudinal (*B* and *C*) images of a hydronephrotic allograft. A lymphocele (*L*) is responsible for the ureteral obstruction. *B*, bladder; *P*, dilated pelvis; *U*, dilated ureter.

Lymphoceles

Lymphoceles develop in approximately 10–20% of transplant recipients (29–31). During routine acquisition of the allograft and during preparation of the recipient's transplant bed, lymphatic vessels are invariably severed around the allograft and within the iliac fossa. If the severed lymphatic vessels are not ligated, or if they fail to reanastomose spontaneously, then lymph may accumulate around the graft. Under these circumstances, a lymphocele may develop, usually 2 to 6 weeks following surgery. The accumulation of lymph in a lymphocele may be exacerbated during a rejection episode, since the engorgement of the graft by edema leads to accentuated transudation of lymph into the transplant bed (29, 31).

Lymphoceles may become larger than the other perinephric fluid collections. Lymphoceles are often lobular in shape (29). Fine stranding may be seen within lymphoceles after 5 days (6). In older lymphoceles, these strands are commonly seen (up to 80% of cases) (29). Lymphoceles may occur anywhere in the extraperitoneal transplant bed (Figs. 15.15 and 15.16). However, they are frequently seen along the inferior margin of the allograft. In this position they may exert a significant mass effect on the iliac vein, ureter, or bladder, leading to leg edema, hydronephrosis, or impaired ability to micturate (30).

Urinoma

Urinoma may occur in the early or late post-transplant period. Reported incidence of urinoma is 3 to 10% (24, 31). Urinoma is a significant complication, since it may lead to wound sepsis, loss of the allograft, and generalized sepsis (32). Early diagnosis is essential.

In the early post-transplant period (during the first postoperative week) the urinoma represents a postsurgical complication with the site of extravasation being most often at the site of the ureteral anastomosis (ureterovesicle, ureteroureteric, ureteropelvic). Later development of urinoma is secondary to either renal biopsy, closed renal injury (incidence 50%), or obstruction, or urinary fistula (incidence 3.1%). Urinary fistula may be caused by either infection or ischemic necrosis (33%). Sonographically, urinomas have a variable shape and are usually seen at the lower pole of the allograft (29) or in the space of Retzius. They seldom demonstrate septations (29). Unlike other perirenal fluid col-

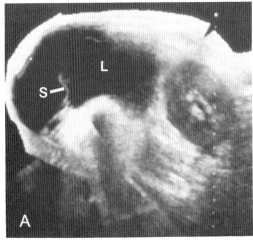

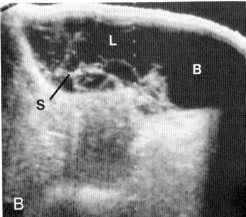

Figure 15.15. Transverse (A) and longitudinal (B) scans of a large lymphocele. The septa (S) are characteristic of a subacute lymphocele (L). B, bladder.

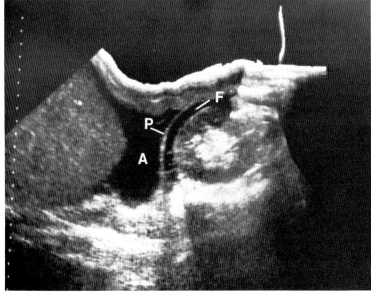

Figure 15.16. Longitudinal supine image. The peritoneum (P) is well seen due to the simultaneous presence of intra- (A) and retroperitoneal fluid (F).

lections, urinomas have a tendency to dissect along tissue planes (Figs. 15.17 and 15.18). Therefore, it is of extreme importance, if a urinoma is suspected, to scan along the flank side as well as scanning the scrotum or labia. In our experience, urine dissection along tissue planes is a characteristic and specific finding for urinoma in a transplant patient. Diagnosis often requires demonstration of urine extravasation by nuclear scintigraphy, excretory urography, or computed tomography. Sometimes a direct aspiration may be necessary (32).

Hematoma

In the immediate post-transplant period hematomas are usually related to technical aspects of the surgical procedure, such as a vascular anastomotic leak. Delayed hematomas are usually related to allograft rupture. While the allograft rupture may be seen during hypertensive episodes, following allograft ischemia, or following renal biopsy (33) or infection, in our experience rupture is most often associated with severe acute allograft rejection. Allograft rupture associated with acute rejection is a life-threatening condition with a high incidence of mortality. In acute rejection, allograft rupture results from the severe, sudden increase in allograft size due to extensive interstitial edema. The site of rupture is often along the superior-lateral margin of the allograft, so called Brodel's line (4). Rupture in this location results in a superiorly placed hematoma.

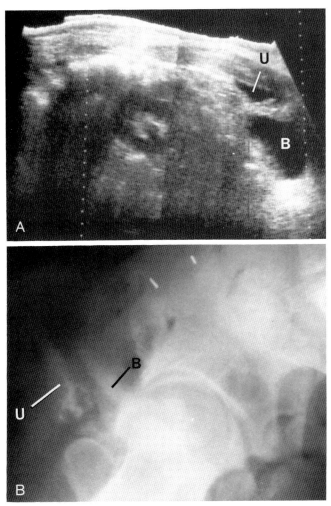

Figure 15.17. *A*, Longitudinal scan demonstrates a urinoma (*U*) anterior to the urinary bladder (*B*). *B*, Lateral projection of delayed excretory urogram demonstrating extravasation of contrast into urinoma anterior to bladder.

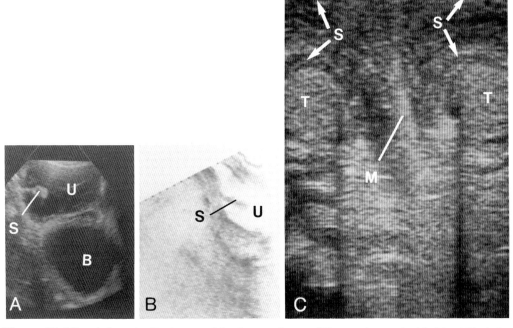

Figure 15.18. *A*, Longitudinal scan with a large urinoma (*U*) anterior to the bladder (*B*). A few septations (*S*) are present. *B*, Longitudinal scan following urine voiding. Urinoma (*U*) has dissected into the space of Retzius. *S*, septations. *C*, Transverse ultrasonogram of patient's scrotum demonstrates marked scrotal wall (*S*) thickening due to dissection of urinoma into the superficial fascia. No hydrocele was present. *T*, testicle; *M*, median raphe.

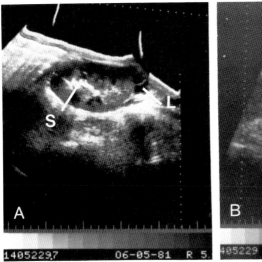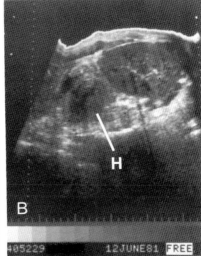

Figure 15.19. Longitudinal scans of allograft showing mild (*A*) and severe (*B*) rejection. Note the sparseness of renal sinus (*S*) fat and the hypoechogenicity of medullary pyramids in mild rejection (*A*). With severe rejection interval decrease in central sinus fat and marked increase in allograft size have occurred. The echogenic mass superior to the allograft is a hematoma (*H*) which resulted from transplant rupture during severe rejection. *L*, lymphocele.

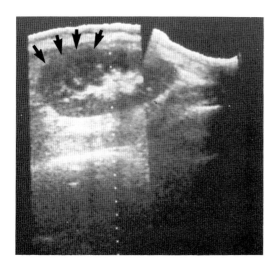

Figure 15.20. Longitudinal scan demonstrates indistinctness of the ventral, superior allograft margin with mild mass effect (*arrows*). This represented an acute intrarenal hematoma following a renal biopsy. Note the similarity of the hematoma and renal cortex in echogenicity.

Sonographically, an acute hematoma may be quite echogenic and may display an echogenicity similar to the surrounding soft tissue. Therefore, fresh hematoma may be difficult to detect sonographically. In this setting only detection of a mass effect allows one to diagnose a peritransplant hematoma (Figs. 15.19 and 15.20). For this reason, static scanning with an articulated arm "B"-scanner is more useful than real-time, since the static scanner can demonstrate a wider field of view and, therefore, is more sensitive in the detection of a peritransplant mass effect. If an acute hematoma is clinically strongly suspected and the ultrasound is unremarkable, then computed tomography is indicated. A hematoma greater than 5 days old undergoes liquification and may develop thick septations. These subacute hematomas are easily detected with ultrasound.

SONOGRAPHIC APPEARANCE OF THE LONG TERM ALLOGRAFT

The ultrasound appearance of the long term renal transplant is largely unknown. Various reports suggest that in chronic rejection the allograft is of normal size and displays increased cortical echogenicity (12–14). Pathological observations seem to support these reports since chronic rejection is characterized by periglomerular cellular infiltration, cortical fibrosis, and a paucity of interstitial edema (34). Confirmation of these sonographic features of chronic rejection awaits further study.

SUMMARY

With recent advances in ultrasound technology, ultrasound can play a major diagnostic role in the evaluation of patients with acute post-transplant renal failure and in patients with perinephric fluid collections. The most significant recent developments have been in the elucidation of the sonographic features of acute allograft rejection.

References

1. Hamburger J, Crosnier J, Bach J, Kreis H: *Renal Transplantation: Therapy and Practice.* Baltimore, Williams & Wilkins, 1981, preface v–x, 187.
2. Morris PJ: Kidney transplantation. *Transplant Proc.* 18:26–32, 1981.
3. Heckemann R, Rehwald U, Jakubowski HD, Donhuijsen K: Sonographic criteria for renal allograft rejection. *Urol Radiol* 4:15–18, 1982.
4. Hricak H, Cruz C, Eyler WR, Madrazo BL, Romanski R, Sandler MA: Acute post-transplantation renal failure: differential diagnosis by ultrasound. *Radiology* 139:441–449, 1981.
5. Ingelfinger JR, Teele R, Levely RH: Renal growth after transplantation: infant kidney received by adolescent. *Clin Nephrol* 156:28–32, 1981.
6. Hricak H, Cruz C, Sandler M, Romanski R, Madrazo B, Levin N, Eyler WR: Sonographic evaluation of the transplanted: a prospective study (abstr). Presented at Radiological Society of North America, 61st Scientific Assembly and Annual Meeting, Chicago, Ill., 1981.
7. Schiff M: Ureter in renal transplantation. *Urology* 12:256–260, 1978.
8. Becker JA, Kutcher R: The renal transplant: rejection and acute tubular necrosis. *Semin Roentgenol* 13:352–362, 1978.
9. Olsen S: Pathology of the renal allograft rejection. In Chung J, Spango BH, Mostafi KF: *Kidney Disease—Present Status.* Baltimore, Williams & Wilkins, 1979, pp 327–355.
10. Brown E, Siegel N, Finkelstein FO: Symptomless acute renal transplant rejection. *JAMA* 239:2256–2258, 1978.
11. Conrad MR, Dickerman R, Love IL, Curry T, Peters P, Hall H, Lerman M, Helderman H: New observation in renal transplants using ultrasound. *AJR* 131:851–855, 1978.
12. Maklad NF, Wright CH, Rosenthal SJ: Gray scale ultrasononic appearances of renal transplant rejection. *Radiology* 131:711–717, 1979.
13. Hillman RJ, Birnholz JC, Busch GJ: Correlation of echographic and histologic findings in suspected renal allograft rejection. *Radiology* 132:673–676, 1979.
14. Hricak H, Toledo-Pereyra LH, Eyler WR, Madrazo BL, Zammit M: The role of ultrasound in the diagnosis of kidney allograft rejection. *Radiology* 132:667–672, 1979.
15. Singh A, Cohen WN: Renal allograft rejection: sonography and scintigraphy. *AJR* 135:73–77, 1980.
16. Frick MP, Feinberg SB, Sibley R, Idstrom ME: Ultrasound in acute renal transplant rejection. *Radiology* 138:657–660, 1981.
17. Harkanyi Z, Jaray J, Alfoldy F, Perner F, Torok I: Echography of renal transplant patients. *Radiology* 21:485–487, 1981.
18. Jafri SZ, Kaude JV, Wright PG: Ultrasound findings in renal transplant rejection. *Acta Radiol (Diag) Stockholm* 22:245–253, 1981.
19. Heckemann R, Rehwald U, Jakubowski HD, Donhuijsen K: Sonographic criteria for renal allograft rejection. *Urol Radiol* 4:15–18, 1982.
20. Hricak H, Romanski RN, Eyler WR: The renal sinus during allograft rejection. Sonographic and histopathologic findings. *Radiology* 142:693–699, 1982.
21. Hricak H, Zammit M, Eyler WR, Farah R: Ureteral peristalsis in the rejecting allograft. Presented at Association of University Radiologists, 28th Annual Meeting, 1980.
22. Leopold G: Renal transplant size measured by reflected ultrasound. *Radiology* 95:687–689, 1970.
23. Hricak H, Cruz C, Eyler WR, Madrazo BL, Sandler MA: Post-transplant renal failure: differential diagnosis by ultrasound—experimental and clinical observations. *Med Ultrasound* 6:1–10, 1982.
24. Delmonico FL, McKusich KA, Cosini AB, Russell PS: Differentiation between renal allograft rejection and acute tubular necrosis by renal scan. *AJR* 128:625–628, 1977.
25. Hricak H, Toledo-Pereyra LH, Eyler WR, Madrazo BL, Sy GS: Evaluation of acute prost-transplant renal failure by ultrasound. *Radiology* 133:443–447, 1979.
26. Palestract AM, DeWolff WC: The pseudostricture of transplant ureteral torsion. *Radiology* 145:49–50, 1982.
27. Balchunes WR, Hill MC, Isikoff MB, Morillo G: The clinical significance of dilatation of the collecting system in the transplanted kidney. *J Clin Ultrasound* 10:221–225, 1982.
28. Schweizer RT, Bartus SA, Kalur CS: Fibrosis of a renal transplant ureter. *J Urol* 117:125–126, 1977.
29. Silver TM, Campbell D, Wicks JD, Lorber MI, Surace P, Turlott J: Peritransplant fluid collection. *Radiology* 138:145–151, 1981.
30. Brockis JG, Hulbert JC, Patel AS, Golinger D, Hurst P, Saker B, Haywood EF, House AK, Van Merwyk A: The diagnosis and treatment of lymphoceles associated with renal transplantation. *Br J Urol* 50:307–312, 1978.
31. Yap R, Mmadrazo B, Oh HK, Dienst SG: Perirenal fluid collection after renal transplantation. *Am Surg* 47:287–290, 1981.
32. Spigos DG, Tan W, Pavel DG, Mozes M, Jonasson O, Capek V: Diagnosis of urine extravasation after renal transplantation. *AJR* 129:409–413, 1977.
33. Rahatzad M, Henderson SL, Boren GS: Ultrasound appearance of spontaneous rupture of renal transplant. *J Urol* 126:535–536, 1981.
34. Hamburger J, Crosnier J, Laure-Helene N: Recurrent glomerulonephritis after renal transplantation. *Ann Ren Med* 29:67–72, 1978.

CHAPTER 16

Renal Puncture Techniques

ROGER C. SANDERS, M.D.

In most of the diseases that the sonographer encounters, a definitive diagnosis is only achieved when tissue is examined by the pathologist. On many occasions the questions the sonographer answers are stages along the path to a definitive answer—Is there really a mass present? Do we have any clues to its pathological nature?—i.e., is it a cyst or a solid lesion? From what primary organ does the mass arise? In many instances a short cut to the diagnosis is possible using puncture techniques. Percutaneous aspiration biopsy and collection drainage techniques using ultrasound guidance have greatly changed the diagnosis and management of fluid and mass lesions in the kidney and prostate.

INDICATIONS FOR PUNCTURE OF THE GENITOURINARY SYSTEM

Renal Cyst

At least 50% of the population over 50 years of age have incidentally found renal cysts at autopsy (1). Therefore, it is not surprising that cysts are common on computed tomography (CT) or ultrasound, and, provided these cysts meet the classical criteria for a cyst by sonography (see Chapter 5), no further diagnostic maneuvers are usually performed at our institution.

Although the sonographic detection of a cyst is usually now considered to be a diagnostic end point since most cysts are benign, we recognize that a small but significant minority of cystic lesions in the kidney represent primary or, much less commonly, secondary neoplasms. Angiography has been shown to be unreliable in the differentiation of benign and malignant cysts (2). CT scanning may be confusing if the cyst is small and a partial volume effect is present. To confirm that a questionable cyst is benign, it is accepted that such a lesion be aspirated percutaneously. Puncture of fluid-filled lesions in the

kidney is reserved for a few unusual situations.

1. A cyst which shows internal echoes along its border or within its lumen should be viewed with suspicion. On some occasions, a subsequent CT scan will show that the cyst is less bothersome than it first appeared by sonography. Of the eight cysts that contained neoplasms that we have seen, all in which a satisfactory sonogram was performed had an irregular wall and internal echoes. On the other hand, a number of cysts which were subsequently shown to be benign had a similar sonographic appearance, in part due to the presence of lobulation and in part due to septa that were incompletely seen.

2. A strong indication for cyst puncture is a CT scan showing a cyst with a density number not that of serous fluid (when a partial volume effect is not confusing the issue). Such cysts should be viewed with suspicion even when the sonogram is reassuring.

3. Certain urological symptoms are of great worry, such as hematuria. In these patients, the finding of a cyst may be an indication for cyst puncture because occasional cysts cause hematuria and a neoplasm has to be excluded.

4. On rare occasions, cysts cause secondary obstruction of neighboring calyces; these cysts should be punctured and ablated so that permanent renal damage does not occur. Certain cysts become so large that they cause local pain. Therapeutic drainage of such a cyst may relieve the patient's symptoms, although generally the pain turns out to be due to a lesion other than a cyst.

5. Whether young patients should undergo a cyst puncture is now debatable since it does not seem as if the incidence of a cyst with neoplasm is any greater in young people than in the elderly. On the other hand, cysts are rare in this age group, and the procedure is benign.

Renal Mass Biopsy

The possibility that a solid mass in the kidney is benign or treatable by medical means exists, although the chances are not high. In some countries, notably Sweden, large series of such masses have been biopsied percutaneously with few or no side effects (3, 4) and with the discovery of an occasional angiomyolipoma or lymphoma. Angiomyolipoma may be diagnosed by seeing a different fat content within a mass on CT; therefore, mass biopsy for possible angiomyolipoma is now less frequently performed, although an angiomyolipoma with a low fat content may be missed. We confine renal mass biopsy to (a) situations in which it is uncertain whether a mass is cystic or solid, (b) where a patient has had a previous neoplasm and now presents with a lesion in the kidney that could be metastatic or could represent a second primary (the treatment of lymphoma, for example, differs markedly from the treatment of hypernephroma), and (c) when the lesion, if malignant, is inoperable (5).

Adrenal Mass Biopsy

Biopsy of lesions in the adrenal gland is no more difficult than biopsy of renal lesions using ultrasound (6) except that the lesion is closer to the diaphragm and, therefore, access may be a little more tricky. A number of incidental adrenal masses have been found on CT examination (7). As a rule these are treated conservatively with relatively frequent follow-up; should there be a worrisome increase in size, a mass biopsy is a simple procedure.

Renal Biopsy

Ultrasound has been shown to be the best method of localizing the kidney for renal biopsy (8). In one trial, biopsies of the kidney were made in 48 patients using fluoroscopy, ultrasound, nuclear medicine, and intravenous pyelography (IVP) as the means of guidance (9). Only ultrasound gave a 100% yield of renal tissue. An identical approach can be used in children (10). Although the technique is essentially the same as that used for an aspiration biopsy of a renal mass, the biopsy needle is so large (14 gauge) it will not pass through some older aspiration transducers. If a modern real-time ultrasound transducer with a lumen large enough to accept the average renal biopsy needle is not available, ultrasound can be used to indicate direction and depth (11–13) but not to follow the needle into the tissues under real-time.

Perinephric Fluid Collection Aspiration

When a fluid collection surrounding the kidney is seen sonographically, it is usually unclear whether it represents an abscess or a hematoma. Therapy varies depending on the nature of the fluid. The simplest method of ascertaining the type of fluid present is to insert a small needle into the collection and withdraw some fluid. This procedure has been found to be essentially without side effects.

Renal Abscesses

If diagnostic puncture of a collection shows that a lesion is an abscess, therapeutic drainage and instillation of antibiotics are now widely performed (14, 15). This technique is effective and usually without side effects. It can be used at the bedside (16), although a large bore catheter and some relatively complex catheter insertion manipulations are required.

Antegrade Pyelography

If a kidney is hydronephrotic and the cause of the hydronephrosis is not apparent on the intravenous pyelogram, there are two possible ways of radiologically displaying the nature of the obstructing lesion. The most commonly used method is a retrograde pyelogram. This procedure is not without hazard and requires considerable technical skill (17). A trend is developing toward the performance of the simpler technique of antegrade pyelography under ultrasonic control (18). In this technique, a needle or catheter is inserted into a dilated renal pelvis and contrast medium shows the upper part of the obstructed system above the stricture (19). A less common indication for antegrade pyelography is the obtainment of fluid from a hydronephrotic pelvis either for culture or cytopathology when it is uncertain whether a mass adjacent to the pelvis is a neoplasm or a benign lesion.

The hazards of antegrade pyelography appear to be fewer than those of retrograde pyelography; normally the procedure is well tolerated by the patient, and unsatisfactory studies are rare.

Percutaneous Nephrostomy

If an antegrade pyelogram shows obstruction of a ureter, a catheter should be left in place because infection is otherwise likely to ensue (19). Additional indications for percutaneous nephrostomy using ultrasound include attempts to dissolve stones by medical means, stone-removing techniques, and stricture dilatation. Although ultrasound is used to aid in the insertion of catheters, the major portion of the procedure is performed under x-ray so that guide wire insertion can be followed fluoroscopically and ideal catheter placement can be obtained.

Renal Transplant

Renal transplants are eminently accessible to renal biopsy (20), antegrade pyelography (21, 22), and percutaneous nephrostomy for the same indications that have been mentioned in regard to the normal kidney. Aspiration of perinephric collections is a particularly common problem in renal transplant patients.

Prostate Biopsy

Ultrasound significantly increases the yield from prostate biopsy if a real-time linear array rectal transducer is used (23, 24). Biopsy can be directed to the area of suspicion rather than on a "blind basis" as is currently the usual practice.

CHOICE OF ASPIRATION TRANSDUCER

Sonography can aid in the performance of percutaneous puncture of a mass or collection in five ways. Should the lesion be relatively superficial, large, and yet not palpable or visible, sonography can be used to define the surface markings and to show the depth to which the needle should be inserted. It is usually then possible to perform the puncture without the aid of an aspiration transducer. If the mass is over 4 cm wide and within 3 or 4 cm of the skin surface, the use of an aspiration transducer is an encumbrance rather than an asset; the procedure is more tedious, a longer needle has to be used, and the transducer has to be resterilized. Such lesions are not uncommon in the kidney because this organ often lies at a superficial level. In most individuals, its posterior margin is between 3 and 5 cm beneath the skin. In muscular or obese individuals, it can be as deep as 8 or 9 cm beneath the skin.

If the mass is moderately large and located relatively close to the skin surface, but one is not absolutely confident that one will be able to hit it percutaneously without guidance (Fig. 16.1), it is useful to have a B-scan transducer available to check the depth and direction once the skin has been cleansed (Fig. 16.2). When the

skin is marked and one has memorized the appropriate direction, the mass is punctured with a needle but without the aid of a transducer. Since the transducer increases the complexity of the procedure, it is only used if fluid or pathological tissue is not obtained on the initial pass. It is no longer necessary to sterilize transducers for this approach since the use of a sterile plastic bag placed around the transducer is equally effective. The sterile bag has gel placed within so good contact is maintained between the transducer and the bag; more gel is placed on the skin between the plastic bag and the patient. In this way a standard B-scan arm or real-time transducer can be used as a guidance system. The B-scan arm is valuable if it is placed so that B-scan dot markers are shown on the screen at the same time as the needle is within the tissue (Fig. 16.1). One then aligns the needle parallel to the B-scan transducer arm axis.

A third technique involves the use of the A-mode aspiration transducer (Fig. 16.3). The puncture of renal lesions is complicated by the considerable respiratory movement that occurs in the kidney. Since the A-mode aspiration transducer is connected to the ultrasound instrument solely by a cable, movement can occur without laceration of the renal tissue once the needle is in place even if the needle has been placed through the aspiration transducer. An A-mode transducer is, therefore, particularly valuable in the kidney when the needle may have to be left in place for some time while fluid is aspirated. A further advantage of the A-mode transducer is that it can be angled small amounts in any direction when the needle is approximately 2 cm into the patient's skin, thus allowing correction of needle placement errors without repuncturing the skin. A B-scan aspiration transducer, when used in contact with the transducer arm, can only be obliqued in the direction that the arm bends. Yet another advantage to the use of an A-mode aspiration transducer during the course of a renal cyst puncture is that one may monitor the size of the cyst as it is aspirated and see how much fluid remains in the cyst and where the needle tip lies in relation to the cyst wall. Following the size of the cyst visually as it deflates is particularly important if one intends to place a sclerosing agent in the cyst; total cyst aspiration is likely to cause the sclerosing agent to extravasate when it is injected, but the less fluid remaining the more likely it is that the cyst will not recur.

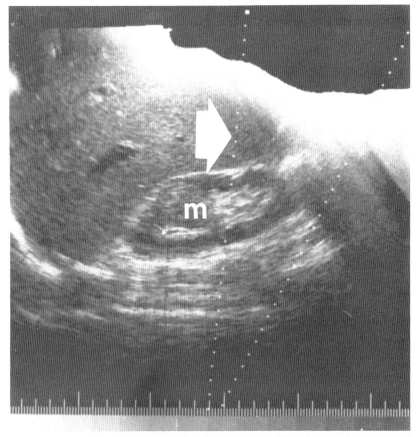

Figure 16.1. Mass (*m*) in the upper pole of the kidney. The dot markers (*arrow*) indicate a potential erroneous needle insertion site.

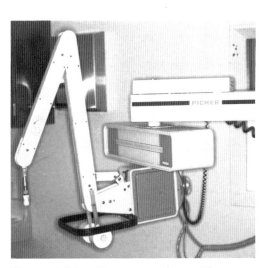

Figure 16.2. B-scan transducer. The transducer is placed above the needle as it is inserted, and the dot marker indicates the correct axis.

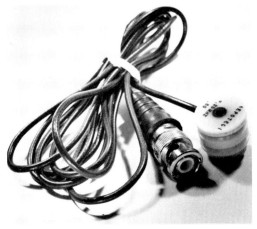

Figure 16.3. A-mode 2.25-MHz transducer with cable. The cable allows the needle to move with respiration.

Provided one is using a transducer of sufficiently high frequency (e.g., 20-gauge with 3.5-MHz transducer), the needle tip can be observed as it relates to the wall of the cyst when fluid is removed from the cyst.

A fourth technique involves the use of a B-scan transducer. These transducers come in two designs. One such transducer has a central hole through it (Fig. 16.4). The advantage of this transducer is that it provides a relatively snug fit for a needle so that, once the needle is placed in the center of the transducer and the mass is located, it is hard for the needle to wander in an oblique direction away from the plotted sonographic course. However, once the needle is in the mass, a rigid set-up is created. The needle, the transducer, and the transducer arm form a single entity, and any renal movement is bound to cause some laceration of the renal parenchyma. The use of this transducer in the kidney for aspiration when fixed to the transducer arm should be considered obsolete.

A second type of B-scan aspiration transducer, known as the "keyhole" transducer, is preferable for the aspiration of small renal lesions if a B-scan technique is to be used (Fig. 16.5). This transducer has a notch throughout its length. Once the needle is in place with its tip in the mass, the needle can be slid sideways away from the transducer and the kidney is then able to move freely. These transducers are ex-

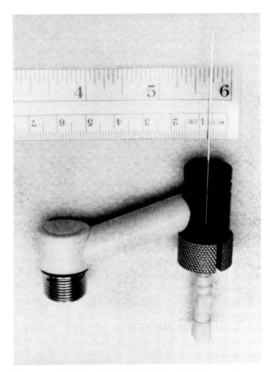

Figure 16.5. A 3.5-MHz keyhole transducer with needle through the keyhole. The cap preventing the needle from moving into the keyhole is rotated slightly to the right.

pensive because it is difficult to make them electrically safe. A disadvantage of this type of transducer is the relative freedom that the needle has to move in an off-axis oblique direction along the line of the keyhole. This defect has been partially corrected in recent keyhole aspiration transducers by the placement of a metal cap on the top of the transducer which rotates so that the keyhole becomes obliterated at least at the most superior aspect of the hole. This cap can be rotated free when the needle is in place so the keyhole becomes patent once more and the needle can be removed. The presence of the keyhole within the aspiration transducer reduces the sensitivity of the transducer so the needle tip is more difficult to see. The 3.5-MHz B-scan aspiration transducer without a keyhole is more sensitive—with this transducer a 20-gauge needle tip can consistently be seen in echo-free fluid.

A cable is available which can be attached to the aspiration transducer enabling one to use the B-scan aspiration transducer in the same way as an A-mode transducer (Fig. 16.6). The

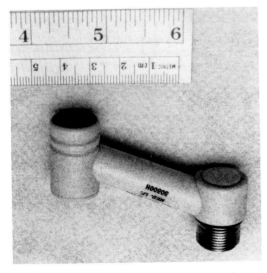

Figure 16.4. A 3.5-MHz B-scan transducer. The hole in the main portion of the transducer is large enough to fit an 18-gauge needle.

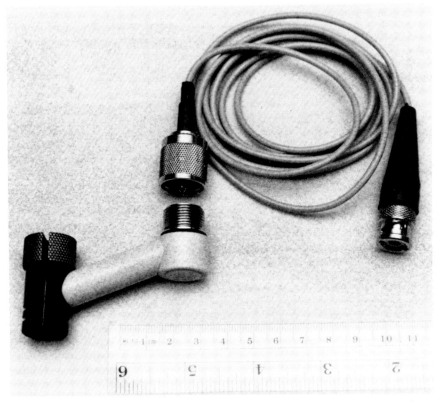

Figure 16.6. Cable adaptor which can convert a B-scan transducer into an A-mode transducer shown with a keyhole transducer.

specific advantage of the B-scan transducer is that, even though one is working in a sterile field, one can perform a repeat B-scan to confirm the localization of the mass without contaminating the puncture site. One can then leave an image on a storage oscilloscope and use B-scan markers to confirm that one is placing the needle in the correct direction (Fig. 16.7). Some air can be injected into tissues as a marker of the site where the biopsy was performed (25). Both the B-scan and A-scan aspiration transducers have to be sterilized between uses; gas sterilization is recommended, but if the transducer is needed urgently, immersion in an antiseptic is possible.

The last technique, now becoming the most common, involves the use of real-time aspiration transducers. Very significant improvements in puncture technique and in needle visualization have occurred since the introduction of real-time aspiration transducers. Constant equipment upgrades have led to even better images. Real-time can be used in several ways.

1. Use of a real-time transducer at right angles to the lesion. This technique can be used if the renal problem is located in a position where one can use the liver or spleen as an acoustic window to view the kidney from an axis at right angles to the needle insertion angle (Fig. 16.8). Such a technique is slightly easier with a linear array real-time system than with a sector scanner because it is easier to orientate oneself to the direction in which the needle is entering the tissues. Usually with a 3.5-MHz, and certainly with a 5-MHz, transducer it is possible to see even a 22-gauge needle throughout its course as long as one can accurately align the ultrasonic beam at right angles to the needle entrance site. The transducer can be in a nonsterile location used by a second operator. Slight movements of the subcutaneous tissues can be seen with a transducer if the needle is moved backwards and forwards as it is inserted. Once the needle entrance site is recognized, careful insertion of the needle into the tissues can be followed by real-time. Whenever the needle is lost to vision,

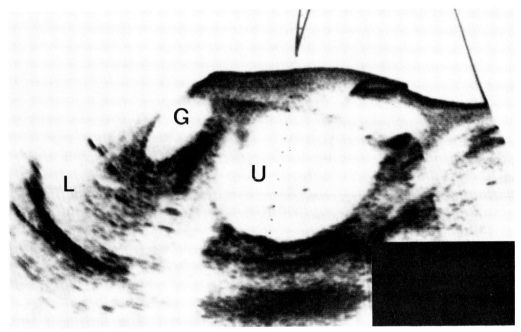

Figure 16.7. Large perinephric collection (*U*) in the right flank (a urinoma) with B-scan centimeter markers showing the site, direction, and depth where the needle will be inserted. *L,* liver; *G,* gallbladder.

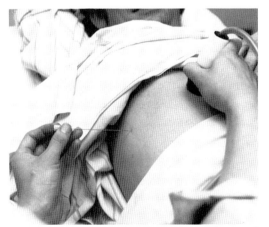

Figure 16.8. The needle is being inserted into the right kidney under guidance of a real-time transducer located on the anterior aspect of the abdomen. With this technique, one can see the needle path of a needle as small as a 22-gauge.

wiggling the needle under real-time will establish its position. Percutaneous nephrostomy insertion using this technique is possible (26).

2. Should it be impossible to visualize the area from a 90° axis because the kidney is not overlain by the liver or spleen, an alternative approach using real-time is to sight the lesion with a real-time transducer within a sterile plastic bag or which has been presterilized, making a mark on the skin at the point where the needle insertion will be made. A sterile plastic bag then has sterile gel placed within it. The bag is placed over the real-time transducer and fixed to the cable with an elastic band or flexible wire, such as a pipe cleaner. To find the ideal site, a linear structure, such as a pen or needle, is placed beneath the real-time transducer and moved, producing an echo-free line on the image until it is directly superior to the lesion; an appropriate mark is then made on the skin with a needle hub or pen top. It is often then possible to view the needle as it enters the tissues if it is inserted at a 45° angle with the transducer also obliqued at a 45° angle (27). This technique is only satisfactory with relatively superficial lesions.

3. A third and preferable technique using a real-time transducer is to have a needle guide attachment to the transducer either in the form of a central slot within the linear array (28) (Fig. 16.9) or as a lever coming off the side (at an oblique angle) of a mechanical sector scan transducer (Fig. 16.10). A preordained needle tract

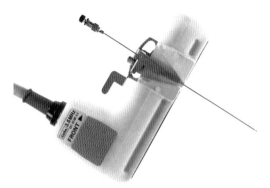

Figure 16.9. Linear array aspiration transducer. The needle can be angled through the central slot. A 22-gauge needle can be seen in tissue during insertion provided it is inserted at a 20° angle.

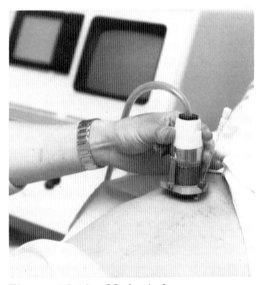

Figure 16.10. Mechanical sector scanner with obliquely offset needle guide. A template on the television screen shows the exact direction that the needle will take.

conforms to a template on the oscilloscope; the transducer can be moved until the plotted tract is aligned with the mass. With either technique it is possible to see the needle throughout its course and to prove that the needle tip has truly entered the lesion (Fig. 16.11, *A–E*). This is of considerable practical value in mass biopsy because a negative mass biopsy might be due to inadequate cytological material, poor cytological technique, or missing the mass. If one proves by direct vision that the needle tip is within the

mass, then one knows that faulty sonographic technique is not responsible for a nondiagnostic puncture.

When drainage of any type is an option, we prefer to perform the study on the fluoroscopy table with the aid of A-mode or real-time because this will allow a subsequent cystogram or insertion of a guide wire and catheter to be performed with contrast. Most real-time systems are portable so the two techniques can be combined.

PRACTICAL DETAILS OF ASPIRATION

The practical details of the performance of an aspiration do not vary a great deal whether an A-mode, B-scan, or real-time transducer is being used. In the first instance, the patient is scanned with gray-scale ultrasound or with real-time, and a decision on the best location for the puncture is made. The ideal position for renal puncture is below the lowest rib, but if this requires a very deep inspiration and the patient is relatively uncooperative and unable to perform the same size inspiration consistently, an inter-rib site on comfortable inspiration or quiet breathing is acceptable provided a small needle is used. Remember that one is puncturing pleura; for this reason, it is not desirable to leave a permanent indwelling catheter at such a site. An oblique angle approach can be used with a B-scan or real-time transducer if a large needle is used. However, with high lesions close to the diaphragm, performance under real-time vision is most desirable. Triangulation techniques can be used if the lesion is close to the diaphragm (29).

Once the site has been chosen, the patient is marked in such a fashion that the puncture site will be visible when the mineral oil has been removed. The easiest method of marking a patient is to take the cap of a pen or hub of a needle and twist it while pressing into the patient's skin so that a small circular indentation is made. Grease pencils and radiotherapy marking dyes are not satisfactory. Once the mineral oil is removed, they also disappear. When a suitable mark has been made, the patient's back is cleaned of mineral oil with either acetone or specific agents which remove mineral oil, such as "Sound Off" (E-Z Em, Inc., Westbury, NY). Standard procedures are adopted to cleanse the patient's back around the puncture site and the puncture site is surrounded by sterile towels.

The equipment for puncture is shown in Figure 16.12. Local anesthetic is then inserted down to the level of the ribs, making sure no air is injected, because this will prevent sound transmission. A small nick is made at the puncture site with a scalpel blade if an 18-gauge needle or larger is used or if a 22-gauge needle is used. The incision is necessary because the skin is by far the toughest point through which the needle passes; without it, a 22-gauge needle will bend, or, if a large needle is used, it may be impossible to push it through the skin. A 20-gauge needle can be inserted through the skin with ease without more pain than local anesthetic injection.

B-scan and A-mode Aspiration Transducers

At this juncture an aspiration transducer may be used. The exact direction and depth are localized with the help of the aspiration transducer. A plastic sleeve is placed over the transducer to keep the field sterile (Fig. 16.13), or a sterile transducer is used. After the appropriate location and depth have been ascertained from the ultrasonic image, a sterile ruler is placed alongside the needle to measure the point at which the correct depth is reached. A needle stop, consisting of a small plastic or metallic bolt (Fig. 16.14), is screwed onto the needle at a level equivalent to the center of the cyst (including the length of the aspiration transducer). The aspiration transducer adds between 2 and 5 cm to the overall length between needle stop and needle tip. The presence of a needle stop allows one to plunge the needle into the patient with a single swift pass. This is advantageous because it means that a renal mass is transfixed rather than displaced into the body as may occur if a more tentative approach is used.

Once the needle has been inserted into an optimal location with the patient holding his breath, an A-mode transducer may be used to see the needle tip lying within the cyst (30). The needle is freed from the transducer if a B-scan transducer is in use. The central stylette is removed, and aspiration of fluid from the needle is facilitated by the use of extension tubing so that free movement of the needle with the kidney can be maintained and respiratory excursion does not cause laceration of the kidney while fluid is being aspirated. This might occur if the needle were directly attached to a syringe. If fluid is not seen dripping back through the needle with an 18-gauge or a larger needle, it is

unlikely that one has succeeded in penetrating the cyst. Although the contents of an abscess or hemorrhagic cyst may not drip spontaneously, they can be aspirated through a 22-gauge needle (31).

There should be a characteristic feeling of "release" as the needle punctures a cyst wall. It is not uncommon for blood to return mixed with cyst fluid or urine initially; eventually the fluid becomes free of blood. It is also possible for the first few drops of cyst fluid or urine to be blood free but for the remainder of the aspirate to be slightly blood contaminated. Either way, the finding that some portion of the aspirate is free of blood and straw-colored is of practical significance since it almost always indicates benignity in a renal cyst. It may be necessary to perform a second puncture if two adjacent cysts are present, or it may be possible to transfix both cysts with a single puncture (32).

Real-Time

Real-time techniques require slight modifications to the procedure described above. If the real-time transducer is being used at right angles to the needle insertion site, the real-time transducer can be in a nonsterile area. One should, of course, be careful not to contaminate the field with the nonsterile real-time transducer, and a second operator is required to use the real-time at the same time that the needle insertion is made. If the needle is being inserted alongside or through the real-time transducer, then a sterile technique is needed. Some real-time transducers can only be gas sterilized, but the more modern ones can be immersed in a sterilizing solution. This is desirable because it means they can be used twice in the course of a day providing they are immersed for several hours between procedures. If the transducer requires gas sterilization and is needed rapidly when unsterile, it can, as has already been mentioned, be used after it has been inserted into a sterile plastic bag. Such a sterile bag technique means that the aspiration transducer with a central slot or a lever at one side cannot be used. In one variant of a sector scanner aspirator attachment, the clamp is placed around the plastic bag and the clamp alone is sterilized. If the needle is being placed through the aspiration transducer, it is best to place the needle tip through the skin prior to aligning the needle with the mass. Local anesthetic is inserted through the slit in the transducer into the skin after lining up the

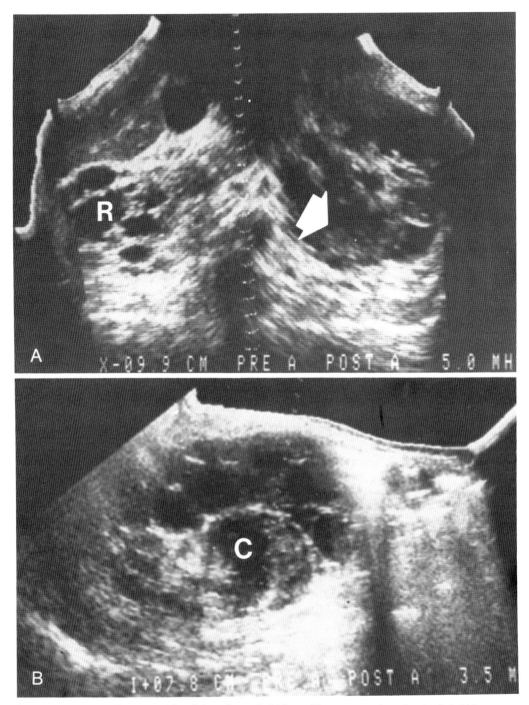

Figure 16.11. *A*, Patient with adult polycystic kidney. Transverse view. In the left kidney area the patient was suffering a good deal of pain. A suspicious cyst can be seen (*arrow*). *R*, right kidney. *B*, Longitudinal view. Left kidney. One cyst (*C*) contains internal echoes suggestive of abscess or hematoma.

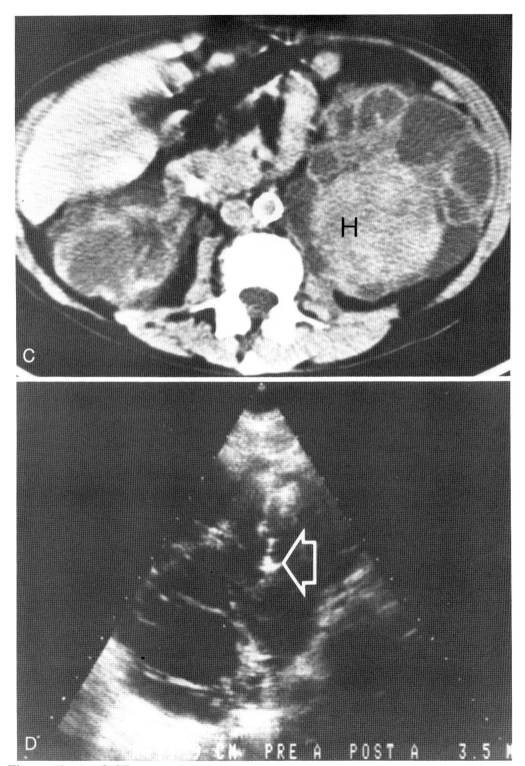

Figure 16.11. *C*, CT scan confirmed that one of the cysts (*H*) contined material with the density number of blood. *D*, Under ultrasound control using the sector scanner transducer guide, a 22-gauge needle was inserted into the infected cyst. The needle can be seen (*arrow*). Some old blood was withdrawn which proved to be infected on culture.

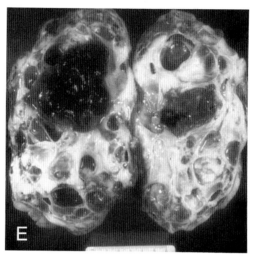

Figure 16.11. *E,* The kidney was removed. The cyst with the infected hematoma within it can be seen.

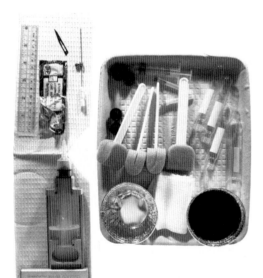

Figure 16.12. Equipment required for performance of an aspiration. Apart from cleansing material and collection bottles, specific instrumentation required includes the aspiration transducer (not shown), extension tubing, a sterile plastic ruler, a needle stop, and a scalpel blade.

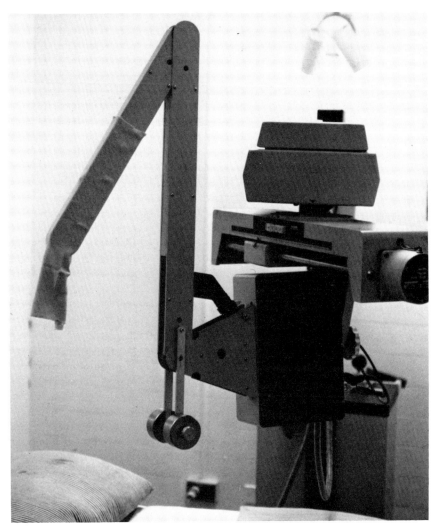

Figure 16.13.   The B-scan transducer arm is covered by sterile tube gauze to prevent inadvertent contamination of the sterile field.

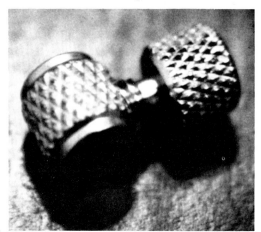

Figure 16.14. Needle stop used to prevent the needle being inserted too far. This allows a swift puncture so the kidney is transfixed rather than being displaced internally.

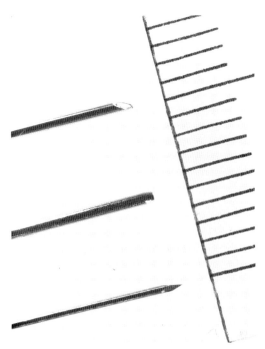

Figure 16.15. Two different 22-gauge needle tips; one beveled and one with a central point. Both have a similar accuracy in obtaining mass biopsy material.

lesion. It is usually simplest to have help with the procedure; an assistant who holds the real-time transducer while a second individual performs the actual insertion.

CHOICE OF NEEDLE

The choice of needle depends on the nature and depth of the lesion that is to be punctured and the type of procedure being performed. A simple renal cyst which is small and located within the kidney is probably best approached with a 20-gauge L.P. needle. Such needles cannot be seen with a 2.25-MHz aspiration transducer but can be seen with a 3.5-MHz aspiration transducer without a keyhole or with real-time systems. If no aspiration transducer is to be used and the procedure is for diagnosis only, a 22-gauge needle is even safer. With this narrow-gauge needle many abscesses have been successfully aspirated. However, in general, if an abscess or hematoma is suspected, a larger needle, such as an 18 gauge, is used. Hematomas are a particular problem because they may be clot filled. The inability to obtain any fluid apart from a small amount of blood should be taken as an indication of the presence of a hematoma if one is certain that the needle is in the center of the cystic area. We generally go up in needle size to 18 gauge before deciding a lesion is a hematoma.

Although a 22-gauge tumor biopsy needle is used for obtaining cytopathological material from mass lesions (Fig. 16.15), a larger needle is used if no diagnosis can be made by the cytopathologist (who should be present at the time of examination). There is no significant difference between the different types of 22-gauge needle tips in practice (Fig. 16.15); the Chiba needle, the tumor biopsy needle, and the Madayag needle are all satisfactory and will give a similar cystological yield (33). We find the Chiba needle is longer and more flexible than the others and, therefore, not so desirable. If necessary, we have used a 16-gauge True Cut needle for renal masses, but one should be confident that the mass is avascular before using such a large needle. Review of a CT scan with intravenous contrast or a previous arteriogram is helpful. The 18-, 20-, or 21-gauge Surecut modified Menghini needle gives good results if the 22-gauge aspiration needle is unsatisfactory. Another needle that we have found of value is the 21-gauge Rotex screw biopsy needle. A plunger attached to the syringe has proved helpful since it not only increases pressure, but it also allows the procedure to be performed with one hand (Fig. 16.16). We have performed at least 10 renal mass biopsies with larger needles without complications.

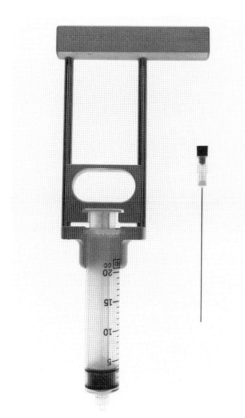

Figure 16.16. A plunger attached to a 20-gauge syringe increases aspiration pressure and allows the procedure to be performed single-handed. A 22-gauge needle is also shown.

ABSCESS DRAINAGE OF PERCUTANEOUS NEPHROSTOMY

If a permanent drainage procedure is being performed for an abscess, lymphocele, or urinoma, a larger size system with side holes and a catheter should be inserted (34, 35). A wide choice of possible systems exists, which are variants on two basic approaches. If the lesion is relatively inaccessible and the puncture tract passes close to potentially dangerous sites, such as the renal hilar vessels, the use of a system which involves a small needle, a guide wire, and a series of dilaters is desirable. In one common system a 22-gauge needle is inserted under ultrasonic localization. After contrast has been inserted into the cyst, collecting system, or collection, an 18-gauge needle is inserted under ultrasonic and fluoroscopic guidance. A 38 guide wire can be passed through this needle. The needle is removed, and a series of dilators, starting with 6 or 7 French and increasing in size up to 8 or 10 French, is used to create a sizable tract along which a pigtail catheter can be pushed. Systems are now available to allow the dilatation of a tract up to a 14 French with the insertion of a Malekot catheter. This is a tedious procedure, and a single stab technique is preferred if the collection is easily accessible. Van Sonnenberg and Ring McLean sump catheters are alternatives which can be used with dilaters, but they are usually used with a single stab insertion technique (14). Such 14 French catheters have multiple side holes and a second sump drain lumen to allow the entrance of air into an abscess while pus is draining out. These systems or the Argyle system, which has a Foley balloon at the end and a double lumen (35), are used in the drainage of abscesses which lie close to the skin without intervening potentially dangerous structures alongside the tract.

As might be expected, percutaneous nephrostomy and abscess drainage are more easily performed under real-time ultrasound control than with a static scanner (36–38). Such techniques have been used in children (38).

PYELOSCOPY

Endoscopic study of lesions of the renal pelvis is beginning to be developed and can be successfully performed under ultrasonic control (39).

CYST FLUID ANALYSIS

There is some controversy as to the value of the various tests that are performed on renal cyst fluid. Most reliance is placed upon the appearance of the fluid. If the fluid is yellow and looks like dilute urine, it is most likely that the cyst is benign. However, there are several recorded examples in the literature of malignant cysts with straw-colored fluid (40–42). If the fluid is consistently bloody throughout the aspiration or chocolate- or green-colored, the chances of neoplasia become much greater. Even if the cytopathology is negative, the patient should be considered a surgical candidate (43). Some patients with bloody fluid within the cyst will have hemorrhagic cysts—a benign condition due to trauma that is indistinguishable from neoplasia prior to surgery (44). In any event, as much fluid as possible is sent for cytopathology. Valuable information can be obtained even if the fluid is mixed with contrast media (45). The cytopathologist centrifuges the fluid to look at shed cells. If the cyst is small, a large volume of fluid cannot be obtained; this is only one of the reasons why the proportion of malignant cysts which show neoplastic cells at cytopathology, even when a neoplasm is later found by other means to be present, is less than 50% (46). The degree of experience and expertise required in a renal cytopathologist is great.

Biochemical tests for neoplasia within the cyst are of limited value. Fat has been found to be increased in conditions other than neoplasia, such as infection, and the test is technically difficult to perform. Lactic acid dehydrogenase (LDH) is elevated in some benign cysts, particularly those that are infected, so it is of limited diagnostic value (46, 47). Biochemical tests are worth performing if there is some doubt as to whether one is in a cyst or a hydronephrotic calyx (Fig. 16.17). Analysis for urea and electrolytes should be performed to make sure that one has not obtained urine. If the patient has a history of pyrexia or recent pyelonephritis, fluid is sent for bacteriological tests to make sure that the cyst is not infected.

Once fluid has been aspirated in sufficient volume for adequate cytopathology and biochemical tests, a decision has to be made as to whether contrast should be inserted in the cyst. If x-rays are to be taken, the cyst should not be aspirated to completion; contrast should be inserted when it is about three-fourths empty. The volume of the cyst should have been estimated prior to the performance of the puncture by using the formula: volume = diameter 3/2, if it is oblong; by a simplified formula for a prolate ellipse, $\dfrac{L \times H \times W}{0.5}$; or $\frac{1}{3}\pi r^3$, if it is circular.

Once fluoroscopy has been performed, the cyst should be aspirated completely because this reduces the likelihood of recurrence. When no more fluid can be aspirated, a further sonographic examination should be made to ensure that the cyst has been completely evacuated and that there are no other cysts adjacent to the initial cyst which were not emptied because the lesion was wrongly considered to be a single cyst and was, in fact, multilocular. If a second or

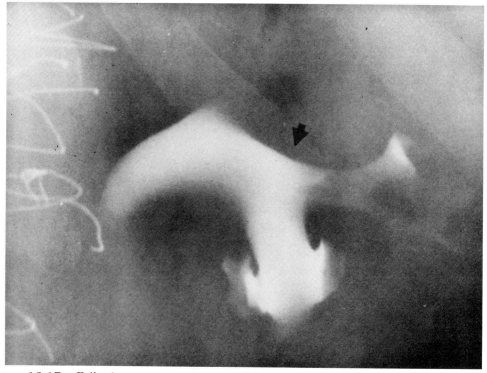

Figure 16.17. Following an apparently successful cyst puncture. Although on aspiration yellow fluid was obtained, contrast was inserted; this outlined the pelvicalyceal system showing the needle was actually in the renal pelvis. The impression of a renal cyst on the collecting system can be seen (*arrow*).

third cyst is discovered, the only practical way to exclude neoplasia is to puncture the other cysts separately.

If the cyst is symptomatic or sufficiently large to be causing mechanical problems to the kidney in the form of obstruction of a calyx or seems about to provoke mechanical side effects, an attempt should be made to prevent its recurrence. Successful permanent cyst "ablation" has now been achieved by placing sclerosing material within cysts or other collections. Ninety-five percent alcohol is one such substance which causes considerable fibrosis. Technique is important if alcohol is being instilled. It is desirable to use a small pigtail catheter (5 or 6 French) rather than a needle so that as much of the cyst contents can be aspirated as possible (48). The pigtail catheter prevents the alcohol from spilling into the surrounding tissues. Alcohol is extremely painful if it escapes outside the cyst. It may provoke fibrosis or even enter into the blood stream, so one must be sure that none leaks from the cyst into the surrounding tissues. Our practice is for the patient to lie still for an hour in the same position as the puncture was performed after alcohol insertion. Another fibrosing material that can be used is Atabrine (otherwise known as Quinocrine). This antimalarial is a potent fibroblast provoker. Results with a solution of this substance and complete aspiration of the cyst have also been impressive and appear comparable to those with alcohol.

CONTRAINDICATIONS AND COMPLICATIONS

Perirenal hematoma formation after renal cyst puncture or mass puncture is difficult to detect unless the patient is subsequently surgically explored; a 0.6% incidence was reported following cyst puncture using ultrasound in Lang's series (49). However, to our knowledge, hematoma formation of any clinical consequence (50) has not occurred following the use of a flexible transducer technique. It is wise to be certain that there is no history of increased bleeding as evidenced by a history of bleeding after tooth extraction, excess menstrual bleeding, easy bruising, etc., but a prothrombin time and platelet count are unnecessary if such a history is normal.

Surprisingly, in Lang's series (49), six (1.18%) patients undergoing cyst puncture under ultrasonic control suffered a pneumothorax. Ultrasonic visualization of a cyst is not possible if lung intervenes between the needle and the cyst. One can only presume that the punctures performed in these individuals did not follow the ultrasonic path.

A theoretical contraindication which has only been recorded once, although reported twice, is tumor implantation along the tract of the needle (51, 52). In a series of 75 cases compared with 73 similar controls in which needle puncture of a hypernephroma was performed, a 5-year follow-up showed a better survival rate among those who underwent needle puncture than the control group (53). As yet, experience is limited with transitional carcinomas of the kidney which seem more likely to give rise to spread along the needle tract, since spread is known to occur from these tumors to surgical incisions.

Insertion of Pantopaque into a cyst can give rise to allergic reactions similar to those seen with excretion urography. Ten percent of patients having Pantopaque inserted reported temperature elevation, and 4% had pain (49). In one patient, a rash developed around the needle site following the insertion of Pantopaque and disappeared only when Pantopaque was resorbed from the cyst. A sterile abscess can develop (54). A potential complication of a needle puncture, which is in practice rare (0.02%), is infection (55, 56). It seems more likely to occur if Pantopaque is inserted (57). Infection has, however, been reported in patients who undergo percutaneous nephrostomy when the catheter is left in place (19). Other complications of percutaneous nephrostomy that have been recorded are clot catheter blockage, urinoma formation (58), arteriovenous fistula, pseudoaneurysms (59, 60), and gross hematuria (61). Trivial hematuria is seen in about 10% of patients (49). Mild pain lasting longer than 3 days occurs in about 10% of patients (62).

FLUOROSCOPY OR NOT

The sonographic puncture of a cyst or of a dilated calyx is usually simple; however, contrast visualization allows views of the wall and more precise delineation of the needle catheter or guide wire site. Real-time ultrasound is a portable technique which should be combined with fluoroscopy so that the advantages of both techniques are available. Fluoroscopic visualization of the kidney is sometimes necessary in difficult cases where the lesion is small and difficult to find by ultrasound alone. It may be easier to perform a fluoroscopic rather than an ultrasonic localization. Extravasation or communication with the collecting system can be detected immediately (63). However, fluoroscopic localization usually requires more time, personnel, and expensive equipment, and it carries a radiation hazard. The relationship of the needle to the lateral and medial wall of the cyst is well shown by fluoroscopy.

Ideally, the same person should perform the puncture procedures under fluoroscopy and sonography so that the appropriate technique can be used in each situation. The major advantage of using sonography is that it indicates the depth of the needle within the cyst. X-ray views are important to establish that one actually is puncturing a cyst and not the renal pelvis (Fig. 16.17) and to visualize the cyst wall and exclude tumor

(Fig. 16.18). A special effort should be made to see the cyst walls fluoroscopically in patients with a history of hematuria or other ominous symptoms, in patients with a sonogram that shows an irregular wall, and in patients in whom the aspiration fluid is other than yellow in color. Nevertheless, in the remaining patients, if we have gone to the trouble of performing a cyst puncture, we inject contrast and take radiographs of the injected cyst since a very few cysts contain straw-colored fluid and yet are malignant (42).

If an antegrade pyelogram is being performed for diagnostic purposes, the nature of the stricture can only be adequately shown by fluoroscopic visualization; catheter insertion into an abscess or for percutaneous nephrostomy can only be accurately placed with fluoroscopy.

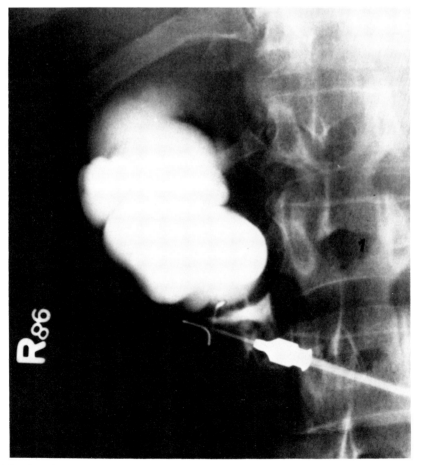

Figure 16.18. Cystogram showing numerous infoldings of the wall of a benign variety. These looked sonographically sinister; each infolding produced echoes.

References

1. Kissane JM: The morphology of renal cystic disease. *Perspect Nephrol Hypertension* 4:31–63, 1976.
2. Meaney TF: Errors in angiographic diagnosis of renal masses. *Radiology* 93:361, 1969.
3. Karp W, Ekelund L: Ultrasound, angiography and fine needle aspiration biopsy in diagnosis of renal neoplasms. *Acta Radiol Diag* 20:649–659, 1979.
4. Lindblom K: Diagnostic kidney puncture in cysts and tumors. *J Urol* 68:209, 1952.
5. Ekelund L: Hypovascular renal tumors: an aggressive diagnostic approach required. *J Urol* 119:566–568, 1978.
6. Heaston DK, Handel DB, Ashton PR, Korobkin M: Narrow gauge needle aspiration of solid adrenal masses. *AJR* 138:1143–1148, 1982.
7. Glazer HS, Weyman PJ, Sagel SS, et al: Nonfunctioning adrenal masses: incidental discovery on computed tomography. *AJR* 139:81–85, 1982.
8. Appel GB, Saltzman MJ, King KL, et al: Use of ultrasound for renal allograft biopsy. *Kidney Int* 19:471–473, 1981
9. Bolton WK, Tully RJ, Lewis EJ, et al: Localization of the kidney for percutaneous biopsy: a comparative study of methods. *Ann Intern Med* 81:159, 1974.
10. Schneider M, Haller JO, Moel DI, et al: Ultrasonic localization for renal biopsy in infants and children. *J Int Am Col Radiol* 2:39–40, 1977.
11. Goldberg BB, Pollack HM, Kellerman E: Ultrasonic localization for renal biopsy. *Radiology* 115:167, 1975.
12. Maxwell DR, Asher WM: Ultrasound localization of the kidneys for closed renal biopsy. *J Clin Ultrasound* 2:279, 1974.
13. Kristensen JK, Bartels E, Jorgensen HE: Percutaneous renal biopsy under the guidance of ultrasound. *Scand J Urol Nephrol* 8:223, 1974.
14. Gerzof SG, Gale ME: Computed tomography and ultrasonography for diagnosis and treatment of renal and retroperitoneal abscess. *Urol Clin North Am* 9:185–193, 1982.
15. Johnson WC, Gerzof SG, Robbins AH, et al: Treatment of abdominal abscesses. *Ann Surg* 194:510–520, 1981.
16. Crass JR, Karl R: Bedside drainage of abscesses with sonographic guidance in the desperately ill. *AJR* 139:183–185, 1982.
17. Lissoos I, van Blerk PJ: Retrograde pyelography and ureteric catheterization. *S Afr Med J* 45:495, 1971.
18. Weinstein B, Skolnick ML: Ultrasonically guided antegrade pyelography. *J Urol* 120:323, 1978.
19. Stables DP, Gilsberg NJ, Johnson KL: Percutaneous nephrostomy: a series and review of the literature. *AJR* 130:75, 1978.
20. Parker RA, Elliott WC, Muther RS, et al: Percutaneous aspiration biopsy of renal allografts using ultrasound localization. *Urology* 15:534, 1980.
21. Turner AG, Howlett KA, Eban R, Williams GB: The role of anterograde pyelography in the transplant kidney. *J Urol* 123:812, 1980.
22. Lieberman RP, Crummy AB, Glass NR, et al: Fine needle antegrade pyelography in the renal

transplant. *J Urol* 126:155, 1981.
23. Hastak SM, Gammelgaard J, Holm HH: Ultrasonically guided transperineal biopsy in the diagnosis of prostatic carcinoma. *J Urol* 128:69, 1982.
24. Rifkin MD, Kurtz AB, Goldberg BB: Prostate biopsy utilizing transrectal ultrasound guidance: diagnosis of clinically non-palpable cancers. *J Ultrasound Med* 2:165–167, 1983.
25. Lee TG, Knochel JQ: Air as an ultrasound contrast marker for accurate determination of needle placement. *Radiology* 143:787–788, 1982.
26. Burnett KR, Handler SJ, Conroy RM, et al: Percutaneous nephrostomy utilizing B-mode and real-time ultrasound guidance: the lateral approach and puncture facilitation with furosemide. *J Clin Ultrasound* 10:252–255, 1982.
27. Rice BT, Crow HC, Bartrum RJ: The tugger technique of ultrasonically-guided percutaneous puncture using a wide-field real-time scanner. *J Clin Ultrasound* 10:299–301, 1982.
28. Montali G, Solbiati L, Croce F, et al: Fine-needle aspiration biopsy of liver focal lesions ultrasonically guided with a real-time probe. Report on 126 cases. *Br J Radiol* 55:717–723, 1982.
29. van Sonnenberg E, Wittenberg J, Ferrucci JT, et al: Triangulation method for percutaneous needle guidance: the angled approach to upper abdominal masses. *AJR* 137:757–761, 1981.
30. Goldberg BB, Pollack HM: Ultrasonically guided renal cyst aspiration. *JK Urol* 109:5, 1973.
31. Elyaderani MK, Skolnick ML: Ultrasonic detection of abdominal abscesses and verification by percutaneous aspiration. In White D, Lyons EA: *Ultrasound in Medicine.* New York, Plenum Press, 1978, vol 4, p 167.
32. Darby RE, Wayne RW: Ultrasound diagnosis of and cyst puncture guidance for a second unilateral renal cyst. *J Clin Ultrasound* 2:295, 1974.
33. Wittenberg J, Mueller PR, Ferrucci JT, et al: Percutaneous core biopsy of abdominal tumors using 22 gauge needles: further observations. *AJR* 139:75–80, 1982.
34. Gronvall J, Gronvall S, Hegedus V: Ultrasound-guided drainage of fluid-containing masses using angiographic catheterization techniques. *AJR* 129:997–1002, 1977.
35. Gerzof SG: Percutaneous drainage of renal and perinephric abscess. *Urol Radiol* 2:171–179, 1981.
36. Heckemann R, Meyer-Schwickerath M, Hezel J, et al: Percutaneous nephropyelostomy under continuous real-time ultrasound guidance. *Urol Radiol* 3:171–175, 1981.
37. Baron RL, Lee JKT, McClennan BL, et al: Percutaneous nephrostomy using real-time sonographic guidance. *AJR* 136:1018, 1981.
38. Babcock JR, Skolnik A, Cook WA: Ultrasound-guided percutaneous nephrostomy in the pediatric patient. *J Urol* 121:327, 1979.
39. Saitoh M, Watanabe H: Ultrasonically-guided percutaneous pyeloscopy. *Urology* 17:457, 1981.
40. Brannan W, Miller W, Crisler M: Coexistence of renal neoplasms and renal cysts. *South Med J* 55:749, 1962.
41. Lang EK: Coexistence of cyst and tumor in the same kidney. *Radiology* 101:7, 1972.
42. Ambrose SS, Lewis EL, O'Brien DP III, et al:

Unsuspected renal tumors associated with renal cysts. *J Urol* 117:704, 1977.

43. Harris RD, Goergen TG, Talner LB: The bloody renal cysts aspirate: a diagnostic dilemma. *J Urol* 114:832, 1975.

44. Jackman RJ, Stevens GM: Benign hemorrhagic renal cyst: nephrotomography, renal arteriography and cyst puncture. *Radiology* 110:7, 1973.

45. Barry JM, Murphy JB, Nassir E, et al: The influence of retrograde contrast medium on urinary cytodiagnosis: a preliminary report. *J Urol* 119:633–634, 1978.

46. Schneider M, Phillips G, Becker J: Sonographically guided cyst puncture. A safe and accurate outpatient procedure. Presented at American Institute of Ultrasound in Medicine Meeting, San Diego, October 1978.

47. Lang EK: The differential diagnosis of renal cysts and tumors. *Radiology* 87:883, 1966.

48. Bean WJ: Renal cysts: Treatment with alcohol. *Radiology* 138:329, 1981.

49. Lang EK: Renal cyst puncture and aspiration: A survey of complications. *AJR* 128:723, 1977.

50. Thompson IM, Kovac A, Geshner J: Ultrasound followup of renal cyst puncture. *J Urol* 124:175, 1980.

51. Buch WH Jr, Burnett LL, Gibbons RP: Needle tract seeding of renal cell carcinoma. *AJR* 129:725, 1977.

52. Gibbons RP, Bush WH Jr, Burnett LL: Needle tract seeding following aspiration of renal cell carcinoma. *J Urol* 118:865, 1977.

53. von Schreeb T, Arner O, Skovsted G, et al: Renal adenocarcinoma: is there a risk of spreading tumor cells in diagnostic puncture? *Scand J Urol Nephrol* 1:270, 1967.

54. Shumaker BP, Pierce JM: Renal cystography: unusual complication. *J Urol* 123:245, 1980.

55. Feldberg MAAM, Th Mali WP: An infected renal cyst. *Urol Radiol* 2:47–49, 1980.

56. Lockhart JL, Wacksman J, deVere White R, et al: Renal cyst puncture and abscess formation. *Urology* 10:98, 1977.

57. Barbaric ZL, Davis RS, Frank IN, et al: Percutaneous nephropyelostomy in the management of acute pyohydronephrosis. *Radiology* 118:567, 1976.

58. Portela LA, Patel SK, Callahan DH: Pararenal pseudocyst (urinoma) as complication of percutaneous nephrostomy. *Urology* 13:570, 1979.

59. Cope C, Zeit RM: Pseudoaneurysms after nephrostomy. *AJR* 139:255–261, 1982.

60. Gavant ML, Gold RE, Church JC: Delayed rupture of renal pseudoaneurysms: complication of percutaneous nephrostomy. *AJR* 138:948–949, 1982.

61. Eckhauser ML, Haaga JR, Hampel N, et al: Arterial embolization of renal allograft to control hemorrahge secondary to percutaneous nephropyelostomy. *J Urol* 126:679, 1981.

62. Plaine LI, Hinman F Jr: Malignancy in asymptomatic renal masses. *J Urol* 94:342, 1965.

63. Raskin MM, Roen SA, Serafini AN: Renal cyst puncture: combined fluoroscopic and ultrasonic technique. *Radiology* 113:425, 1974.

CHAPTER 17

Intraoperative Localization of Renal Calculi with Ultrasound

FLOYD A. FRIED, M.D.

During the past 50 years the operative management of renal calculi has made impressive strides. The importance of removing all calculi when operating for renal stones has been clearly demonstrated (1–3). The incidence of additional stone formation has been reported to be 23% if residual stones are left behind, whereas the recurrence rate is 8 to 12% if "complete" removal is achieved (4). Nonetheless, the adequate detection of calculi intraoperatively has remained a knotty problem and has provided the stimulus for a variety of ancillary intraoperative aids. The nephroscope has been advocated, but its use may be severely limited by poor visibility when bleeding is encountered (5, 6). In addition, blood clot may further impede visibility and hide small calculi. Intraoperative radiographic techniques were developed during the 1930's and thus far have become the standard for intraoperative stone localization. Unfortunately, obtaining high quality intraoperative films has proved to be a frustrating problem in many institutions. Further radiographic modifications, such as the development of grids to localize the renal segment containing the calculus and the use of mammography film, have increased the value of radiographic techniques, but the problems of improper exposure and lengthy intervals awaiting the development of films are problems familiar to all urologists. In addition, x-rays are limited in that one gets a two-dimensional picture. In 1943, Dees (7) published a technique for removing small calculi from the renal collecting system using a fibrin clot. For many years coagulum pyelolithotomy could not be performed because of the Food and Drug Administration's prohibition of the use of pooled human fibrinogen because of the problem of serum hepatitis. Coagulum pyelolithotomy has recently become popular with the availability of cryoprecipitate as a source of fibrin. The procedure is a valuable technique in removing small and oftentimes un-

suspected calculi from the kidney (8). Limitations of the coagulum technique include the inability to use coagulum in patients with a small intrarenal pelvis, the obvious inability to remove calyceal stones larger than the infundibuli with which they communicate, and the difficulty of using this technique once the collecting system of the kidney has been opened. One must also be aware of the potential complication of pulmonary embolus when performing coagulum pyelolithotomy. Factors such as the degree of renal obstruction and the amount of renal bleeding may be important in permitting the entry of thrombogenic components into the circulation. It is prudent to use low concentrations of thrombin and to avoid overdistention of the collecting system (9).

The use of ultrasound in urology is now well established. Important uses in the urinary tract include the determination of renal size, detection of hydronephrosis, and distinguishing between renal cysts and tumors. Ultrasound offers the major advantage of having no known deleterious effects and being noninvasive (10). The application of ultrasound to the problem of intraoperative localization of stones is eminently reasonable. The substantial physical differences between the surface of the calculus and the surrounding kidney account for a strong reflection of sound at the surface of the stone and characteristic distal acoustic shadowing which enables stones to be detected clearly by ultrasound.

Schlegel et al. (11) first reported use of intraoperative ultrasound to detect calculi in 1961. The instrument used was an A-mode which displays a graph of the amplitude of ultrasound echoes and the distance between objects in the path of the ultrasound beam (Fig. 17.1). In this early study, A-mode intraoperative ultrasound was used in nine patients. The calculus was demonstrated in each case. There were three

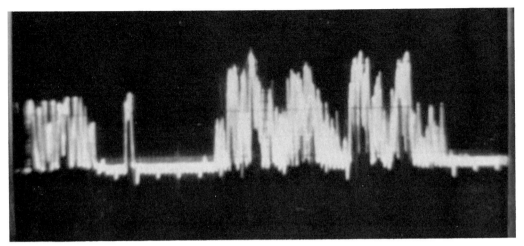

Figure 17.1. Ultrasonic A-mode scan. Echo strength is indicated by the vertical height of the wave form and depth by the distance from the left-hand margin.

false positive studies which were attributed to prominent fat deposits or possible calcifications in the papillae. Schlegel pointed out the value of this technique, particularly in the small intrarenal pelvis, which prevented localization of stones by conventional methods (11). In view of this early success, it is somewhat surprising that the procedure did not gain in popularity for several years.

The development of the B-mode ultrasound scanner offered a major advantage because it provided an anatomical display of the organ being scanned. The image produced is a cross-sectional or longitudinal picture which is produced by the return ultrasound echoes (Fig. 17.2). The more familiar anatomical display of the B-mode scanner is a major factor in its increasing acceptance and popularity. In addition, the development of smaller scanning heads and real-tme scanners, which give a dynamic ultrasound image, have made intraoperative renal ultrasound scanning for the localization of stones a valuable adjunct in stone surgery.

Cook and Lytton (12) have demonstrated the practicality of intraoperative stone localization with ultrasound. Using an instrument initially designed for ophthalmological use, the Bronson ophthalmic B-scan probe with a frequency of 10 MHz, these authors found good discrimination of stones 2 to 3 mm in diameter at depths of 2 to 2.5 cm from the renal surface (12). Others have reported similar favorable results and have noted that this technique has the ability to identify radiolucent calculi (13).

Work from our laboratory in porcine kidneys

was designed to define the limits of ultrasound in localizing intrarenal calculi. In these studies the porcine kidney into which zero, one, two, or three human calculi were placed was radiographed and studied by ultrasound. The unit originally used was a Picker 80-L Static Scanner which produced a static B-scale image. We found a real-time scanner to be better suited for this work and used an ADR Real-Time Dynamic Scanner equipped with linear array transducers of 3, 5, and 7 MHz. The 7-MHz transducer provided a reasonable compromise of discrimination, penetrance, and field size. The ultrasonographer involved in this study had no knowledge of the size, number, location, or composition of stones in each kidney. These observations demonstrated that stones as small as 2 mm could consistently be identified and that the composition was not a factor in detecting the stone (14). The in vitro stone model used was of great help in familiarizing the surgeons with the sonographic appearance of the kidney as well as the appearance of calculi seen by the ultrasound scanner.

TECHNIQUE

Most real-time ultrasound scanners currently available in a hospital are suitable for use in the operating room. We now use an ATL Mk300 real-time scanner which has a 5-MHz short focused transducer. This instrument is easily transported on a cart which also holds a video monitor and a videotape recorder and permits video recording of the procedure (Fig. 17.3). The

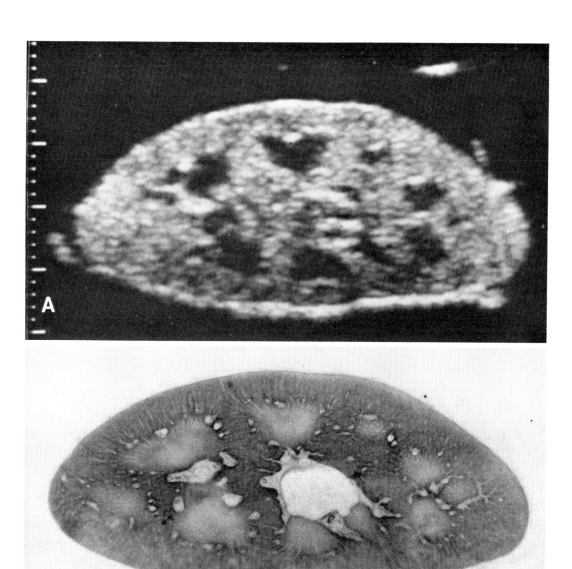

Figure 17.2. Comparison of ultrasonogram (A) and identical anatomical cross-section (B) of the kidney. This in vitro study shows the characteristic echo pattern seen in vivo. The cortex has a "speckled" echogenicity and medulla is sonolucent. Vessels and pelvicalyceal structures return bright echoes.

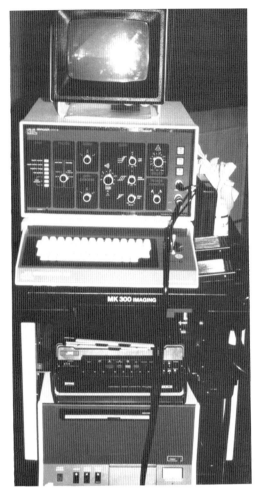

Figure 17.3. Ultrasound scanner with video monitor (*top*), character generator (*keyboard*) for entering patient name, etc., and videotape recorder with camera mounted on cart allow easy transportation of unit.

probe size is small enough so that it can easily be placed in the operative field (Fig. 17.4).

Sterilization of the probe is no longer necessary since we now use a XOMED sterile arthroscope drape with corner cut off to cover the probe cord (Fig. 17.5). The unsterile transducer and cord are draped as follows. A member of the surgical team placed a large (size 8) glove over his already gloved hand and grasps the probe (Fig. 17.6), pulling the outer glove back over the probe head, a drop of transmission gel having previously been placed over the window of the transducer (Fig. 17.7). The XOMED arthroscope drape with the corner cut off is passed over the transducer head (Fig. 17.8). The opening of the arthroscope drape is secured to the gloved transducer by wrapping a sterile rubber band around the drape and transducer head. The arthroscope drape is then drawn over the cord until that segment of cord which is in danger of contaminating the sterile field is covered (Fig. 17.9). The probe head covered by the slightly stretched sterile glove is placed in contact with the kidney capsule using additional sterile transmission gel to make a good contact with the kidney surface. The image is displayed on a 12-inch video monitor with a grid calibrated in centimeters, permitting accurate measurement of the depth of the stone from the kidney surface.

The kidney is then systematically scanned from pole to pole. Once a stone is identified, its depth is determined on the video monitor and a 22- to 25-gauge spinal needle is passed along the edge of the probe in the direction of the stone. The needle, which is easily seen on the video monitor, is advanced to the stone. A urological unit is now available that is equipped with a

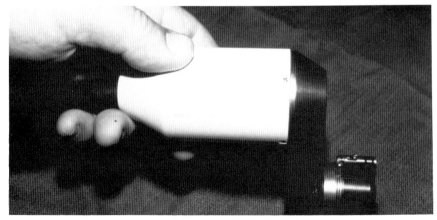

Figure 17.4. Five-megahertz short focused transducer is small enough to scan a kidney easily through a flank incision.

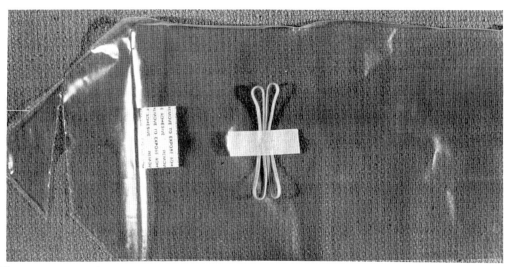

Figure 17.5. XOMED arthroscope drape. The corner is cut off as shown to permit the probe head to fit through the opening.

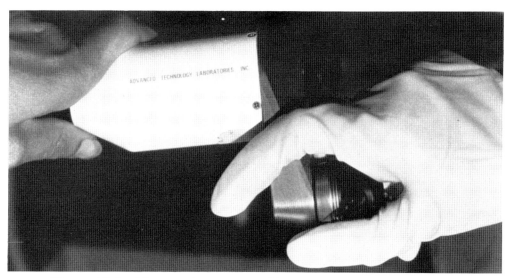

Figure 17.6. The transducer is grasped by the surgeon's double-gloved hand.

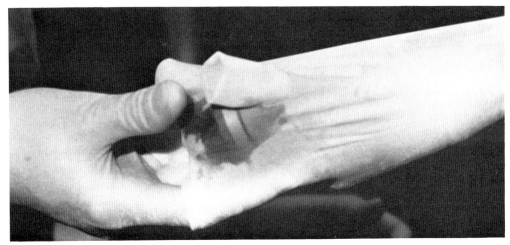

Figure 17.7.   The outer glove is pulled back over the transducer.

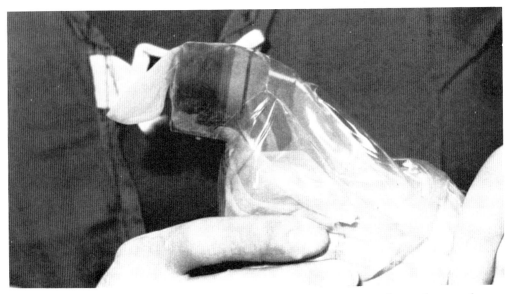

Figure 17.8.   The arthroscopic drape with its corner cut off is passed over the transducer.

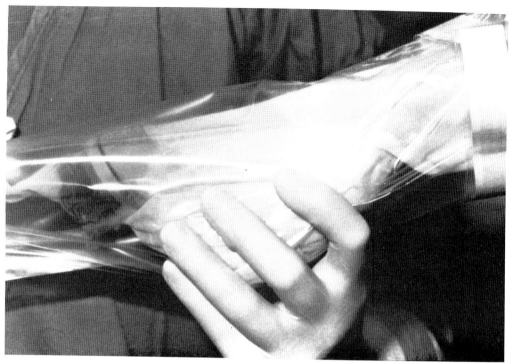

Figure 17.9. The arthroscope drape is pulled over the transducer cord, thereby covering transducer and cord with the sterile drape.

needle guide. This permits a needle to be passed in a groove alongside the probe so as to intercept the stone at the selected depth. A small nephrotomy is made using the needle as a guide, and the stone is removed.

As in all techniques, B-mode scanning to detect stones intraoperatively has some limitations. Confusing images may at times be produced by scar and large vessels. With practice, the ultrasonographer and urologist can usually distinguish these soft tissue echoes from stones, because stones, due to their higher density, produced brighter echoes which persist at low gain and intensify at high gains (Fig. 17.10). Most important, there is a distinctive lack of echoes distal to the stone which is referred to as acoustic shadowing. Acoustic shadowing persists when produced by a stone if the gain is increased. Once air has been introduced into the collecting system, confusing images may result. In our experience, air artifact can be minimized by flooding the collecting system with sterile saline solution. The presence of acoustic shadowing at high gain usually can distinguish stone

from other sources of echoes. Finally, it was mentioned earlier that calculi as small as 2 mm can be detected. However, fragments of smaller size may not be reliably seen with ultrasound. Intraoperative ultrasound at present is not a substitute or replacement for x-ray monitoring, but it is definitely a helpful adjunct that, when combined with x-ray, can hasten the detection and removal of renal calculi. A final x-ray of the kidney is mandatory before concluding that all calculi and fragments within a kidney have been successfully removed.

ILLUSTRATIVE CASES

Case 1. A 25-year-old woman with a 7-year history of renal stones was operated upon 18 months earlier for right renal calculi. Preoperative films localized the stones in the lower pole. The surgeon was unable to locate the stones. Intraoperative nephroscopy was of no help, and the procedure was terminated. The patient continued to have right flank pain and was referred

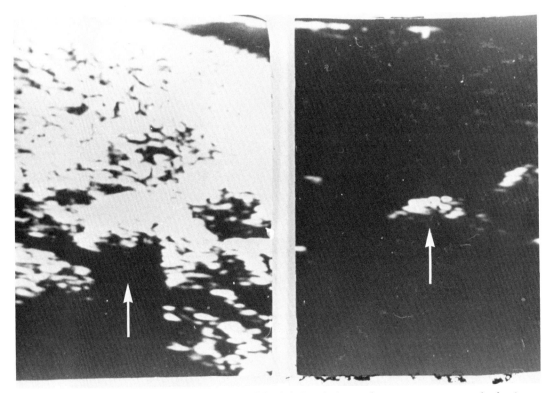

Figure 17.10.   Shadowing and persistence. The *left-hand picture* demonstrates strong shadowing at high ultrasonic gain (*arrow*). When the gain is reduced (*right-hand picture*), cortical echoes disappear and the stone echo persists (*arrow*).

to our institution. Radiographs again demonstrated two or three calculi in the right lower pole (Fig. 17.11*A*). The patient was explored through the previous flank incision. Dense scar was encountered, and the cortical surface of the kidney was exposed with difficulty. Intraoperative ultrasound scan clearly demonstrated the calculi (Fig. 17.11*B*). A 22-gauge spinal needle was passed to the stones, and then a second needle in a different plane of the planned nephrostomy incision was passed to the stone. A 3- to 4-cm nephrotomy incision was made, and the underlying collecting system was opened into the calyx containing the calculi, which were removed under direct vision. Subsequent films showed no further stone.

Case 2. A 43-year-old woman was first diagnosed as having pyelonephritis 18 months prior to admission. Repeated episodes resulted in her referral to our institution. An excretory urogram showed no visualization of the left kidney, which was obstructed by a 2-cm upper ureteral stone and several possible smaller stones in the col-

lecting system of the left kidney. The right kidney had a large staghorn calculus. A left ureterolithotomy and coagulum pyelolithotomy were performed, and her recovery was uneventful. Three weeks later a right anatrophic nephrolithotomy was performed under appropriate antibiotic coverage.

Intraoperative ultrasound scans made after mobilization of the kidney demonstrated the large stone (Fig. 17.12, *A* and *B*). The kidney was cooled, its blood supply was cross-clamped, and an anatrophic nephrolithotomy was performed. After removal of all visible calculi, a repeat ultrasound study was performed, and a stone fragment was identified. This was confirmed by an intraoperative x-ray (Fig. 17.13, *A* and *B*). With the aid of intraoperative ultrasound, the fragment was easily found and removed. Further x-rays showed no further stone present.

Case 3. A 49-year-old male with a 15-year history of left-sided renal calculi presented to the emergency room with an episode of left renal

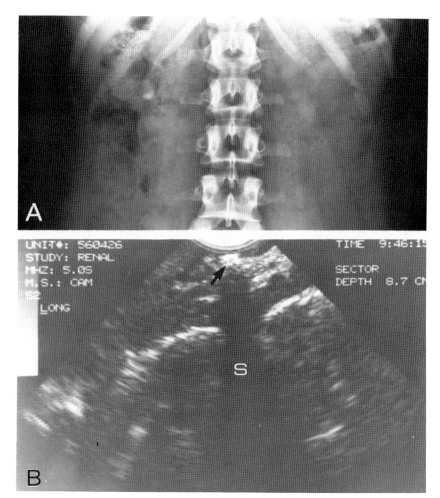

Figure 17.11.   Case 1. *A*, Abdominal film showing left renal calculi. *B*, Intraoperative ultrasound demonstrates strong echo created from renal stone (*arrow*) with echo-free shadow beneath stone (*S*).

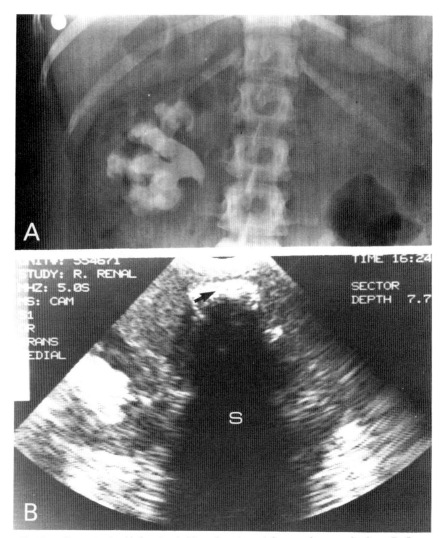

Figure 17.12. Case 2. *A*, Abdominal film showing right staghorn calculus. *B*, Intraoperative ultrasound prior to removal of staghorn calculus demonstrates prominent echo (*arrow*) and large area of shadowing beneath the stone (*S*).

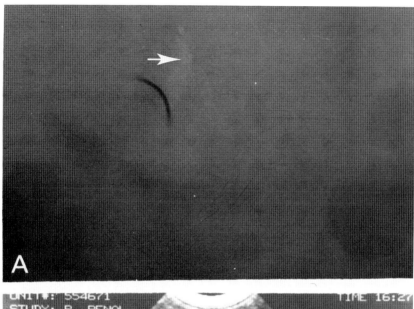

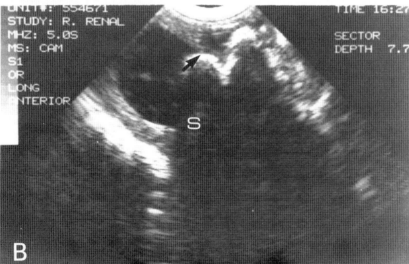

Figure 17.13. Case 2. *A*, Intraoperative film poorly shows remaining stone fragment (*arrow*) after removal of staghorn calculus. *B*, Intraoperative renal ultrasound study demonstrates remaining stone (*arrow*) and acoustic shadow beneath stone echo (*S*).

colic. An intravenous pyelogram revealed one calculus in the proximal left ureter and two calculi in the collecting system of the left kidney (Fig. 17.14*A*). A left proximal ureterolithotomy was performed. A coagulum pyelolithotomy was attempted and recovered one of the two renal calculi. The kidney was further mobilized, and then an intraoperative ultrasound scan was performed (Fig. 17.14*B*) The calculus was readily identified, and, using two 22-gauge needles as a guide, a small nephrotomy was made and the

stone easily removed. An intraoperative x-ray showed no further calculi.

In our experience, most renal calculi 2 mm or larger in diameter can be readily identified using intraoperative ultrasound. To perform this study properly the kidney must be adequately mobilized so that the entire renal surface can be scanned. It is helpful to gain experience by scanning cadaveric or suitable animal kidneys implanted with stones because this will greatly facilitate the use of this technique in the oper-

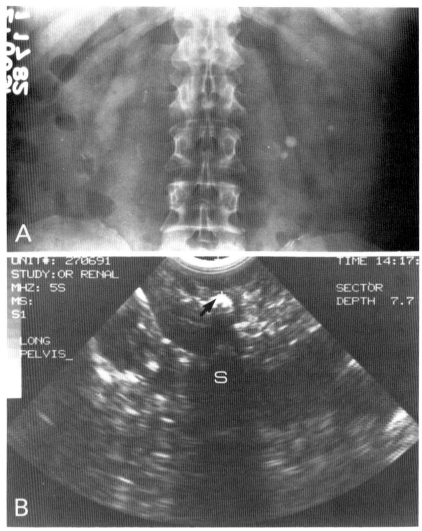

Figure 17.14.   Case 3. *A*, Abdominal film demonstrates three calculi in left kidney and proximal ureter. *B*, Intraoperative renal ultrasound study demonstrates stone in collecting system of kidney (*arrow*) with characteristic acoustic shadow beyond stone (*S*).

ating room. It should be emphasized that intraoperative ultrasound should be used in conjunction with x-rays rather than as a substitute for them.

Finally, brief mention of the use of ultrasound as an aid in the distinction between radiolucent filling defects of the renal pelvis and intrarenal collecting system should be made. Mulholland and co-workers (15) found that conventional, nonoperative ultrasound studies detected radiolucent calculi in nine patients by the presence of acoustic shadowing behind the echo-dense area. In their experience with three other patients having renal pelvic filling defects for non-

calculous disease, the characteristic acoustic shadowing was absent (15). Our experience in two cases suggests that intraoperative ultrasound is useful in distinguishing radiolucent stones from other noncalculous lesions.

References

1. Oppenheimer GD: Nephrectomy vs. conservative operation in unilateral calculous disease of the upper urinary tract. *Surg Gynecol Obstet* 65:829, 1937.
2. Williams RE: Long-term survey of 538 patients with upper urinary tract stone. *Br J Urol* 35:416, 1963.
3. Singh M, Marshall V, Blandy JP: The residual

renal stone. *Br J Urol* 47:125, 1975.

4. Singh M, Chapman R, Tresidder GC, Blandy JP: The fate of the unoperated staghorn calculus. *Br J Urol* 45:581, 1973.
5. Miki M, Inaba Y, Machida T: Operative nephroscopy with fiberoptic scope: preliminary report. *J Urol* 119:166, 1978.
6. Wilbur HJ: The flexible choledochoscope: a welcome addition to the urologic armamentarium. *J Urol* 126:380, 1981.
7. Dees J: The use of intrapelvic coagulum in pyelolithotomy. *South Med J* 36:167, 1943.
8. Patel VJ: The coagulum pyelolithotomy. *Br J Surg* 60:230, 1973.
9. Pence JR II, Airhart AR, Novicki DE, Williams JL, Ehler WJ: Pulmonary emboli associated with coagulum pyelolithotomy. *J Urol* 127:572, 1982.
10. Taylor KJW: Current status of toxicity investigations. *J Clin Ultrasound* 2:149, 1974.
11. Schlegel JU, Diggdon P, Cuellar J: The use of ultrasound for localizing renal calculi. *J Urol* 86:367, 1961.
12. Cook JH, Lytton B: Intraoperative localization of renal calculi during nephrolithotomy by ultrasound scanning. *J Urol* 117:543, 1977.
13. Marshall FF, Smith NA, Murphy JB, Menon M, Sanders RC: A comparison of ultrasonography and radiography in the localization of renal calculi: experimental and operative experience. *J Urol* 126:576, 1981.
14. Stafford SJ, Jenkins JM, Staab EV, Boyce I, Fried FA: Ultrasonic detection of renal calculi: accuracy tested in an in vitro porcine kidney model. *J Clin Ultrasound* 9:359, 1981.
15. Mulholland SG, Arger, PH, Goldberg BB, Pollack HM: Ultrasonic differentiation of renal pelvic filling defects. *J Urol* 122:14, 1979.

CHAPTER 18

Use of Ultrasound in Radiotherapy

DAMON D. BLAKE, M.D.

An explanation of the potential role of ultrasound imaging in the practice of radiotherapy requires an understanding of the various functions involved in the planning and carrying out of a patient's treatment course. The elements of a course of radiation therapy include a number of categories of services provided by the radiation therapist, the radiation physicist, the radiation dosimetrist, and radiotherapy technologists (1). In the following outline there are many points at which ultrasound imaging can be useful:

I. Consultation—includes decision whether patient is suitable for radiation therapy, determination of the role of radiation therapy in relation to other modalities (e.g., surgery or chemotherapy), and providing guidance in additional work-up needed to initiate therapy.

II. Treatment Planning Process—generally includes determination of:

Treatment goal: palliation versus curative intent.

Tumor localization: treatment volume determination and establishment of the patient's external contour.

Type of radiation to be used: energy of beam, number of treatment portals, indications for use of radioactive implants.

Need for special devices or techniques: wedge filters, beam blocks, tissue compensating filters—all of which shape or alter the distribution of the radiation within the treatment volume.

Patient immobilization techniques: to assure day-to-day reproducibility of treatment.

III. Radiation Dosimetry—entails the calculation of radiation dose within the treatment volume. Depending upon the complexity of the beam arrangement, this may require dose calculation only at a few points, or the graphic presentation of computer-generated isodose distribution throughout the volume irradiated, displayed within an accurate cross-section contour of the patient. Precise localization of the tumor extent and of vital normal structures must also be displayed within the contour, since the radiation tolerance of those normal tissues often determines the maximum dose which can be delivered to the tumor.

IV. Treatment Management—during the actual treatment course requires a continuing assessment of the patient's progress. This is not only in regard to his state of health, but also relative to the technical aspects of the treatment. Field check films are often redone at intervals to ensure that proper skin portals are maintained. Reimaging of the tumor may be indicated as it reduces in size in response to treatment, allowing a reduction in treatment volume and/or a change in dose.

V. Assessment of Maximum Response to Treatment—often requires reimaging of the tumor at the end of treatment or at an appropriate interval thereafter. Sometimes this information is helpful in making decisions about subsequent management, such as the need for surgery or chemotherapy.

VI. Patient Follow-Up—is a necessary and informative part of a course of radiation treatment. Not only is it vital to the management of the patient's disease, but it also provides invaluable data about late results and effects on the tumor and normal tissues. Not infrequently, a reimaging of the original tumor area is called for, or perhaps a look at sites of potential disease recurrence (e.g., the retroperitoneal space or the para-aortic nodes).

PRINCIPLES OF RADIATION THERAPY

The goal in radiation therapy treatment is to deliver an adequate dose to all the tumor, while exposing as small a volume of normal tissue as possible to as low a dose as possible. The radiation tolerance of the particular normal tissues in question frequently is the limiting factor which determines the maximum tumor dose. Accurate definition of the tumor and its relationship to nearby vital normal structures can often make it possible to construct a treatment plan which will allow a tumoricidal dose to be delivered without an excessive dose to normal tissues.

The radiation therapist refers to the *tumor volume* as the volume containing just the neoplastic tissue, whereas the *treatment volume* contains also a variable amount of normal tissue, through which the radiation passes before and after reaching the tumor. The amount and kind of normal tissue necessarily included in this treatment volume are determined by the location and extent of the tumor volume, the modality of radiation being used, and the arrangement of the treatment beams, special blocking devices, etc. The maximum allowable radiation dose to the treatment volume depends upon, among other things, the size of the volume and the kind of normal tissue in question.

It is apparent then, that precise knowledge of the tumor location and extent and its relationship to critical normal tissues assumes great importance in treatment planning. In the past, this kind of information has been pieced together from the limited imaging studies available to supplement the information gained from physical examination of the patient and the use of cross-sectional anatomy texts. The final result often left something to be desired in terms of accuracy and precision. In their Research Plan for Radiation Oncology (2) the Committee on Radiation Oncology Studies identified the problem of uncertainties in tumor localization as a critical issue in the goal of uncomplicated local tumor control.

THE NEED FOR ULTRASOUND

Much of the progress made in radiotherapy in recent years has been the result of a broad base of improvements rather than any major "breakthrough." These include increased knowledge of the malignant diseases, better training of the radiotherapy "team," and improved instrumentation for treatment planning and delivery of treatment. The application of the computer to treatment planning has had a major impact on the methods of calculating radiation dose and

depicting its distribution within the tissues of the treatment volume. However, methods for similarly depicting the patient's anatomy and tumor location were not available until recently. The ability of ultrasound and computed axial tomography scanning to produce an accurate cross-section outline of the body and at the same time to image the tumor and critical structures in that plane, has provided an important ingredient in treatment planning.

There is not much logic in applying the talents of a radiotherapist, radiation physicist, dosimetrist, and computer to produce a sophisticated display of dose distribution for a treatment plan—unless the confines of the tumor are well demonstrated. In one study of a group of 51 patients with large abdominal or pelvic tumors, 61% were shown by ultrasound examination to have extension of tumor beyond the confines of previously set radiation therapy ports (3).

The question as to which patients need ultrasound imaging for aid in planning and treating has to be answered on an individual basis. Some of course, do not need it at all; others may need only a simple outline contour. The other end of the spectrum includes the patient who needs body contours at several levels, containing a display of accurately localized tumor and pertinent vital organs. This may include precise localization of both kidneys in prone and supine positions. Repeat imaging of tumor and kidneys may be indicated during a long treatment course to ensure continued reproducibility of the treatment plan or to reduce the treatment volume as the tumor shrinks.

An outline of the possible uses of ultrasound imaging in the course of a radiotherapy program is shown in Table 18.1.

Table 18.1.
Uses of ultrasound in radiotherapy practice

A. Treatment planning
   1. Patient contour
   2. Measurements for dosimetry
   3. Tumor localization
   4. Staging disease
   5. Critical organ localization
   6. Therapy field placement
B. Tumor response
   1. Regression rate during treatment
   2. Regression maximum
C. Follow-up
   1. Persistence or local recurrence
   2. New disease sites

OTHER TUMOR IMAGING METHODS

There are, of course, other methods or modalities for tumor imaging, which are either in use or being developed (4):

Conventional transverse axial tomography

Arteriography

Radionuclide tumor imaging (technetium liver, bone, and brain scans; gallium scan; radioselenium pancreas scan; radioiodine thyroid scan; renal scan)

Simultaneous radionuclide subtraction scanning

Multiplane isotope tomography

Emission transaxial reconstruction tomography

Nuclear magnetic resonance (NMR)

Radiolabeled antibodies for tumor imaging

Computed axial tomography (CAT or CT scan)

Many of these methods can provide very useful diagnostic tumor information and oftentimes help in tumor detection and staging. However, CT scanning is the only method listed which can rather consistently provide the range of treatment planning data needed (5–7). There is a wide area of overlap between CT scanning and ultrasound scanning in terms of their ability to provide the information needed. Each has its limitations and advantages in certain circumstances. Ideally, both methods of imaging should be available to the radiotherapist, since there are times when CT scanning would be preferred. Fortunately, the strong points of the two modalities tend to complement each other. Thus, CT scanning is generally effective in the very obese abdomen, where ultrasound often encounters problems in imaging. Bowel gas also may prevent satisfactory intra-abdominal imaging with ultrasound but does not hinder CT. Other conditions which may require the use of CT scans include those instances in which bone or air prevents penetration of the ultrasound beam. Because of the generally excellent quality of the images of CT scans and the associated tissue density data available from the scans, it is becoming commonplace to use them in many of the larger treatment planning facilities (8, 9).

There are several features of the ultrasound modality which often make it the method of choice for obtaining treatment planning information. It is a harmless, noninvasive procedure of relatively low cost, with ready availability to the patient, generally without need for preparation before scanning. The inherent flexibility of the method makes it easy to obtain scans in a variety of planes as needed and in a short period of time. It is also the simplest and most direct means of correlating images of deep structures with external skin landmarks. In the situation where either method could provide the required information, ultrasound may be preferable because of the features listed in Table 18.2.

TREATMENT PLANNING PROCEDURE

Visualization of the tumor with the ultrasound beam is done either to check the coverage of treatment skin portals already laid out or for

Table 18.2.
Comparison of ultrasound and whole body CT in abdominal and pelvic imaging for radiation therapy purposes

	Ultrasound	Body CT
Instrument cost	Medium	High
Procedure cost	Medium	High
Availability to patient	Fair to good	Probably poor
Flexibility	Good	Poor
Radiation exposure	No	Yes
Invasive procedure	No	Sometimes
Operator skills required	Yes	No
Image formation time	1 to several seconds	2–20 seconds
Contour, any	Good	Fair to good
Bowel gas interferes	Yes	No
Imaging obese patient	Fair to poor	May be good
Imaging thin patient	Good	Poor to good
Tissue density data	No	Yes

the purpose of initially setting up the skin fields. If indicated, the images of the tumor and the pertinent normal organs can be depicted within the contour and recorded on either a Polaroid print or a film transparency. This may then be enlarged to life size by merely projecting the scan with an overhead projector (transparency) or "opaque" projector (Polaroid print).

If the scan information is to be entered into a computerized treatment planning system, the dosimetrist traces the image with a graphic digitizer either from the small print itself (Fig. 18.1*A*) or from the enlarged projected image (Fig. 18.1*B*). Other nongraphic data are entered via the computer terminal keyboard.

With the computer programmed with dosimetry data from the specific high energy therapy machine being used (Telecobalt, linear accelerator, Betatron, etc.), a graphic representation of the radiation beam for each therapy port can be displayed on the cathode ray screen (Fig. 18.2). On the screen the beams are placed in proper orientation with a contour of the patient made at the level of the tumor, and the computer program will provide a composite of the radiation distribution summated from all treatment ports. The computer program takes into account the alteration of the beam by such things as: different field sizes; a beam striking the body surface obliquely rather than straight on; irregular body surfaces within the treatment port; and, finally, planned alterations provided by wedge-shaped radiation-absorbing filters placed within the treatment beam. The final image includes the patient's contour along with position and size of treatment portals, the outline of the apparent tumor-bearing volume and pertinent critical normal organs, and the composite distribution of radiation dose from all treatment portals. A computerized print-out of this image on paper (hard copy) in accurate life size is then produced by a digital plotter (Figs. 18.3 and 18.4).

INSTRUCTING THE ULTRASONOGRAPHER

Because the kinds of information needed for purposes of treatment planning tend to differ from the usual diagnostic ultrasound information, it is imperative that the ultrasonographer be properly instructed in the special requirements and techniques. Until that has been accomplished, a member of the radiotherapy team should be in attendance during the scanning.

For treatment planning purposes the sonographer must be concerned not so much with details of the internal structures of organs and masses as with precise location and relationships. Sometimes the use of "leading edge" or "bi-stable" mode is preferable to gray-scale imaging in outlining a structure. Current scanning machines allow one to switch back and forth easily between these modes.

The scanning instrument should be calibrated at frequent intervals in order to maintain the degree of accuracy needed for therapy planning purposes and reproducibility of scan images made at different times. With reference to measurements made from scans done on a scan converter unit, the centimeter marker should be recorded *in the region of and close to the plane and direction of* the measurement. A measurement made horizontally across the image cannot be referred to a centimeter marker recorded vertically in the scan, because there is distortion due to the TV mode of scan converter screens.

Scans should be properly identified and precisely labeled as to direction and tilt of the plane and relationship to external landmarks (such as scars, umbilicus, pubis, xiphoid, midline, etc.). This is for information purposes and possible future attempts to reproduce them. For proper labeling of scans refer to the official recommendations drawn up by the Standards Committee of the American Institute of Ultrasound in Medicine (AIUM) (10). In some cases, for optimum clarity, it is desirable to indicate the scan planes and skin landmarks on a drawing of the external body surface (Fig. 18.5).

The use of the optimum transducer for the particular imaging problem (i.e., frequency, diameter, focus length) requires that a good selection be available. For obtaining contours on irregular or sharply curved skin surfaces, a small diameter transducer is helpful.

OBTAINING THE BODY CONTOUR

The standard method for obtaining a radiation therapy patient's body contour at the level of interest formerly consisted of molding a lead wire or a strip of plaster of Paris around the body and then transferring it to a sheet of transparent paper (Fig. 18.6). The tumor and pertinent critical organs were then drawn in, their size and location being deduced from whatever information was available, plus the use of cross-sectional anatomy books. This time-consuming

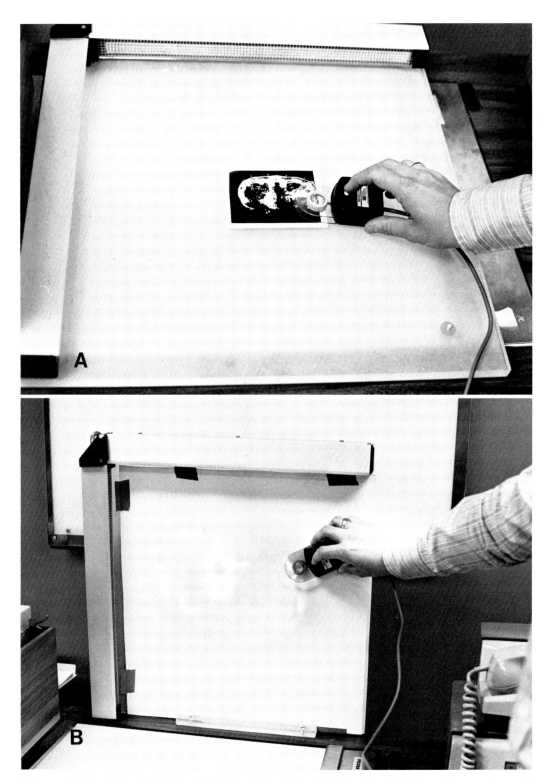

Figure 18.1. *A*, Sonic digitizer in horizontal position. A Polaroid print of an ultrasound scan is laid on the digitizer, and the patient's contour and other pertinent structures are traced from the image with the Graf Pen. This enters the graphic information into the treatment planning computer, which then displays this information on the cathode ray screen. *B*, The sonic digitizer can also be placed in the upright position, so that the ultrasound or CT scan image can be projected onto it life size. The correct amount of enlargement is determined by using the centimeter marker on the scan. Tracing with the Graf Pen from this large image is somewhat more accurate than tracing directly from the original Polaroid.

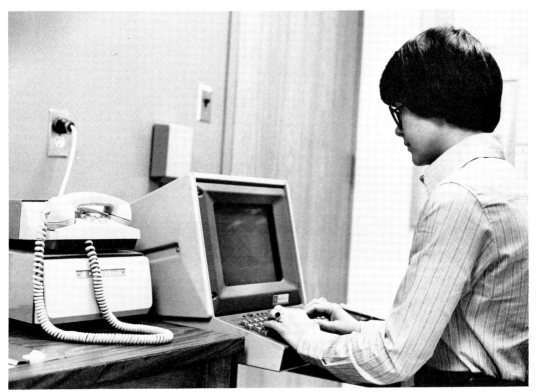

Figure 18.2. The dosimetrist enters nongraphic data into the computer via the keyboard of the computer terminal pictured here. A computer-generated treatment plan is seen on the cathode ray display screen.

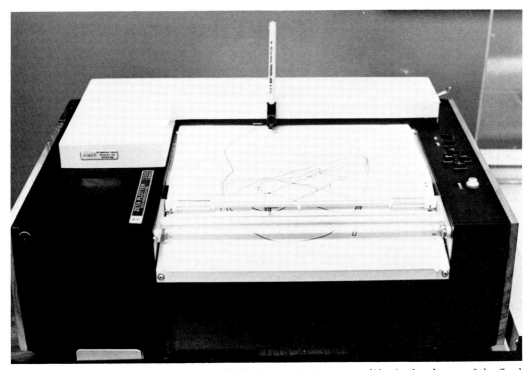

Figure 18.3. The incremental plotter (digital plotter) prints out a life-size hard copy of the final approved treatment plan as it appears on the cathode ray display screen.

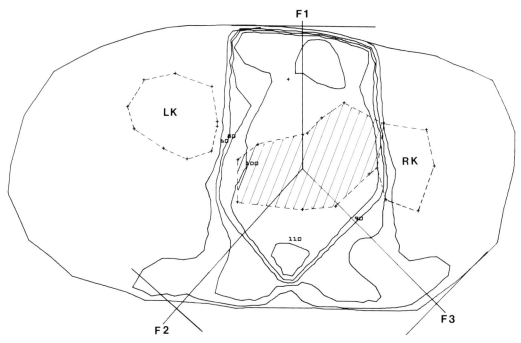

Figure 18.4. Computer-generated treatment plan. This "hard copy" life-size print-out was produced by the digital plotter in Figure 18.3. It depicts the dose distribution from a three-field (*F1, F2, F3*) treatment plan for the tumor (*shaded*) while sparing the kidneys (*RK, LK*). The body cross-sectional contour and the location of the tumor and kidneys were provided by ultrasound scanning. The format of the ultrasound image lends itself well to computerized treatment planning.

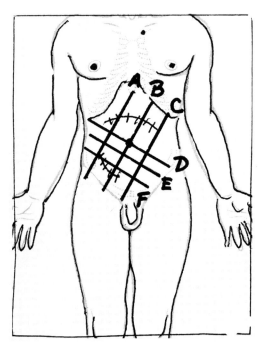

Figure 18.5. Body outline showing the location and direction of six different scan planes (*A* through *F*). Also shown are two scars and the umbilicus—used as landmarks. The use of such drawings is helpful when the pertinent scans are in other than transverse or sagittal planes.

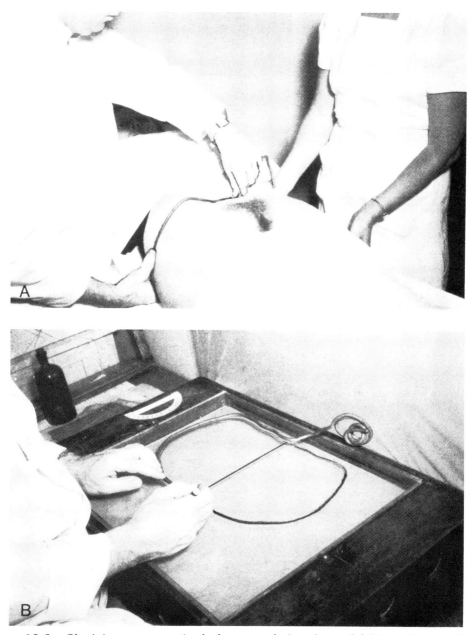

Figure 18.6. Obtaining a cross-section body contour before the availability of ultrasound or CT imaging. *A*, Lead wire or a strip of plaster of Paris was molded around the body and then traced (*B*) on a sheet of treatment planning paper. The accuracy of this method was limited.

procedure can now be done quickly with an ultrasound scan and with far greater accuracy.

Certain precautions need to be taken in this apparently simple procedure. If only the contour is needed, without display of deep structures, the gain can be turned down to eliminate internal echoes. Care has to be taken not to depress the tissues with the transducer, thus reducing the accuracy of the contour. Also, when the location of a skin landmark or therapy field is to be indicated on the contour (either by registering the centimeter marker line or by lifting the transducer off the skin), the center of the transducer face must be exactly over the landmark point. The scan table surface on which the patient is lying should also be indicated. This will correspond to the therapy treatment couch surface in the treatment planning. Of course, the patient should be in the same position for scan as he will be for his treatment, and this includes the position of the arms (alongside the head or down by the side). Considerable move-

ment of chest or abdominal skin can occur with change in arm position. Generally, the contour is made at the level of the center of the treatment field, but other planes may be needed, too. Figure 18.7 demonstrates the change in configuration of the contour between prone and supine positions. The shape of the contour at the entrance site of a treatment port significantly af-

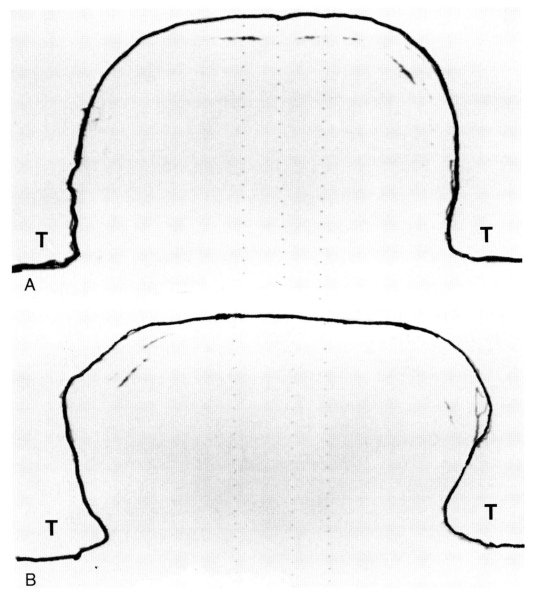

Figure 18.7. Body contour obtained with ultrasound scan. *A*, Supine. *B*, Prone. The gain is turned down to eliminate internal echo information. Note the change in configuration between prone and supine, making it necessary to use the prone contour for posterior fields and the supine contour for anterior fields. The table top is routinely recorded (*T*) for treatment planning purposes.

fects the distribution of radiation in the treatment volume; therefore, the appropriate contour should be used for anterior or posterior ports.

KIDNEY LOCALIZATION (11)

In abdominal tumor irradiation, the normal organ most often of concern in treatment planning is the kidney (one or both). The known radiation dose tolerance in terms of preventing radiation nephritis varies with how much of one or both kidneys are irradiated. Therefore, precise localization is often needed for purposes of shielding all or a part of one or both kidneys. This usually requires the projection of the kidney outline onto the skin surface. While the kidney can be localized by radioisotope scans or by reference to intravenous pyelogram (IVP) radiographs, we have found that the ultrasound technique is clearly most accurate and associated with the fewest potential errors (Fig. 18.8). Localization is done with the patient in treatment position (prone or supine) and with the arms in treatment position. Since the kidneys move significantly with respiration, and since the patient is in a state of *passive expiration* for the majority of the time during quiet respiration, that is the kidney position which should be drawn on the skin. The kidney also moves in changing from prone to supine position, so a prone localization will not suffice for anterior treatment beams (12). It is advisable to recheck the kidney localization once in a while during a treatment course of several weeks, since the skin marks sometimes have a tendency to shift as they are remarked from time to time. A hand-held real-time scanner is a quick way to check this, although it is not very suitable for doing the initial detailed localization.

When a kidney has to be within the treatment volume because of the proximity of malignant tissue, the radiation dose to the kidney can be kept within tolerance limits by introducing a "kidney block" in the radiation beam. Generally this requires blocking only in the *posterior* treatment beam and not in the opposing anterior beam. The first step is to do a prone scan and mark the outline of the kidney on the skin. The location of the central axis of the treatment beam is also marked on the skin. A thin sheet of transparent Plexiglas or a cleared x-ray film is placed on the patient's back, and the skin marks are traced on it. The subsequent steps have to do with determining the proper size block to be made and its proper location within the treatment beam (13). This includes correct-

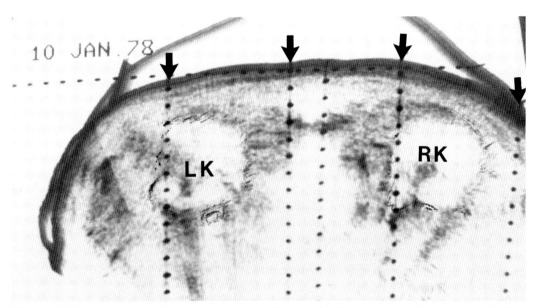

Figure 18.8. Kidney localization, comparing ultrasound with isotope renal scan method. This prone transverse sonic scan demonstrates the true positions of the kidneys (*LK* and *RK*), which do not jibe with the skin marks (*arrows*) placed at the time of isotope renal scan kidney localization. Errors like this are not likely to occur when using *ultrasound* to project the kidney location onto the skin surface.

ing for parallax which occurs as a result of the central axis of the treatment beam not being directly over the kidney.

PROSTATE TREATMENT PLANNING

There are several methods of localizing the prostate gland for radiation treatment including standard transverse CT scans (14, 15), transverse and longitudinal abdominal sonic scans (16), and even a digital rectal technique (17) in which a wire device is taped to the examining rectal finger and used to mark the cephalad and caudad margins of the gland on the anterior skin. There are times when the prostate gland cannot be adequately visualized with angled transverse and longitudinal abdominal scanning, with a full bladder. This is especially apt to be true with the obese patient or one who has had a recent lower abdominal or suprapubic incision. In that case, before deciding to switch to CT for localization of the gland, it is worth trying a longitudinal mid-line scan that is carried down into the perineum. The perineal portion of the scan will frequently fill in the image of the prostate, demonstrating its cephalocaudad and anteroposterior extent. This technique is particularly useful if a direct perineal treatment port is to be used. The scan would be done in the lithotomy position, coinciding with the radiation therapy treatment position (Fig. 18.9). If lateral ports are to be used, the image obtained on the longitudinal mid-line scan is sufficient to locate the ports, providing the scan was obtained with the legs flat.

TESTICULAR TUMORS AND RETROPERITONEAL NODES

Following surgical removal of a seminoma of the testicle, the para-aortic node regions are generally treated through anterior and posterior ports. This can usually be done with a field narrow enough to fit between the kidneys without problem. However, if there are any enlarged nodal masses, kidney localization may be indicated as well as localization of the retroperitoneal masses themselves (Fig. 18.10). When treating these large nodal masses—especially in the case of radiosensitive tumors, such as seminoma and lymphoma—serial scans during the treatment course may demonstrate sufficient shrinkage to allow reduction in treatment field size (Figs. 18.11 and 18.12).

CHEST WALL AND ABDOMINAL WALL TUMORS

Tumors within the wall of the thorax or abdomen are apt to be either metastatic or locally recurrent (e.g., a renal carcinoma recurrent in the flank incision). These superficial tumors are treated either straight-on with a single radiation port, or tangentially with two opposing beams. In either case, contour and tumor imaging is helpful. With a single port it is necessary to know the margins of the gross disease (which often exceeds the palpable boundaries) (Fig. 18.13) and the depth or thickness of the mass. Tangential treatment planning requires additional information (Fig. 18.14) in order that proper beam angles, field separation, and dose calculations can be made. Ultrasound provides this information very nicely (18).

RENAL TUMORS

Planning for treatment of the primary site of a renal tumor calls for a contour at appropriate levels, containing the tumor localization and showing its relationship with the spine and diaphragm and opposite kidney. If it is a right-sided tumor, the liver should also be imaged. Treatment of these tumors may entail a fairly complex arrangement of multiple radiation fields and special devices such as beam blocks and wedge filters, in order to limit the radiation dose to the opposite kidney, spinal cord, and liver. The computerized treatment planning system is a great help in optimizing the dosimetry in a complex problem of this sort.

BLADDER TUMORS

The bladder is easily imaged providing it contains fluid. The bladder base is not as easily visualized as the remainder, and one may have to incorporate information from IVP or cystogram. Also one must keep in mind how full or empty the bladder will be during treatment (usually empty). This becomes especially important if a small treatment volume is to be used and if multiple field arrangements (e.g., three-field, four-field box) are planned. A Foley bag pulled down against the base of the bladder can readily be seen on sonic scan and helps to localize the base.

RENAL TRANSPLANT

Radiation therapy is often given to a transplanted kidney when evidence of active rejection

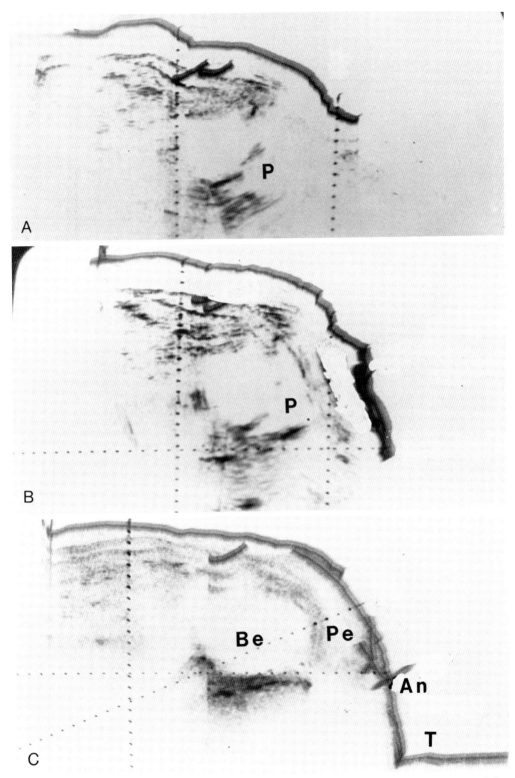

Figure 18.9. Prostate localization for treatment planning. *A*, Longitudinal mid-line transabdominal scan has failed to visualize the caudal extent of the prostate (*P*). However, with the patient in lithotomy position (*B*) the lower portion of the gland has been filled in by adding direct perineal scanning along with abdominal. *C*, This is a similar scan in a patient who has had a prostatectomy and is to receive radiation to the prostate bed via a perineal field. *An*, anus; *Pe*, base of penis; *T*, table top; *Be*, bladder.

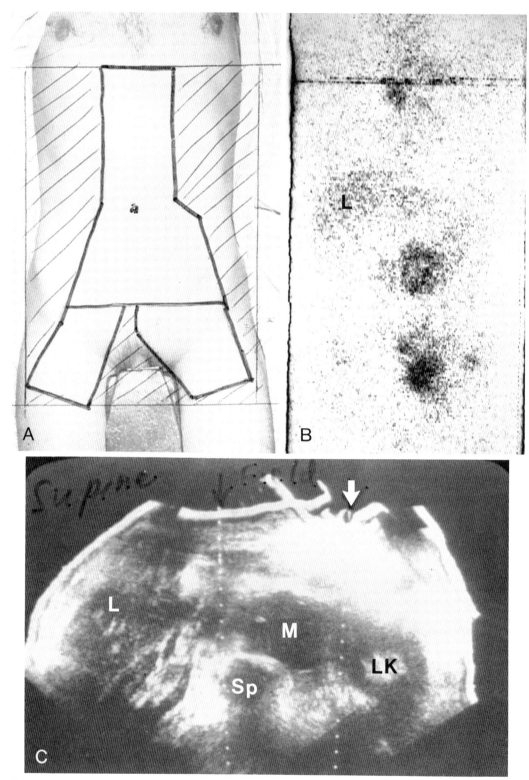

Figure 18.10. Seminoma of the left testicle, postorchiectomy. The tentative anterior treatment portal was set up as shown in *A* to encompass a palpable left lower quadrant metastatic mass. Subsequent gallium scan (*B*) shows metastatic nodes in right mediastinum and left para-aortic areas as well. Supine sonic scan (*C*) shows the para-aortic mass (*M*) to displace and somewhat overlap the left kidney (*LK*). Therefore, the left margin (*arrow*) of the field was widened to include the kidney, and a kidney block was placed in the beam of the posterior field. *L*, liver; *Sp*, spine.

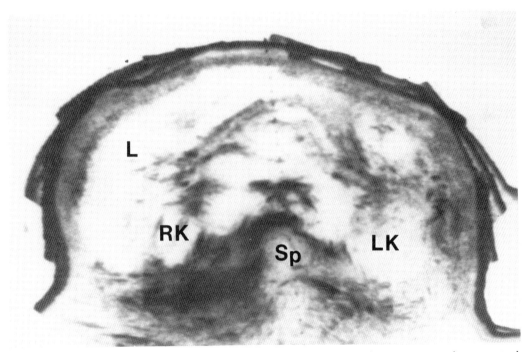

Figure 18.11.   Transverse supine upper abdominal sonic scan demonstrates a large central lobulated node mass (lymphosarcoma) and a smaller 3 × 5 cm mass in the left anterior abdomen, overlying the left kidney (*LK*). The right kidney (*RK*) is displaced laterally. Although this disease is relatively sensitive to radiation, it will be necessary to use a left kidney block in the posterior treatment beam to reduce the dose to that organ. Repeat scans during the treatment course may allow reduction in field size and may show a need for a change in location of the kidney block as the tumor shrinks. *L*, liver; *Sp*, spine.

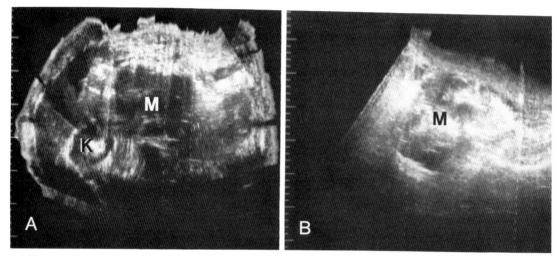

Figure 18.12.   Upper abdominal metastatic mass from renal cell carcinoma previously treated by left nephrectomy. Supine transverse (*A*) and longitudinal (*B*) sonic scans and transverse CT scan (*C*) clearly demonstrate the location of the mass (*M*) and its relationship to the remaining right kidney (*K*). The CT scan has a "starburst" artifact caused by the presence of metallic surgical clips. The row of catheters of unequal length which is projected over the right abdomen in the abdominal film (*D*) is a cumbersome method of figuring out the level at which each CT cut was made. These are shown in cross-section on the skin (*C, arrows*). The two sonic scans provide the three-dimensional limits of the mass and its relation to the kidney and skin surface such that a treatment plan can be developed.

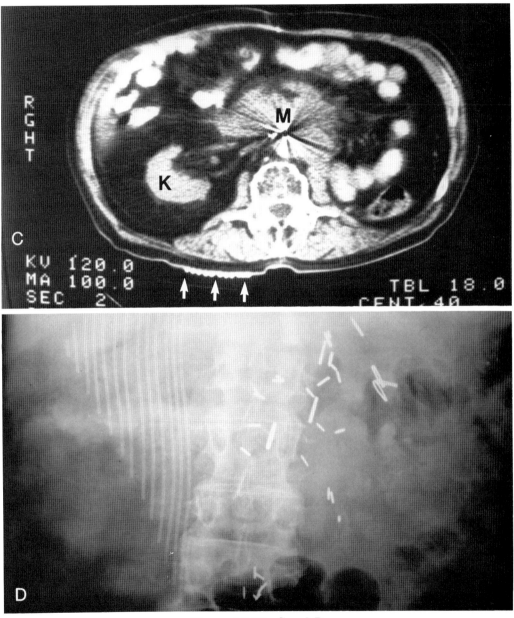

Figure 18.12, *C* and *D*.

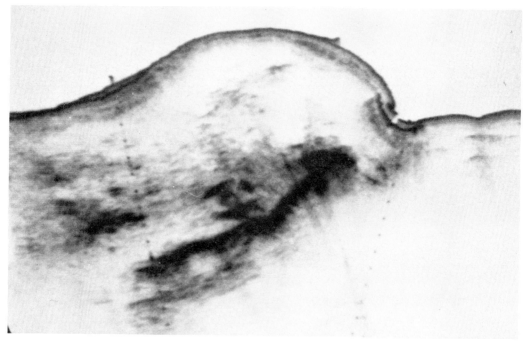

Figure 18.13.   Sonic scan of abdominal wall metastatic tumor. The centimeter markers indicate the location of the skin marks for a single straight-on radiotherapy field, which was initially set up by palpation only. The scan shows that the tumor actually extends 5 or 6 cm beyond one of the field margins.

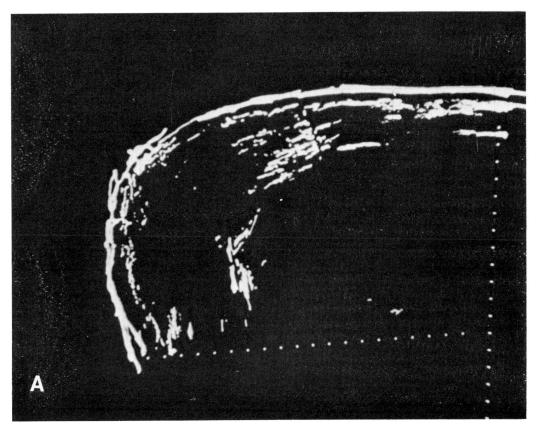

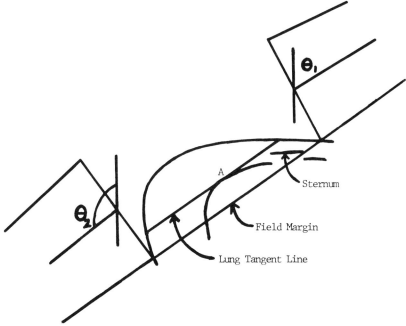

B

Figure 18.14. *A*, Sonic scan of chest wall made for treatment planning and dosimetry purposes. The chest wall tissues are to be treated with opposing tangential radiation beams. The junction of the centimeter marker line with the skin indicates the point at which the edge of the beam strikes the skin. The large echo-free area (*right*) is lung tissue. This scan was made with "leading edge" (bi-stable) mode. *B*, Pertinent information from the sonic scan in *A* is used for dosimetry calculations. It also demonstrates the amount of lung in the irradiated volume.

appears. Although the radiation dose used is relatively small and would not constitute a hazard to the normal tissues in that region, one would like to confine the radiation to the kidney as much as possible. Also, the depth of the organ from the anterior skin surface is useful information for dose calculations. Ultrasound is a simple, consistently effective method of getting the location, size, and depth even in the immediate postoperative period (Fig. 18.15).

On occasion a pararenal fluid collection may be unexpectedly demonstrated when the transplanted kidney is scanned (19). This finding is of real importance to the transplant surgeon, who must take appropriate measures to manage this complication.

CONCLUSION

A growing number of radiotherapists are reporting the value of ultrasound and CT imaging in the planning, management, and response assessment of radiation treatment (20–24). The application of the computer to radiation treatment planning provided the means for highly accurate and sophisticated calculation and display of dose distribution in complex treatment plans. However, until the arrival of these two imaging modalities, the weak link in the chain of data input has been the demonstration of the extent of the disease and its anatomical relationship to vital normal structures. We now have the means of providing this vital information in the majority of cases in which it is needed. The development of both ultrasound and CT imaging will certainly continue at a rapid pace, bringing still further applicability in the practice of radiation oncology. At the present time the choice between the two modalities often goes to ultrasound—based on its advantages of flexibility, absence of radiation exposure, availability, cost, and noninvasiveness.

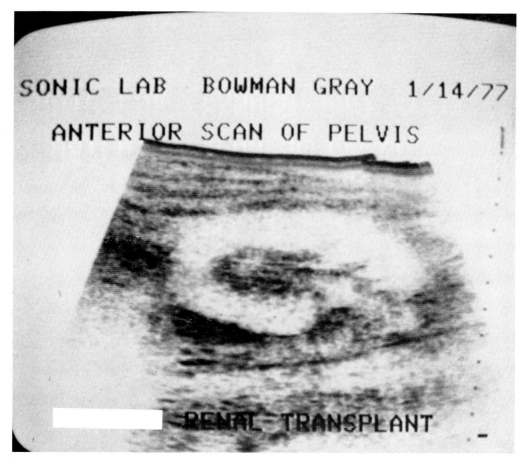

Figure 18.15. Renal transplant in right lower quadrant. Scan is along the long axis of the kidney. Note the echo-free cortex and echogenic collecting system and the absence of any perirenal fluid collection. The anterior surface of the kidney is only 2 cm beneath the skin.

References

1. Bogardus CR Jr, Buchanan WD, Fuller DE, Travis JN, Wizenberg MJ: Standard nomenclature for the conduct of a course in radiation therapy. *Appl Radiol* 6:113, 1977.
2. Research Plan for Radiation Oncology. *Cancer,* suppl 37:2031, 1976.
3. Carter SJ, Denney JD, Tesh DW, Marty R, Davis MC: Ultrasonic evaluation of radiation therapy ports. *J Clin Ultrasound* 5:103, 1977.
4. Maruyama Y: *New Methods in Tumor Localization.* Lexington, University of Kentucky Press, 1977.
5. Stewart JR, Hicks JA, Boone MLM, Simpson LD: Computed tomography in radiation therapy (Report of the Committee on Radiation Oncology Studies Subcommittee on CT Scanning and Radiation Therapy). *Int J Radiat Oncol Biol Phys* 4:313, 1978.
6. Jaffe CC, Simonds BD: Computed tomography and ultrasound of the abdomen: diagnostic implications of the imaging process. *Appl Radiol* 7:81, 1978.
7. Brascho D: Radiation therapy planning with ultrasound. *Radiol Clin North Am* 13:505, 1975.
8. Battista JJ, Van Dyk J, Rider WD: Practical aspects of radiotherapy planning with computed tomography. *Clin Invest Med* 4:5, 1981.
9. Spanos WJ Jr, Hogstrom KR: An overview of radiation therapy planning systems. *Appl Radiol* 11:69, 1982.
10. American Institute of Ultrasound in Medicine standard presentation and labeling of ultrasound images. AIUM Standards Committee. *J Clin Ultrasound* 5:103, 1977.
11. Sanders R, Hughes B, Hazra T: Ultrasound localization of kidney for radiation therapy. *Br J Radiol* 47:196, 1974.
12. Ball WS, Wicks JD, Mettler FA Jr: Prone-supine change in organ position: CT demonstration. *AJR* 135:815, 1980.
13. Reitan JB, Skretting A, Aas M, Stafto S: A simple method for localization and shielding of organs in a diverging radiation treatment beam. *Br J Radiol* 53:802, 1980.
14. Brizel HE, Livingston PA, Grayson EV: Radiotherapeutic applications of pelvic computed tomography. *J Comput Assist Tomogr* 3:453, 1979.
15. Pilepich MV, Prasad SC, Perez CA: Computed tomography in definitive radiotherapy of prostatic carcinoma. Part 2. Definition of target volume. *Int J Radiat Oncol Biol Phys* 8:235, 1982.
16. Lee DJ, Leibel S, Shiels R, Sanders R, Siegelman S, Onder S: The value of ultrasonic imaging and CT scanning in planning the radiotherapy for prostatic carcinoma. *Cancer* 45:724, 1980.
17. Kademian MT, Asp LW, Glassner J: A new device for prostate localization in radiotherapy treatment planning. *Radiology* 135:522, 1980.
18. Ekstrand KE, Dixon RL, Blake DD, Raven M: The calculation of dose distribution for chest wall irradiation using B-mode ultrasonography. *Radiology* 111:185, 1974.
19. Nesbit R, Blake DD, Ekstrand KE, James PM Jr: Lymphocele following renal transplantation: value of ultrasonography in diagnostic and follow-up studies. *South Med J* 69:303, 1976.
20. Munzenrider JE, Pilepich M, Rene-Ferrero JB, Tchakarova I, Carter BL: Use of body scanner in radiotherapy treatment planning. *Cancer* 40:170, 1977.
21. Banjavic RA, Zagzebski JA, Wiley AL, Tolbert DD: A projection system for effective utilization of ultrasound echogram information in radiation therapy. *Radiology* 116:731, 1975.
22. Denney JD, Carter SJ, Tesh DW, Marty R: Evaluation of abdominal and pelvic tumors in radiation therapy: efficacy of diagnostic ultrasound. *Appl Radiol* 6:145, 1977.
23. Brascho DJ, Shawker TH: *Abdominal Ultrasound in the Cancer Patient.* New York, John Wiley & Sons, 1980.
24. Paling MR, Shawker TH, Dwyer A: Ultrasonic evaluation of therapeutic response in tumors: its value and implications. *J Clin Ultrasound* 9:281, 1981.

Suggested Readings

Banjavic RA, Tolbert DD, Zagzebski JA: Ultracomp: a computerized operating system for effective radiotherapy treatment planning. *Appl Radiol* 6:135, 1977.
Blake DD: Ultrasonography in the practice of radiotherapy. *Appl Radiol* 8:112, 1979.
Carson PL, Wenzel WW, Avery P, Hendee WR: Ultrasound imaging as an aid to cancer therapy. I and II. *Int J Radiat Oncol Biol Phys* 1:119, 335, 1975.
Gorham J: Relationship between ultrasound and computed tomography in whole-body scans. *Appl Radiol* 7:129, 1978.
Kratochwil A: Treatment planning. *Clin Diagn Ultrasound* 6:167, 1981.
Sanders R, James AE: *Principal and Practice of Ultrasonography in Obstetrics and Gynecology,* ed 2. New York, Appleton-Century-Crofts, 1980.
Sternick ES, Lane FW, Curran B: Comparison of computed tomography and conventional transverse axial tomography in radiotherapy treatment planning. *Radiology* 124:835, 1977.

CHAPTER 19

Dynamic Evaluation of the Lower Urinary Tract

ROLFE D. WHITE, M.D.
DAVID L. WILLIAMS, M.D.

Lower urinary tract function requires a sequence of changes in normal anatomy and anatomical relationships coordinated by a series of voluntary and involuntary movements. These changes do not lend themselves to easy analysis. Currently, radiological techniques are utilized to define these anatomical relationships.

Lower urinary tract dysfunction may be complex, at times having a multifactorial etiology. In addition to the history, physical examination, and basic laboratory tests, urodynamic testing and radiological evaluation are frequently indicated. Urodynamic testing may include cystourethroscopy, cystourethrometrics, uroflowmetry, urethral pressure profiles, and electromyography. Radiological procedures include the intravenous pyelogram, cystometrogram, distention urethrogram, voiding cystourethrogram, and bead chain cystourethrogram. Some of these studies may be replaced or augmented by dynamic real-time ultrasonography performed in a hospital, clinic, or office setting (Fig. 19.12). Portable ultrasound units may even be taken to the patient's bedside or the operating room. High resolution real-time transducers can give the clinician information which previously was less easily obtained (1). Mass production has brought the cost of real-time ultrasound equipment to a level affordable by many clinicians and small hospitals.

This chapter describes how dynamic real-time ultrasonography may rapidly, safely, and accurately be utilized to augment the evaluation of the patient with lower urinary tract symptoms. The illustrations presented were obtained with the portable Advanced Diagnostics Research Model 2130 Linear Array Scanner, Model 2140 Sector Scanner, and Model 4000 Sector/Linear Array Scanner (Fig. 19.1).

URINARY INCONTINENCE

Urinary incontinence is a common entity which may require a detailed urodynamic evaluation in order to define the precise etiology and best mode of therapy (Table 19.1).

True anatomical stress incontinence is the most common etiology of incontinence in women; however, bladder instability and various types of neurogenic incontinence are also encountered. In children, urinary incontinence may be the result of primary enuresis, neurogenic bladder dysfunction, lower tract obstruction, or other causes (2). The incidence of urinary incontinence in hospitalized elderly patients has been reported to be from 13 to 49%. Although the majority of these patients have some degree of uninhibited neurogenic bladder dysfunction, there may be other etiologies or complicating factors involved (3).

True anatomical stress urinary incontinence is caused by loss of support to the bladder and the urethrovesical junction. Tanagho has effectively demonstrated how simple cystography may supply important information which will aid in the diagnosis and, if appropriate, the surgical correction of this disorder. With the patient lying supine, lateral cystourethrograms are done at rest and with the Valsalva maneuver. Tanagho has described the normal posterior descent of the urethrovesical junction (UVJ) to be between 0.5 and 1.5 cm. A female patient who has not had prior bladder surgery, but who has true anatomical stress urinary incontinence (SUI), should demonstrate a greater measurable descent. If not, this diagnosis should be reconsidered (4; E. A. Tanagho, personal communication, 1983). A modified version of this technique can be applied using portable real-time ultrasonography (6). Ultrasound evaluation of 110 normal female volunteers and over 50 patients with true anatomical stress urinary incontinence confirmed Tanagho's cystographic findings of a measurable descent of the urethrovesical junction (see Table 19.2).

In a typical ultrasound study, the patient arrives for the examination with a full bladder and

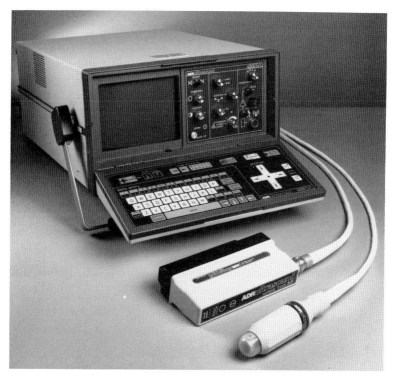

Figure 19.1. ADR 4000 S/L real-time ultrasound system.

Table 19.1.
Evaluation of urinary incontinence

History	Ultrasound
Physical examination	Intravenous pyelogram, voiding cystourethrogram, bead cystogram
Urinalysis	
Urine culture	Uroflowmetry
Cystometrics	Urethral pressure profile
Cystourethroscopy	Electromyography

Table 19.2.

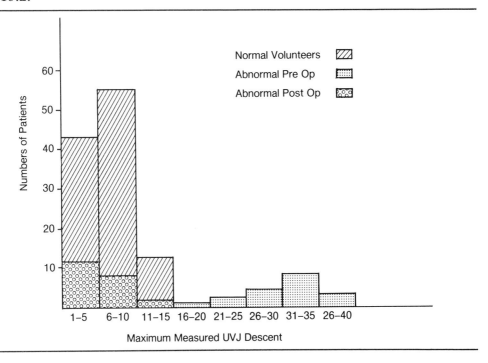

assumes the supine position. The sector or linear array transducer is positioned mid-ventrally and aimed caudad beneath the pubic symphysis (Figs. 19.2 and 19.3) (5). If the urethrovesical junction cannot be positively identified, a clamped 6 or 8 French soft plastic pediatric feeding tube is introduced through the urethra into the bladder (Figs. 19.4 to 19.6). This catheter is used because it conforms well to the urethra and is associated with minimal, if any, discomfort. Other catheters may be utilized if ultrasonography is performed with simultaneous urodynamic studies. Approximately one-third of these patients require no retention of the catheter, as manual oscillation of the catheter allows the sonographer to rapidly locate the UVJ with the transducer. The patient is then asked to perform the Valsalva maneuver. Descent of the UVJ is measured with electronic calipers from its resting position to the point of maximal descent or to the point that the UVJ is lost on the scanner TV screen (Figs. 19.7 to 19.9). A record of the examination is obtained with a Polaroid or videotape technique.

Difficulties can be encountered in obese patients with linear array transducers because with the Valsalva maneuver the recti displace the transducer, preventing proper visualization of the UVJ. The UVJ may be obscured by pubic symphysis shadowing. However, in such patients with true SUI, the bladder base can almost always be followed to a descent of greater than 20 mm, and, thus, a significant anatomical defect can be adequately demonstrated. The new small sector transducers aimed caudad beneath the pubic symphysis allow the sonographer a better view of the UVJ during these maneuvers (Figs. 19.2 and 19.3). Their improved resolution also more frequently allows identification of the urethra without catheterization.

The majority of patients with significant SUI have a bladder base descent of more than 30 mm. Twenty of these patients have had retropubic colpocystourethropexys with absorbable suture material performed with the same technique. Preoperatively, all had more than 15 mm of UVJ descent (Figs. 19.8 to 19.10). All were evaluated again over 3 months after their sur-

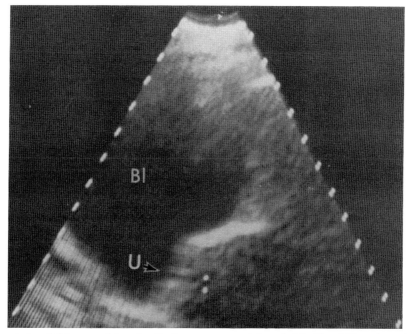

Figure 19.2. Mid-ventral longitudinal sector scan of female bladder (*Bl*) and urethra (*U*).

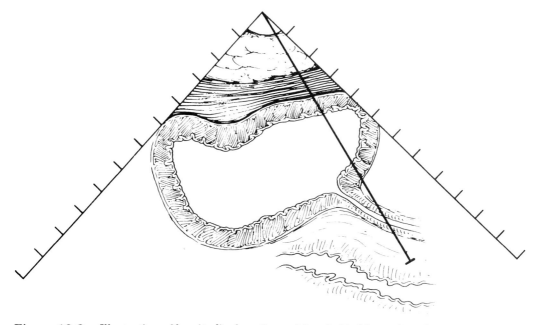

Figure 19.3. Illustration of longitudinal sections of female bladder and urethra in Figure 19.2.

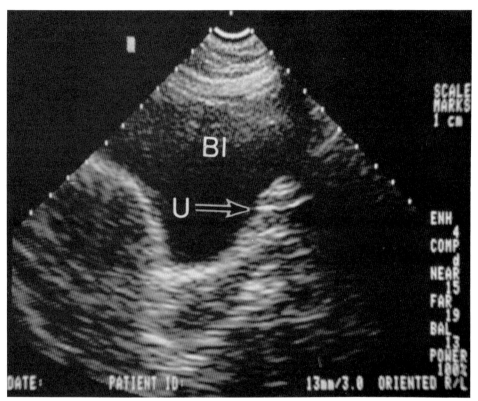

Figure 19.4. Mid-ventral sector scan of bladder (*Bl*) and urethra (*U*) with 7 French pediatric feeding tube within the urethra (*arrow*).

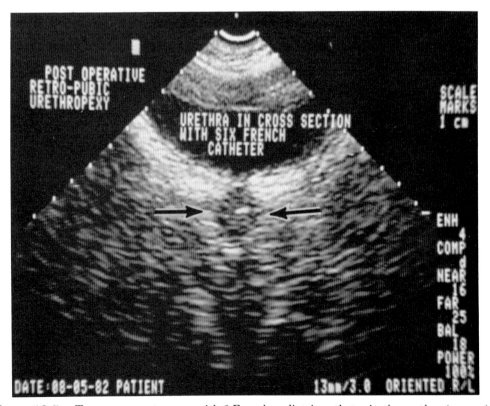

Figure 19.5. Transverse sector scan with 6 French pediatric catheter in the urethra (*arrows*).

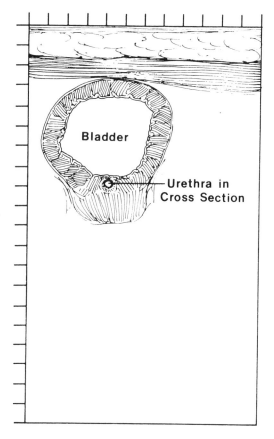

Figure 19.6. Transverse diagram of bladder and urethra.

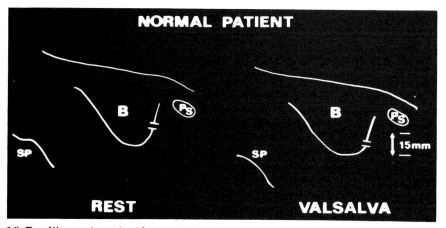

Figure 19.7. Illustration of mid-ventral longitudinal scan showing minimal descent of bladder and urethrovesical junction in normal continent patient.

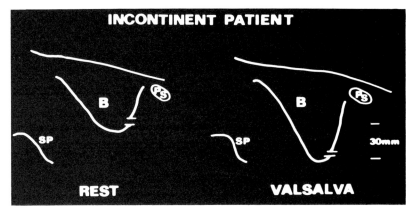

Figure 19.8. Illustration of urethrovesical and bladder descent of over 15 mm in a patient with anatomical stress urinary incontinence.

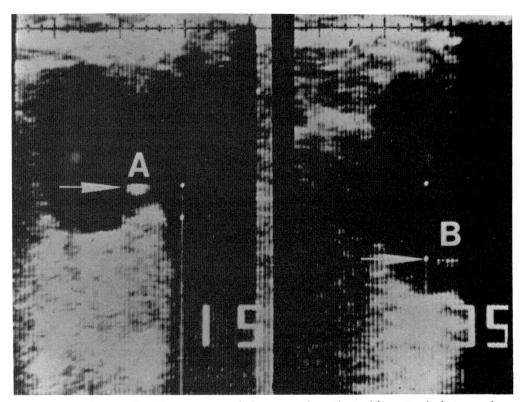

Figure 19.9. Longitudinal linear array real-time scan of a patient with anatomical stress urinary incontinence. *A*, Bladder and ureterovesical junction with 6 French pediatric feeding tube within the urethra at rest. *B* shows descent of the bladder and urethrovesical junction of over 35 mm with Valsalva maneuver, indicating anatomical stress urinary incontinence.

gery. All now have less than 15 mm of descent and are totally continent (6) (Fig. 19.11).

Bladder instability, detrusor dyssynergia, or motor urge incontinence are terms used to describe a condition which is not uncommon in children, in reproductive-age women, and in the elderly. Accurate diagnosis requires cystometric evaluation which may be augmented by dynamic ultrasonography. Many urodynamic laboratories followed abnormal screening carbon dioxide cystometrics with indirect or direct water cystometrics. If a continuous electronic microtip

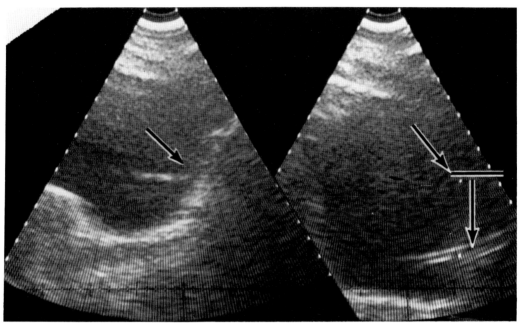

Figure 19.10.   Longitudinal sector scan of patient with anatomical stress urinary incontinence. *left* Bladder and ureterovesical junction with a 6 French pediatric feeding tube within the urethra at rest (*arrow*). *right* descent of the bladder and urethrovesical junction of over 35 mm with Valsalva maneuver, indicating anatomical stress urinary incontinence. The arrows show original position of the urethra and the position adopted when the Valsalva maneuver was performed.

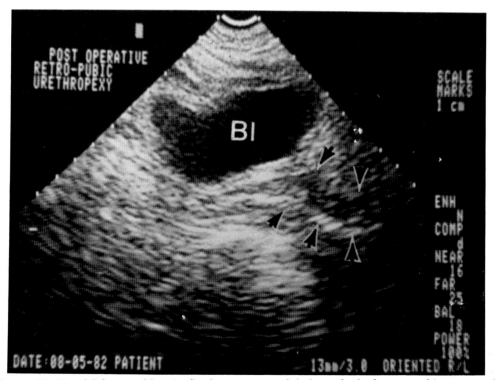

Figure 19.11.   Mid-ventral longitudinal sector scan of patient who had a retropubic cystourethropexy (same patient as in Fig. 19.17). Note that vaginal suspension of bladder (*Bl*) and urethra has flattened the bladder base and elevated the anatomical position of the urethra.

transducer capability is not available, simple water cystometrics may be performed utilizing a catheter, bottle of sterile water, intravenous tubing, and manometer (7). Pressures are measured in 50- or 100-ml increments as the bladder is filled with the patient in a standing or supine position. Uninhibited detrusor contractions may be evoked with simple filling, heel bouncing, coughing, or straining in a patient with bladder instability. Such contractions may be visualized by continuous ultrasound monitoring even though measurements are only being taken at incremental points during filling (Figs. 19.12 and 19.13). Such contractions can easily be recorded by videotape. Synchronous electronic cystourethrometrics and dynamic ultrasonography can be simultaneously recorded, as is currently being performed with fluoroscopy in some urodynamic laboratories.

It must be emphasized that ultrasonography is not a method to diagnose bladder instability or neurogenic bladder dysfunction; however, it can be used to augment other necessary urodynamic studies. It is an ideal noninvasive bedside or office tool to evaluate these problems and others in bedridden elderly patients, small children (2), and spinal cord-injured patients (8). It has, for such patients, the advantages of being portable and not requiring repeated catheterization (Table 19.3). It also can be used frequently at a minimum of expense and time to assess various treatment modalities.

BLADDER VOLUMES

Portable real-time ultrasonography can be used for the rapid evaluation of bladder volumes in patients that might otherwise require difficult or repeated catheterization (9, 10). It is partic-

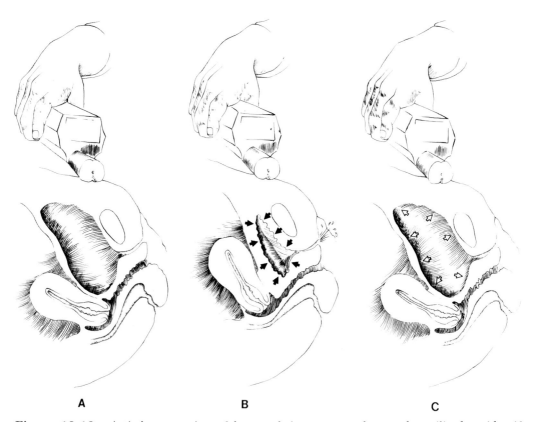

A   B   C

Figure 19.12. Artist's conception of how real-time sonography can be utilized to identify abnormal detrusor contractions. The examination can be performed with the bladder filled from above or below (i.e., via a transurethral catheter).

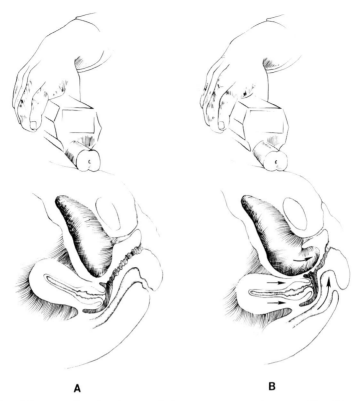

A B

Figure 19.13. Diagram showing how real-time sector scanning may identify pelvic relaxation in the female. Cystoceles can be easily visualized with sector scanning during a Valsalva maneuver.

Table 19.3.
Comparison of real-time ultrasound and radiographic studies for evaluating stress urinary incontinence

	Real-Time Ultrasound	X-rays
Instrument cost	Low to medium	High
Space requirement	Less	More
Procedure cost	Medium	High
Availability to patient	Fair to good	Fair
Flexibility	Good	Poor
Radiation exposure	No	Yes
Invasive procedure	Less	More
Operator skills	Less	More
Time	Less	More
Bowel gas interference	Yes	No
Imaging obese patient	Fair to poor	Good

ularly helpful in neonates, children with voiding difficulties, spinal cord-injured patients, women in labor, and the elderly (8, 11). it is also a useful tool for the bedside estimation of residual urine in both male and female patients who have undergone surgery on or around the lower urinary tract.

A mid-line sagital scan is most frequently used for this technique. The dimensions of the bladder are measured and the volume of the bladder calculated by a geometric formula. Initial catheterization for true volume improves the accuracy of subsequent scans since bladder shape and size can vary markedly, particularly after surgery or in pregnant patients. Real-time ultrasound is a superb teaching tool for bladder training in patients with neurological dysfunction. Parents, as well as adult patients, can be shown, at the bedside or toilet, the effectiveness of a good Credé maneuver. On labor, pediatric, geriatric, and even medical-surgical wards, a rapid "glance" with a portable real-time ultrasound machine can save unnecessary and uncomfortable catheterization. Unit nurses can be quickly taught how to use these simple small machines for this purpose. Such portable machines are now available in the labor and delivery area and radiology departments of most larger hospitals.

Dynamic ultrasonography is now being utilized as a test of renal function to evaluate bladder volume in the fetus. Intravenous furosemide given to the mother will cause the normal fetal bladder to fill. This and subsequent fetal voiding can be assessed by dynamic ultrasonography. Urethral obstruction, posterior uretheral valves, and the "prune-belly" syndrome have been diagnosed after dynamic ultrasonography of the fetus (12).

Bladder identification and evaluation constitute an important application of dynamic real-time ultrasound in the neonatal unit. Such equipment may assist in diagnosing anuria or an abdominal mass and in obtaining a urine specimen suprapubically.

Assessing bladder volumes and residual urine with portable real-time ultrasonography, as well as review for abnormal contractions and vesical mobility, can be easily done with simultaneous cystometric studies in both children and adults (2, 6).

VESICOURETERAL REFLUX

Dynamic ultrasonography, in preliminary studies, appears to be an alternative method with which to evaluate vesicoureteral reflux (8, 13).

The patient is placed in a supine position. An 8 French catheter is introduced into the bladder. Vesical turbulence is created by rapidly drawing Cysto-Conroy (20%) in and out of the bladder through a 19-gauge needle. Microbubbles visualized within the renal collecting system by the real-time transducer verify reflux. Similar information to that gathered by voiding cystourethrography and radionuclide cystography is obtained. Since vesicoureteral reflux in children frequently resolves without surgery, it can be used to follow such patients in an office or clinic setting without the radiation exposure, intravenous contrast material, and expense of a voiding cystogram. It can also be recommended as an alternate method of following this problem in spinal cord-injured patients. Dynamic ultrasonography, in addition to being able to evaluate the renal parenchyma for size and scarring, can also circumvent the bowel gas and fecal material which is so often a problem in the radiological evaluation of these patients (9).

DIVERTICULA

Urethral diverticula may occur in as many as 3 to 4% of adult females. Although these patients may be asymptomatic, some have dysuria, frequency, urgency, and postvoid pain and dribbling. Although diagnosis may be suspected by palpation, cystourethroscopy and radiographic studies are usually required (Fig.19.14). The radiographic studies are most important; frequently, such diverticula are missed by endoscopy or are complex in their size, location, and number. Choice of therapy depends on this information.

Two of the most important procedures for the diagnosis of urethral diverticula are voiding cystourethrography and retrograde distention urethrography. Visualization depends on the filling of the diverticulum with a liquid contrast medium. Preliminary studies reveal that similar information may be obtained utilizing dynamic real-time ultrasonography. The advantages of this technique over radiographic studies are numerous. As newer real-time transducers with improved resolution are brought into everyday use, more of such diverticula may be visualized. Small sector transducers are superior in demonstrating the entire urethra (Figs. 19.2, 19.4, and 19.5).

The retrograde distention urethrogram, although rather difficult and time consuming to perform may provide information superior to the voiding cystourethrogram (Fig. 19.15). This technique has been modified for use with dynamic ultrasonography (Figs. 19.16, 19.17, and 19.18). A double balloon catheter occludes both ends of the female urethra. Water is then injected under pressure into the urethra through

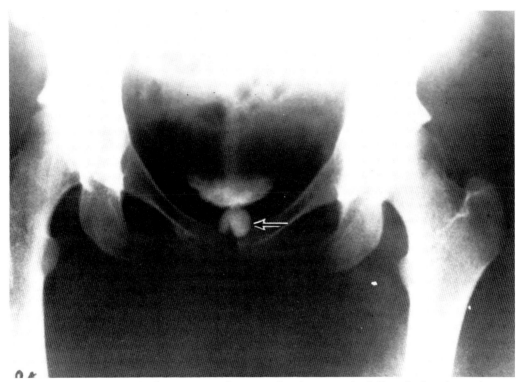

Figure 19.14.   Voiding cystourethrogram showing a urethral diverticulum (*arrow*).

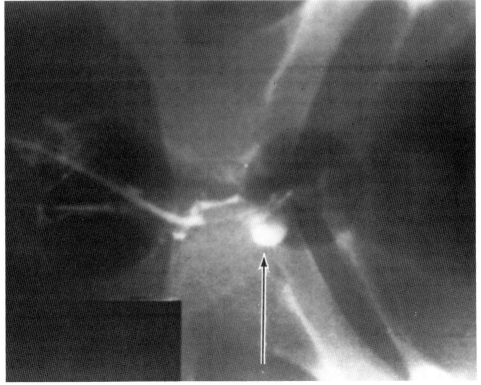

Figure 19.15.   Double balloon urethrogram illustrating a urethral diverticulum (*arrow*).

another lumen in the catheter while the entire length of the urethra is examined sonographically (14) (Figs. 19.17 and 19.18). The advantage of this technique is that pressure may force the water through a small opening into a diverticulum that may not have filled on voiding cystourethrography. Diverticula filled with pus or urine may be visualized with ultrasound but not

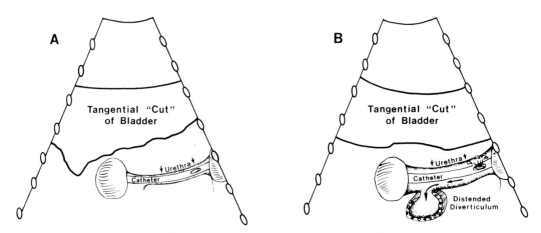

Figure 19.16. Schematic drawing of urethrogram technique. *A*, Catheter before injection of normal saline. *B*, Urethra and urethral diverticulum distension following injection of saline into the urethrogram catheter.

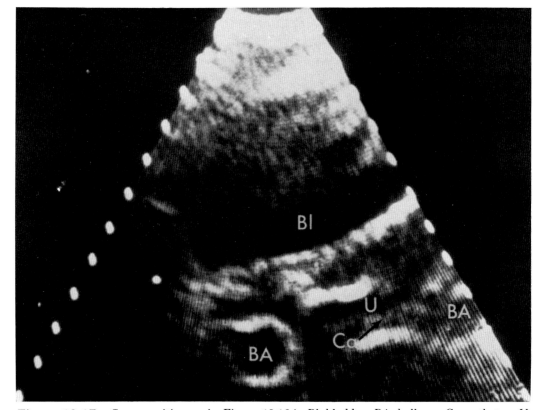

Figure 19.17. Same position as in Figure 19.16*A*. *Bl*, bladder; *BA*, balloon; *Ca*, catheter; *U*, urethra.

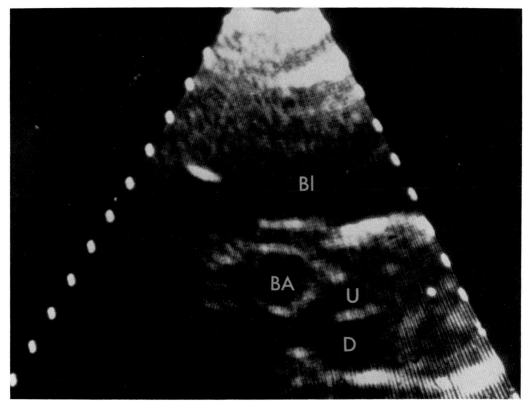

Figure 19.18.   As in schematic drawing in Figure 19.16*B*. *Bl*, bladder; *BA*, balloon; *U*, urethra; *D*, diverticulum.

with conventional x-ray equipment. There are, however, several disadvantages. At the present time, transducer resolution with portable real-time units prevents the imaging of very small diverticula. Markedly obese patients are technically difficult to scan. Only an anterior-posterior view of a diverticulum may be obtained by the above techniques. It is, therefore, possible to miss a diverticulum or portion of one beneath the catheter or urethra. Early work with oblique and vaginal imaging indicates that these problems may soon be solved. The above technique is also useful in the evaluation of periurethral and perivesical cysts which may not communicate with the urinary tract (Fig. 19.19).

Dynamic ultrasonography also is useful and practical for the evaluation of bladder diverticula (Figs. 19.20 to 19.22). Viewing the bladder with ultrasound during the filling and emptying may yield clinically valuable information about entities such as nonopaque stones within a diverticulum. Simultaneous cystoscopic instrumentation and dynamic sonography may also

assist the surgeon in assessing depth, content, and related anatomy.

We predict that a simple real-time ultrasound voiding cystourethroscopy will, in the future, enable one to diagnose many urethral and vesical abnormalities in patients with lower urinary tract symptoms.

OTHER ABNORMALITIES

Not infrequently, the female patient with SUI may also have symptomatic pelvic relaxation or other pelvic abnormalities which may influence the preoperative evaluation and even the choice of surgical procedures. While dynamic ultrasonography is not a substitute for a thorough bimanual and speculum examination of the pelvis and perineum, it has, on many occasions, demonstrated other abnormalities during the evaluation of the urinary tract. Ovarian cysts, uterine myomata, endometriosis, uterine malignancy, pregnancy, hematocolpos, and pelvic abscesses have all been associated with lower urinary tract dysfunction. The new sector trans-

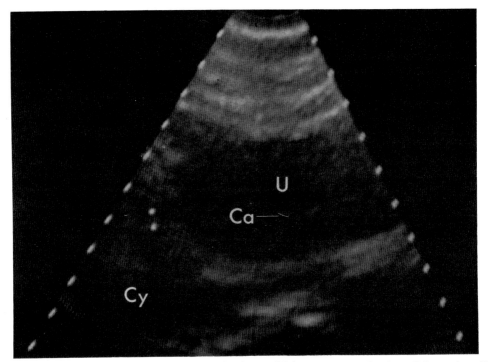

Figure 19.19. Sonogram showing periurethral cyst (*Cy*) not communicating with urethra (*U*). *Ca*, double balloon catheter in the urethra. The urethra has been distended with saline.

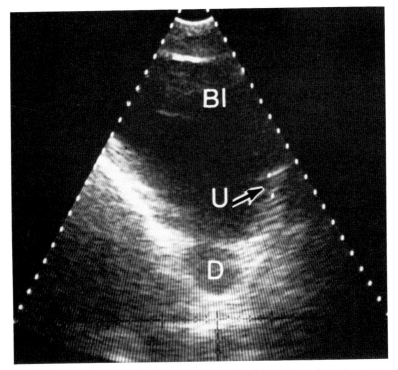

Figure 19.20. Mid-ventral longitudinal sector scan of bladder (*Bl*) and urethra (*U*) with bladder diverticulum (*D*).

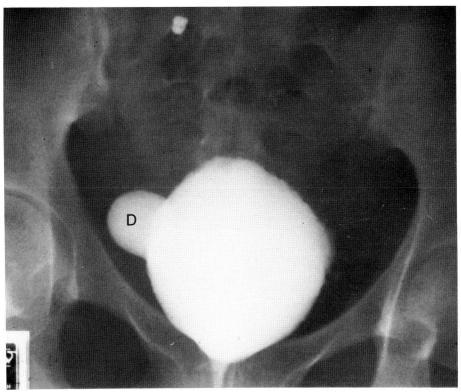

Figure 19.21.   Cystogram with bladder diverticulum (*D*) in female with stress urinary incontinence.

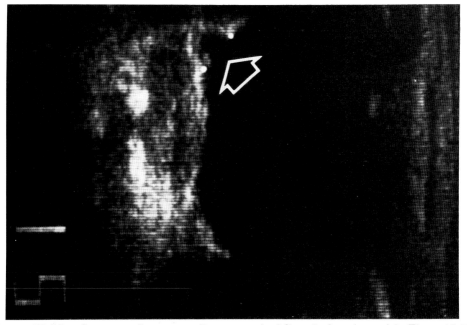

Figure 19.22.   Sonogram (transverse linear array) of diverticulum (*arrow*) in Figure 19.21.

ducers also frequently allow the clinician to view a significant cystocele and even uterine prolapse (Fig. 19.13). It must be emphasized that real-time ultrasonography is not the preferred method for making the above diagnoses; however, such equipment may supply information to the clinician to indicate that further evaluation is necessary.

SUMMARY

Dynamic real-time ultrasonography, when accompanied by a detailed history and physical examination, as well as other important laboratory tests, may significantly aid the clinician in the evaluation of the bladder, urethra, and urethrovesical junction in the patient with lower urinary tract symptoms.

References

1. Lee JKT, Baron RL, Melson L, et al: Can real-time ultrasonography replace static B scanning in the diagnosis of renal obstruction. *Radiology* 139:161, 1981.
2. Rabinovitch HH: Urinary incontinence in children. *Med Times* 110:5s, 1982.
3. Portnoi V: Urinary incontinence in the elderly. *AFP* 23:151, 1981.
4. Tanagho EA: Simplified cystography in stress urinary incontinence. *Br J Urol* 46:295, 1977.
5. White RD, McQuown D, McCarthy TA, et al: Real-time ultrasonography in the evaluation of urinary stress incontinence. *Am J Obstet Gynecol* 15:138, 235, 1980.
6. White RD, Williams DL: The evaluation of the lower urinary tract with real-time ultrasonography. Accepted for publication by *Am J Obstet Gynecol*.
7. Lapides J: *Fundamentals of Urology*. Philadelphia, WB Saunders, 1976.
8. Brandt TD, Neiman HL, Calenoff L, et al: Ultrasound evaluation in the urinary system in spinal cord injury patients. *Radiology* 141:473, 1981.
9. Holmes JH: Ultrasonic studies of the bladder. *J Urol* 97:654, 1967.
10. Pedersen JF, Bartrum RJ, Grytter C: Residual urine determination by ultrasonic scanning. *AJR* 125:474, 1975.
11. Harrison NW, Parks C, Sherwood F: Ultrasound assessment of residual urine in children. *Br J Urol* 67:805–814, 1976.
12. Cooperberg PL: Abnormalities of the fetal genitourinary tract. In Sanders R, James AE: *Principles and Practice of Ultrasound in Obstetrics and Gynecology*. New York, Appleton-Century-Crofts, 1980.
13. Kessler RM, Altman DH: Real-time sonographic detection of vesicoureteral reflux in children. *AJR* 130:1033, 1982.
14. White RD, Williams DL: The demonstration of urethral and bladder diverticula with real-time sonography. Submitted for publication.

Index